A
TEXTBOOK
OF HEALTH EDUCATION

by the same author
A TEXTBOOK OF HEALTH EDUCATION (first edition)
(co-authored with Denis Pirrie)

A
TEXTBOOK
OF HEALTH EDUCATION

FOR
STUDENTS IN COLLEGES OF EDUCATION,
TEACHERS AND HEALTH EDUCATORS

A. Dalzell-Ward

CHIEF MEDICAL OFFICER
HEALTH EDUCATION COUNCIL,
FELLOW AND MEMBER OF COUNCIL, ROYAL
INSTITUTE OF PUBLIC HEALTH AND HYGIENE

TAVISTOCK PUBLICATIONS

First published in 1974
by Tavistock Publications Limited
11 New Fetter Lane, London EC4P 4EE

Typeset by Preface Limited, Salisbury
Printed by T. & A. Constable Ltd, Hopetoun St, Edinburgh

© A. J. Dalzell-Ward, 1975
SBN Hardback 0 422 74550 2
Paperback 0 422 74560 X

Distributed in the USA by
HARPER & ROW PUBLISHERS, INC.
BARNES & NOBLE IMPORT DIVISION

Dedication

To the many colleagues, at home and abroad, in the several professions contributing to the practice of health education, whose work has made this book possible.

Contents

List of Figures

List of Tables

Acknowledgements

The author and publishers would like to thank the following for permission to reproduce the various figures and tables in the text:

The Editor of the *Journal of School Health* (USA) for two tables from J. D. Osman 'Nutrition Education: Too Much, Too Little, or Too Bad?'; the Comptroller, HMSO, for 'Schedule of Vaccination and Immunizations' from *Immunization against Infectious Diseases*; tables 1.6, 1.11. 11.6, and 1.10 from *On the State of the Public Health*; and for a table from L. M. Watson, 'Studies of Health Education Methods' *Sc. Hlth. Bull.*; the Office of Health Economics for a figure from *Medicine and Society*; the editor of the British Medical Journal for two figures from A. J. King 'Failure to Control Venereal Disease' and a table from the leading article of the *British Medical Journal* 26 May 1973; the Editor of *Community Medicine* (now the *Health and Social Service Journal*) for a questionnaire on drug dependence from W. J. Wigfield 'Survey of Young People's Attitudes to Drug Abuse'; the Editor of the *Practitioner* for a table from A. M. W. Porter and D. M. McCullogh 'Counselling against Cigarette Smoking: A Controlled Study from General Practice'; English Universities Press for a table and a figure from N. T. J. Bailey *Statistical Methods in Biology*; Longmans for a table from M. Rutter, J. Tizard and K. Whitmore *Education, Health and Behaviour*; Pitman Medical Books for two figures from *Smoking and Health Now*, Report of the Royal College of Physicians; and Dr H. D. Chalke for three figures on the consumption of potable spirits, beer, and wine.

Foreword

This edition of the Textbook has been written primarily to meet the needs of students at colleges of education who are preparing for the Teachers' Certificate. It is hoped that it will also be of value to professional health educators who are involved in team teaching in schools. The needs of the pupils have also been borne in mind as health education in schools is no longer limited to information about human biology and guidance concerning problems of the moment. Health education is highly relevant to the life in the community outside school and also to the future needs of the children who will live a substantial part of their adult lives in the twenty-first century. The character of the social and political changes in the twelve years that have elapsed since the publication of the first edition and the pace of change has made it imperative to change radically not only the content, but the format of this book. Therefore divisions into general principles and health education in school, biological and sociological bases etc., now seem artificial and in conformity with modern educational trends an attempt has been made at integration of the content. The reader should be able to meet the biological, behavioural and communication aspects in every section and, where applicable, administrative and economic considerations are also included. This will place the subject on the same plane as other subjects in the curriculum of the College of Education where administrative, historical, social and philosophical aspects of education are studied.

Health education has passed through its own identity crisis and is now entering an era in which its value to the promotion of health is generally recognized. The prominent landmarks in the last twelve years are the Report of the Cohen Committee which led to substantial governmental investment in health education, the acceptance of health education as an optional subject in Part II of the B.Ed. examination in the University of London, the promotion of professional training and curriculum development by the Health

Education Council, the projects of the Schools Council, and the establishment of a diploma course in the University of Leeds by the joint efforts of the Institute of Education, Department of Social and Preventive Medicine of that University and the Health Education Council. On the professional and academic plane there has been an increasing contribution from social scientists who have produced a large body of research.

The general public has also become much more conscious of the importance of the prevention of illness and the mass media have played an important part in removing emotional barriers to public discussion on matters such as sexual behaviour, drug abuse, smoking, and alcoholism – to name prominent matters of public concern at the present day. One would need only to cite the Abortion Act, and the provisions for the supply of contraceptives to all under the reorganized National Health Service, as evidence of radical changes in public opinion since 1962.

The reorganization of the National Health Service which came into operation in 1947 is also relevant to health education needs. This marks the commencement of a new phase in health care which is of an evolutionary character. There is an interest in the public as 'consumer' – a radical change from the traditional passive role of the 'patient'. In order that our future citizens will be equipped to play their part in the democratic processes of decision-taking they should have a grasp of the general principles on which the National Health Service operates. In the meantime Britain has entered the EEC, and in all the other member countries health education is supported nationally and practised widely, although using different kinds of agency. It is appropriate therefore that reference should be made from time to time to Europe, and this has been provided for.

I am indebted to many colleagues for their advice and help during the course of drafting and editing the manuscript, in particular to Mr C. A. P. Noseworthy M.B.E. who read the entire text, offered many helpful suggestions, and gave valuable assistance in the compilation of bibliography and lists of audio-visual aids. He also contributed the notes which are appended to the chapter on the school health service. Dr G. S. Wigley, Dr Isobel Smith, Dr F. Tait, and Mr L. G. Wallace kindly read the chapter on the school health service and offered many helpful suggestions which have been incorporated. Mr G. L. C. Elliston gave advice on the restructured National Health Service, and Dr H. D. Chalke O.B.E. provided the charts for the section on alcohol.

A. J. D-W

CHAPTER 1

Why health education in schools?

Historical Background

In 1779, Johann Peter Frank, a German physician, commenced the publication in Mannheim of four volumes of a work entitled *System einer vollstandingen medicinische Polizey*. The title of this work, curiously translated *Medical Police*, announced a treatise on public health policy, and it is an understatement to say that it was much in advance of its time. Frank advocated the supervision of the health of school children, laid down programmes for school meals and specifications for school furniture and also urged the instruction of boys and girls in hygiene, including sexual hygiene. Regular medical inspection was an important part of the programme. The significance of Frank's thinking lies not in the superficial resemblance to the school health service of the present day, but in that it was the first declaration that the health of school children should be included as part of the educational process. The aims of education have generally been considered to be concerned with intellectual and social development. The idea that children's health should be part of the responsibility of a school has been accepted only in recent times. The idea that prevention of illness and the promotion of health and general well-being could be achieved partly by what is somewhat erroneously termed, 'health education', has been accepted even more recently.

It is remarkable that Frank could have had such ideas at a time when the scientific, economic, social and political scene was so under-developed that such ideas could not have been put into effect. The techniques of medical examination were rudimentary, and could detect disease only so gross that it would have been obvious to everybody. Investment in State education had not yet begun in most countries in Europe — the small kingdoms of the German States being a notable exception. The practice of education itself was entirely authoritarian and had neither the advantage of the discoveries of the relationship of child development to the educational process, nor a recognition of the child's human rights at school. Frank himself was overtly authoritarian, so much so that it is doubtful if even in his own day, he could have been taken seriously. His choice of the word, 'police', in the title of his work, is significant. Frank believed that the police were the solution to every problem, including a situation where physicians fell out with each other over a diagnosis! In such a case he said the police should be present. Such were the weaknesses in Frank's programme which was never implemented to any degree, but this does not diminish the genius that could anticipate the twentieth century educational scene.

There is a long time-lapse between Frank's treatise and the setting up of the school health service in Britain in 1907, but there is a distinct thread of continuity between the two.

Economic, Social, and Sanitary Developments

As regards the United Kingdom, the year 1776 is identified as having the greatest significance for economic, social, and sanitary development. In Glasgow Adam Smith published the first economic treatise — *Wealth of Nations* — and in London, Jeremy Bentham published the *Fragment of Government*. In the same year, Captain James Cook, FRS, received the Copley Medal of the Royal Society in recognition of his having completed successfully a voyage around the world with a loss of only three members of the combined crews of his small fleet. These three events are inter-related. Adam Smith pointed the way to a science of economics, the application of which would result in the economic growth of a community in which, eventually, surpluses could be invested in health and social services. Bentham, a Utilitarian, pointed the way to scientific methods of administration, i.e. decision-taking as a result of the collection and analysis of information. It was a lack of scientific direction that handicapped the efforts of philanthropic societies in the eighteenth century and early nineteenth century. Transition from the administration of charity to a community-orientated system of support for the unfortunate depended upon the development of scientific administration. [1]

A Pioneer in Public Health

Cook's achievement was in the field of public health. The term, public health, means the policy which an authority adopts in order to safeguard the health and promote the well-being of the members of its community. In Cook's case, his community consisted of the personnel in the ships under his command. These men were living under the most adverse conditions that could be imagined. The mortality rate and the frequency of serious crippling injury and destruction of health were notorious. When Anson returned at the same time from a similar voyage, it was reported that he had had to replace the majority of his crew. This endows Cook's achievements with the scientific status of a controlled experiment. The measures which Cook adopted to preserve the health of his men were very simple. He had the lower decks ventilated by rigging wind sails, and he shortened the hours of watch. The latter anticipated measures undertaken in the twentieth century in the industrial health field. He made provision for the drying of clothes when men had been exposed to the weather, and he planned his voyage in such a way that the regular intake of fresh foods was possible at each port of call.

The measures adopted by Cook also introduce the concept of health education. It is true that this was of an extremely harsh and brutal kind. In the National Maritime Museum at Greenwich, where there is an exhibit illustrating Cook's voyage around the world, it is recorded that one man refused to eat fresh meat and was flogged. It is significant that measures designed to improve conditions, and which might be considered to improve the attractiveness of life on board ship, were resented by at least one individual. Nowadays in the field of health education, we still encounter great difficulties with individuals or small minorities. Some people refuse innovations in diet or mode of living and do not seem to be open to intellectual argument. Cook's work also illustrates the indivisible nature of administration and health education.

At the beginning of the twentieth century ideas concerning the preservation of the health of school children began to be formulated in educational policy. The weakness of any reforms or advances produced by one individual is that they may not necessarily work in other hands, and that they will not be tested. They are therefore seldom useful for public policies on a large scale. When, however, such ideas can be sifted by discussion in committee and evaluated, then they form useful material for public policy. Such a process was undertaken by the members of two important governmental committees in Britain in 1903 and 1904 respectively.

Governmental Committees

In 1903, the Royal Commission on Physical Training produced its report, a fact that is rather obscured by the brilliance of the work of another committee, the Inter-departmental Committee on Physical Deterioration which reported in 1904. [2] Nevertheless, the two are related. Frank believed that boys and girls should have regular, supervised, physical exercise. Physical training, a term now supplanted by the more enlightened physical education, was recognized as an important aspect of the educational process from its beginning. However, as regards health education, it is the

Inter-departmental Committee with which we are concerned. Its curious title derives from the fact that it was set up in response to public alarm that the nation was undergoing a process of physical deterioration. Army recruitment to the Boer War campaigns introduced medical examination and the doctors undertaking the examination rejected large numbers of men on account of the presence of organic disease, chronic infections, poor physique and under-nourishment. The problem which started as a military one, gradually spread to being a matter of general concern involving not only the War Office Authorities, but also those concerned with the general welfare and well-being of the people. These included educationalists, and, together with other leading experts, they gave evidence to the Committee which completed its work in the record time of twenty-six days. Such speed, coupled with precision of judgment and complete rightness of thinking as has subsequently been shown, should be an example to statutory committees of the present day.

Blueprint for the Twentieth Century

There are two exceptional features of this Committee. First it was composed entirely of civil servants, men of education and long experience in administration who nevertheless had no particular specialist knowledge of the subject. They were objective assessors of the information they were given. Second, they changed their terms of reference, [3] and no one seems to have rebuked them. Had they not changed their terms of reference, they would not have been able to produce what was a blueprint of public health and social services for the remainder of the century. So many reforms were advocated, that even today all of them have not yet been implemented. They identified childhood and the years during school as being of vital importance for the building of physical health. Characteristic of the times, mental health did not concern them, nor behavioural disorders, which are nowadays a preoccupation of school medical officers.

The Committee reinforced Frank's views expressed 120 years previously that the supervision of the health of children should be part of the educational process. Their major recommendation in this field was the setting up of a school medical service, as it was then called, and in fact this came into being in 1908 under the provisions of the Education (Administrative Provisions) Act of 1907. Although the term health education does not appear to have been used as early as this, the Committee recommended that girls be given instruction in nutrition and domestic science and both boys and girls in the care of the teeth and the dangers of alcohol, and that physical education be provided. A school meals programme for needy children was recommended with due care being taken for the nutritional quality of the meals provided. The Committee was impressed with the importance of good nutrition and it was recommended that the Local Government Board should fix standards of purity for all food and drink. The Committee was also concerned with the effect of fatigue on school children, and over all was preoccupied with the important point that children who were sick or under-developed physically could not benefit from the education provided for them.

The school medical service, later to be transformed into the school health service — the significant difference will be appreciated later — is unique as being a true integration between the practice of medicine and the educational process. This is a realization of Frank's ideal but it is important to realize that the thought behind it was not entirely medical; it represents a partnership between medicine, politics, and administration.

In its early days, and indeed even until 1948 in many cases, the school medical service provided a substitute for the family doctor. The National Health Insurance Act came into operation only in 1911, and even then, coverage for medical care extended only to wage-earners, not to their families. Therefore, the school medical service was preoccupied with the detection of organic disease, tuberculosis, orthopaedic defects, and nutritional disorders which were then treated either in hospitals or at special clinics. It is significant that specialist clinics for treatment of diseases of the eyes and the ears appeared very early, reflecting the importance of the sensory input to the learning process. Similarly, orthopaedic clinics and hospitals were developed because of the crippling effects of rickets, developmental deformities, and bone and joint tuberculosis.

The school medical service, however, was never intended only for ascertainment of defect and provision for its treatment.

Partnership between Medicine and Education

The administration of the service was delegated by the central government to local education authorities and it was they who appointed the medical and nursing staff, mainly full-time, to carry out the clinical work in the schools and special clinics. For the most part, the local education authorities were also health authorities, and the Medical Officer of Health whose duties were the supervision of the community's health became also the Principal School Medical Officer. By appointing full-time medical and nursing staff, the opportunity was afforded for the latter to work more closely with teachers, so that there began a mutual exchange of experience and information, doctors and nurses learning more about the educational process, and teachers learning more about medicine, health, and disease.

raining of the teacher in health education started on this
1 concentrated even until fairly recent times upon the signs
ould enable the teacher to detect defects early and to
heir ascertainment and treatment, or on the other hand, to
organize the classroom environment so as to compensate for the
handicap. Infectious diseases were an important problem before the
advent of immunization and the general raising of living standards,
so that teachers were expected to know the quarantine and
exclusion periods for the various notifiable infections.

A link with Frank's idea about design of the benches on which
children should sit at school was the provision of building
regulations, including lighting, heating, and ventilation requirements, so that the environment of the classroom was maintained at
a level, so far as possible, to prevent cross-infection, and to promote
the bodily comfort and visual and auditory acuity necessary for the
learning process.

If the school medical service had stopped at this point, it would
have achieved little in the improvement of the positive physical and
mental health of children now enjoyed at the present day. Health
education for the parent and the individual child was an extension
of the traditional clinical activities of the school medical officer
and nurse. Teachers who attended the medical inspections became
interested in counselling problems, and group health education in
the form of talks to groups of parents and to the children
themselves was a natural development.

It is from such beginnings that the modern, relatively sophisticated practice of health education began. The term itself is
admittedly unsatisfactory and even erroneous. There is continual
debate and discussion about the nature of both health and
education, although the definition of education seems to produce
more agreement at the present day. The authoritarianism of Frank,
and even that of the Inter-departmental Committee, has been
replaced by a philosophy in which an educational environment is
created which enables the pupil to learn. In the field of health,
however, so rapid is the pace of change that aspects which were
once a matter for health education disappear and new problems
take their place. The economic growth anticipated by Adam Smith
has resulted in what is called, usually pejoratively, the affluent
society.

The Affluent Society

There are two sides to this coin, and affluence is by no means to be
despised. Problems of personal hygiene, nutrition, and housing have
been largely solved by the rise of the standard of living. There is the
exception of the pockets of poverty which still exist, particularly in
the case of the so-called problem families. One has only to compare

the countryside of Hardy's time with the countryside of today with the benefit of electricity, mobility that makes social life possible for all, and the whole world brought into the home by the use of television. There can be few people who would seriously wish to go back to the miseries suffered by Tess or the 'Woodlanders'. Cleanliness, good order, comfort, amenities, and the regular stimulation of intellectual and social interests are all basic to the promotion of health, and are made possible for a large majority of people in the Western democracies. It is significant that studies in health education in the Eastern European countries [4,5] reveal a pattern of life which resembles the consumer society to an increasing degree.

Preoccupation with helping people to improvise and to compensate for lack of standards is now outmoded. We have new problems that sometimes arise from affluence itself. How to tackle these, without at the same time depreciating the standard of living, presents a difficulty. Thus we have mental health problems created by the intense competitiveness stimulated by the natural desire to enjoy the amenities of living. Even some of those who are successful are now threatened by redundancy as a streamlining of industry by amalgamation into larger and larger units becomes necessary to maintain its profitability. Problems resulting from the retirement from an active occupation are now being given serious attention, and quite apart from the stress imposed by working life in a modern industrial society, there is the overall problem of violence and general insecurity. We have yet to evaluate the effects of mass communication which now bring violence and extreme distress into every home. The impact of disaster upon the human mind constitutes one of the little recognized mental health problems today.

We are also faced with problems of pollution and the need for conservation of our environment. An increasing tempo of industrial production brings with it waste-materials that have to be disposed of. Modern agriculture disturbs ecology. The encroachment on space and amenities by the increasing use of road transport and the problem of noise are important aspects of environmental hygiene. These are clearly areas of community responsibility, but they are also areas of personal responsibility, and here, health education in the school aims at introducing a dialogue on personal responsibility for health.

Affluence has raised the standard of living to the point where many elementary health problems have virtually disappeared. It has also made possible a greater degree of self-indulgence by a larger number of people. Over-fatigue in the search for pleasure, abuse of drugs, including alcohol, the smoking of tobacco, the abandoning of regular exercise, and the consumption of diets providing greatly superfluous calories are all problems of the affluent society. The position is complicated by the fact that so many adults seek medical treatment for the results of over-indulgence. It may well be that in the twenty-first century, it would be possible to over-indulge with impunity. There may be a pill to mitigate the toxic effects of tobacco and excess of alcohol, or even to overcome the effects of a rise in blood cholesterol which leads to arterial disease. Any value-judgment on this issue must be a personal one; if technological advances achieve such results, then undoubtedly the majority of people will wish to benefit from them. In the meantime we have no such benefits and in the prevention of lung cancer, alcoholism, and diseases associated with overweight, health education is the most important measure.

The Twenty-first Century

It is worth while considering what kind of world the child who is entering school today will live in in the early part of the twenty-first century. There will be the overall problem of population, and this at present, although in a sphere of personal responsibility, is rapidly becoming accepted as in the area of community responsibility. With the complete dissociation between sexual intercourse and procreation, and the growing acceptance by society that sexual intercourse as part of a relationship between two people need not necessarily be sanctioned by legal or religious ties, the traditional pattern of marriage will change. It is likely that there will be fewer marriages, but those that are contracted will be on a sound basis in that they will be entered upon from the point of view of a satisfying permanent relationship with sexual activity coming second.

The days when early marriage was necessary in order to regularize sexual activity have now virtually gone. It has been predicted that the average European in the twenty-first century will marry at least twice and he will undergo retraining for at least one change in occupation. The emotional trauma associated with the break-up of marriage and its effect upon children may well be one of the mental health problems to be faced by health education. There is already a blurring of the feminine and masculine roles and this may well merge into a situation where in some cases the roles may be reversed. Although a few women have undertaken a completely non-sexual role, the majority of women are seeking to integrate the sexual and nonsexual aspects, i.e. their domestic and career roles, rather than choosing exclusively one or the other.

Biological Engineering

The application of biological technology to practical living has already produced some radical changes in society, and we may expect these to increase. Contraceptive techniques are now so well established as to hardly need mention, but experiments in the field of fertility on the other hand have now gone far beyond artificial insemination by a donor, and include the possibility of the implantation of a fertilized ovum in a host, or even the extra-corporeal cultivation of a human being. The discovery of the chemical composition of living material, DNA, has also introduced the question of what is called genetic engineering. This means the deliberate interference with the process of reproduction so that undesirable genes can be eliminated, and desirable genes incor-porated in the build-up of a new person.

Applied biology is already being employed in such practical activities as space travel, high-altitude flight, supersonic flight, and undersea exploration. None of these activities would be possible without the application of the principles of human physiology which recognize that man, being adapted for life on the earth, needs to take with him, artificially contrived, a micro-climate if he intends to leave the earth's atmosphere. Thus, temperature, pressure, oxygen-tension, and the effect of gravity on the body are all taken into account in the design of vehicles and clothing.

Forming Judgments

These topics are relatively 'safe', in that they do not threaten emotional security or produce a challenge to traditional values that are contained in the other developments mentioned above. More-over, the ordinary citizen is never required to form judgments or to take decisions on space travel or various modifications of aviation. He tends to be impressed with the journalists' accounts of these activities, just as he tends to be overawed by the journalists' accounts of heart transplants, genetic engineering, and other so-called marvels of modern science.

Already the individual is faced with difficult decisions resulting from genetic counselling. Up to the present the decision has been to avoid having children if there is a calculable risk of the hereditary transmission of a serious defect. The introduction of amniocentesis, i.e. the sampling of amniotic fluid early in pregnancy in order to detect chromosomal abnormalities, imposes a graver decision on married couples. This procedure is able to detect the abnormality that is responsible for Down's syndrome — known popularly as mongolism. If the test is positive then abortion would be recommended. It has been forecast in the USA that if amniocentesis was practised as a screening procedure in the case of expectant mothers who were known to be at risk of having children with this defect, and if a positive result was followed by abortion then, by the end of the century, the incidence of subnormality would be reduced by 50 per cent.

are faced with the use of abortion not in the personal
a woman who has an unwanted pregnancy, but in the
interest. The pregnancy may well be desired and the
...ul need to have confidence in the advice offered and the
...rage to take the necessary action. How can they do this unless
well informed and equipped with a critical judgment on biological
matters? If we are to preserve a democratic society all citizens of
able mind should be equipped to form value-judgments upon
information received, and should be able to analyse and assess the
quality of scientific information. The aims of health education in
schools include equipping the future adult to form such judgments.
With the voting age now being lowered to eighteen, it will not be so
long after leaving school, and perhaps in many cases before leaving
school, that an opportunity for a practical application will be
offered.

The defence of the mind against propaganda and misuse of the
mass media, or even against the unintended misrepresentation by
over-zealous journalists, lies in attitudes reinforced or modified by
knowledge. Health education is much more than the popularization
of science, or even the imparting of information. It is concerned
with the formation of attitudes which are favourable to personal
and community health, and the change of attitudes, if these are not
satisfactory. In some cases, it may even be the reinforcement of
attitudes.

Trends in School Health Education

Health education in schools today therefore must necessarily be
much more sophisticated and wider in scope than the simple lessons
in hygiene and deportment which characterized the early manuals
and codes of practice. It will concern every teacher in the school,
and this is in conformity with the policy of the Department of
Education and Science, which does not favour the appearance of
health education on the time-table as a curriculum subject.
Nevertheless, a good case can be made out for the appointment of
specialist teachers in secondary schools, who can act as co-
ordinators of health education throughout the whole school.

There is intense activity in the field of curriculum development
at the present time. The Schools Council, the Nuffield Science
Project, and the Health Education Council are all engaged in
curriculum development in health education. In the meantime, the
Central Department has kept pace with developments in the field of
health and education from the time that the first handbook of
health education was published by what was then the Board of
Education. These 'pamphlets' — they are in fact substantial
booklets — are intended as a guide for teachers, and they do not lay
down syllabuses or codes of practice. The field of health education

from the infant school until school-leaving age, as well as at colleg of further education, colleges of education and in adult education are covered in the most recent edition published in 1968. [6]

Successive editions of this important handbook have shown that mental health, behaviour, and the general life-experience of the child are more important than any rigid code of hygiene practice. This means that the methodology adopted for health education should be biased towards active participation methods and group activities, as well as learning by the undertaking of projects.

Responsibility for Health Education

We have already suggested that health education should not be confined to the needs of the school. This was the view of the members of the Cohen Committee on Health Education who stated in their report: 'The contents of the schools' health education syllabus should be broadly based, aiming at giving the child such knowledge as would equip him to face the social and health problems he will meet in later years.' [7]

In the schools a member of the staff appointed as a co-ordinator of health education can discharge the following functions: responsibility for the care and maintenance of health education resource materials; acting as a contact within the school for Inspectors and the Authority's advisers; liaison with outside organizations and specialists; convening meetings of members of staff who are involved in the health education programme; and initiating projects.

The school, moreover, is part of the greater community, and health education has already been very well developed as a branch of preventive and social medicine. For many years health visitors have been engaged in health education as part of their duties in the maternal and child health services. Public health inspectors have been responsible for the education of food-handlers as well as the general public in the principles of food hygiene. They have also employed health education methods in other departments of their work of environmental control. Both of these professional groups have received training in the techniques of group work, and in many areas they have been welcome as visitors to schools to share in the team teaching of health education.

A number of local education authorities are compiling, or have compiled schemes for their schools. Examples are Gloucestershire, Birmingham, and Wiltshire.

The advent of the health education officer has been responsible for the further development of health education in the local authority services. These officers are trained and experienced professional workers who combine skills in organization of a public relations character with background health knowledge, and in some cases research skills. They have provided leadership for the further development of health education and have inspired their colleagues in the public health service to take more and more interest in this aspect of preventive medicine.

Again, the Cohen Committee had this to say about health educators:

'a Health Educator has:

(i) Special skill, based partly on training and partly on experience in identifying the difficulties, including the psychological difficulties, which prevent individuals taking some health action or adopting some healthy habit.

(ii) Special skill in deploying techniques.
These techniques involve approaches to community leaders and others, the use of group discussion, and the use, not only of the mass media, but of all appropriate publicity instruments.

(iii) Basic knowledge about ways to promote health.

(iv) A particular capacity because of the qualifications above, for drawing up master programmes for health education which unify the efforts of many, and make those of each individual more effective.

(v) Some capacity to evaluate the work which has been done.'

The report of the Cohen Committee on Health Education in 1964 recognized the importance of health education in the public health service and its recommendations led to the strengthening of the central provision for co-ordination, research, and experiment which is intended to encourage regional activities. With the unification of the National Health Service in 1974, the health education functions of the local health authorities, which have been the main source of health education during the last twenty years, have been absorbed by the area health authorities and specialist officers have been designated for responsibilities in health education.

The health education services of the area health authorities and the school health service can work closely together. A conference held at Loughborough in 1967, sponsored by the Association of Teachers in Departments of Education, the Society of Medical Officers of Health (now the Society of Community Medicine), and the Central Council for Health Education (which was wound up in 1968 and incorporated in the Health Education Council), reaffirmed the partnership between education and medicine and made several practical recommendations as to how this could be implemented. [8] Whereas the doctors and nurses in the school health service fully appreciate that the task of teaching must be left to the trained professional teacher in the classroom, there still remains scope for co-operation between the two professions, and teachers will find the staff of the school health service valuable allies. They will also find the health educators employed by the area health authorities helpful from the point of view of providing facilities for the practice of health education in the school.

Aims and Purpose

Academically, it has been difficult to establish health education as a discipline in its own right. It is eclectic, and this means that all kinds of specialists will claim that the subject is really theirs. When its aims and purpose are fully understood however, it will be seen that the eclectic nature of the content is by no means a barrier to its acceptance as a subject in its own right. In the University of London, it is possible to take health education as an optional subject in Part II of the Bachelor of Education degree.

Although the Report of the 1904 Committee was in favour of health education in schools the position as regards the training of teachers in this subject is very patchy. Some colleges of education offer the subject in the curriculum as a foundation course while in many it is an optional subject. In some colleges the subject can be studied both as a foundation course and at a more advanced level as an option. This situation prevails despite the fact that all teachers are teaching health education whether they are aware of it or not. It is fully comprehensive in colleges where the health needs of the students themselves are taken into account, as well as their needs as future teachers.

The aims and purpose of health education have undergone radical changes in thinking during the last twenty years. In 1954, an expert committee on health education of the World Health Organization defined health education simply in the following terms. [9] Its aims were:

1. To ensure that the community accepted health as a valued asset.
2. To equip individuals with knowledge and skills and to influence their attitudes in such a way as to help them to solve their own health problems.
3. To promote development of health services.

For many years these aims seemed applicable to every community in the world, although necessarily the emphasis was different, according to the stage of social and economic development. There has been some hesitation however about the second of these aims. There has always been the suspicion that health education was attempting to make people their own physicians. Nevertheless there is a growing recognition in the medical profession that many conditions presented for diagnosis and treatment are preventable, and would not have occurred if people had adopted certain forms of behaviour. The most obvious of these of course is the vast amount of respiratory disease caused by smoking.

Profound changes in the training of doctors are envisaged which will introduce a more preventive outlook into medical care. A working party set up by the British Medical Association [10] reported in 1970: 'The primary physician (i.e. general practitioner) should have commitments to the field of preventive medicine and health education.' The Royal Commission on Medical Education [11] recommended that the future training of doctors should include training and teaching methods and instruction in the behavioural sciences and psychology. This anticipates a changing role for the physician in the future society, and we can see 'future society' in this respect when we look at developing countries such as those in Latin America, where a completely new concept for the medical school has arisen. Here, the medical student is being trained in the community as opposed to being trained in the hospital ward and is sharing the training with the student nurse.

Some authorities have expressed the opinion that in the future people can be educated to undertake the treatment of minor disorders for themselves. A child entering school today therefore will be one of these citizens of the future who would be expected to take more personal responsibility for minor ailments, and to be able to make a judgment as to when professional advice is necessary. This is already an important aspect of parent education, as it is the mother who usually makes a diagnosis of illness, and makes a decision as to whether a doctor should be called.

The widening scope of health education has been recognized by a more recent expert committee report of the World Health Organization. [12] The definition now offered is lengthy; it runs into more than a hundred words. Health education according to this view can be differentiated between that which takes into account the total life-experience of an individual, and that which is concerned with formal campaigns for the tackling of immediate public health problems. It is stated that health education concerns all those experiences of an individual group or community that influence beliefs, attitudes and behaviour with respect to health. Planned or formal efforts on the other hand aim at stimulating and providing experiences at times, in ways, and through situations leading to the development of the health, knowledge, attitudes, and behaviour that are most conducive to the attainment of the individual, group, or community health.

The School's Concern

It is clear that the school is concerned with both aspects of health education. In the first place, the child can learn through his own personal experiences, and this is certainly true of the human

biology aspect of the content, and secondly, experien
contrived, and this is particularly applicable to a seconda
education. If we take as an example the field of sex edu
physical experiences of children at the time of puberty c
to explain the biological nature of sexual developme
puberty questions of personal responsibility can be studied by the
use of group methods. Experiences can be contrived in which the
pupils project themselves into life-situations in which they must
make decisions.

Health education in schools today is very much preoccupied with
questions of sexual behaviour, venereal disease, contraception, drug
abuse, and smoking. There is also the beginning of an interest in the
problems of alcoholism. To a great extent, this concentration on
problem-centred health education has been forced on the schools
by public opinion. It is generally believed that these problems
should not be approached in isolation, and that they should form
part of a general curriculum of health education in which there is a
thorough understanding of human biology and ecology as well as
the social pressures and attitudes having a bearing upon behaviour.

The programme for health education in schools, therefore,
should be a balanced one, and should be comprehensive, and we
should not lose sight of the fact that health education is one of the
important factors in psychosocial evolution, which will bring about
changes in society. It should also be borne in mind that one of the
aims of health education is to guide people in making suitable
choices and there is usually a wide range of choice within the area
that can be considered to be healthy behaviour. Authoritarianism
and dogmatism have no place in modern health education. The aim
is not to bully people into health as Frank would have liked to have
done, but rather to liberate them from unnecessary fear and
anxiety, and to help them to develop their utmost potential.

QUESTIONS

1. Should the main aim of health education be to either: (i) change society
   (ii) equip the individual to realize his potential or (iii) make the individual
   conform to society?

2. What problems of conscience and ethics are raised by the technological
   applications of biology?

3. How would you try to convince an interviewing committee that health
   education should be included in the school curriculum?

4. Comment on the statement 'Health education is being taught in every
   school whether the staff realise it or not.' Does the current health education
   programme of your college, or department, equip you sufficiently to
   become involved in a school's programme? Would you care to suggest how
   it may be improved?

REFERENCES

1. Simon, J. (1895). *English Sanitary Institutions*. London: Longman.
2. *Report of Interdepartmental Comittee on Physical Deterioration* (1904). London: HMSO.
3. Dalzell-Ward, A. J. (1957). 'The Twenty-six Days and After'. *Pub. Hlth.* 71:49.
4. Federal German Centre for Health Education (1972). *Health Education in Europe*: viii:137. Geneva: Int. J. Hlth. Educ.
5. Reti, E. (ed.) (1972). *Recueil de travaux de recherche et méthodologiques sur l'éducation sanitaire* 1967—1968. Budapest: Centre d'éducation sanitaire.
6. Department of Education and Science (1968). *Handbook of Health Education*. London: HMSO.
7. Report of a Joint Committe of the Central and Scottish Health Services Councils (1964). *Hlth. Educ.* London: HMSO.
8. Education and Medicine — a Partnership in Health Education (1968) (symposium of papers by various authors read at the Conference at Loughborough 1967). *Publ. Hlth.* 82:153—72.
9. World Health Organization (1954). *Report of Expert Comittee on Health Education*. Technical Report Series No. 89. London: HMSO.
10. British Medical Association (1970). *Primary Medical Care*. Report of a Working Party.
11. *Report of the Royal Commission on Medical Education* (1965). London: HMSO.
12. World Health Organization (1969). *Research in Health Education*. Report of a working Group. Technical Report Series No. 432. London: HMSO.

FURTHER READING

Bacon, L. (1964). 'Health Education and the Schools'. *Hlth. Educ. J.* 22:216.
Campbell, A. V. (1972). *Moral Dilemmas in Medicine*. Edinburgh and London: Churchill-Livingston.
Galbraith, J. K. (1970). *The Affluent Society*. 2nd. ed. Harmondsworth: Penguin.
Messenger, S. E. G. (1971). 'The Need to maintain and improve the Status of Health Education in Colleges of Education'. *Hlth. Educ. J.* 30 (1):21.
Read, D. A. (ed.) (1971). *New Directions in Health Education*. London: Collier-Macmillan.
Tones, B. K. (1973). 'The Educational Needs of Health Educators'. *Hlth. Educ. J.* 32 (1):69.

CHAPTER 2

Sources of personal well-being

The second of the two definitions of health education with its reference to 'total' experience is directly relevant to the various factors which are known to be responsible for physical, mental, and social well-being. Although many causes of disease have been recognized, there has been a tendency for some pioneers in health education to believe that there was a single cause of health. Thus they have emphasized the importance of diet, clothing, or specialized regimes to which they have severally ascribed reasons for their own health and longevity. In the light of our contemporary knowledge of physiology and the effect of social and environmental forces, such a simplification cannot be accepted. It is no longer profitable to pursue the study of man in separate compartments. The former division into biological and social aspects is as artificial as the division of man into a physical, intellectual, and emotional being. Health education has made a considerable contribution towards the acceptance of man as 'indivisible'.

The earlier definition of health education referred to the individual's capacity to solve his own health problems. This requires self-knowledge just as the community's capacity to solve its health problems calls for knowledge of the needs of its members and of their attitudes and behaviour towards health and disease.

Homeostasis

As regards the individual's make-up, when we examine the fundamentals we are confronted with phenomena that are universal. Setting aside differences due to variations in the human race — size, colour, intellectual and physical capacities, language and social customs, the internal environment is common to all. By the internal environment is meant those physiological conditions, levels, gradients, and regular fluctuations that must be maintained in a state of constancy for life to go on and for a sense of well-being to be experienced. Claude Bernard, [1] the French physiologist who discovered this principle, wrote a hundred years ago, 'Man in health is a piece of constancy, living, and moving in a world of variables,' while J. S. Haldane (father of JBS) said at the turn of the century, 'The maintenance of the internal environment must be regarded as the essential condition of free and independent life'.

Walter B. Cannon [2] a distinguished American physiologist coined the term 'homeostasis' to describe this phenomenon on which depends the daily life of everyone. Homeostasis means that there is a natural tendency to return to the *status quo*. A major part of our organic apparatus is concerned with homeostasis which operates through the various body systems under the control of the nervous system aided by the hormones of the endocrine system.

The Basic Mechanism

The basic mechanism operates in the following way: as a result of external (and sometimes internal) stress an 'error' is caused. This is then corrected by a compensatory change in the internal environment in order to correct the error. Sometimes there is over-correction and another 'error' occurs which is corrected in turn. Although to the outward eye the body remains stable and there is seldom any change of sufficient intensity to reach consciousness, an intensely dynamic process operates in order to maintain the necessary equilibrium.

This homeostatic principle has been used in technology by the invention of the 'feedback'. The earliest form of feedback was the thermostat but with the discovery of electronics innumerable devices have been introduced in order to maintain the stability of dynamic systems – the automatic pilot, for example, or even the automatic gearbox. It is therefore easier to explain physiological homeostasis in terms of feedbacks. The nervous system maintains control of the organic systems by feedbacks which feed impulses into the network and so to the various controlling centres. Feedbacks occur also through physio-chemical systems operating at all interfaces and on the surface of membranes. Here the feedback is sensitive to chemical gradients or to osmotic pressure or to hormone levels.

Maintenance of Body Temperature

The maintenance of the body temperatures at a level of about 37 °C is the prime example of homeostasis. For the preservation of well-being and for optimum physical and intellectual performance, the body temperature must not vary too much or for too long from its normal level. In extreme cases death will ensue if the temperature rises to extreme levels – heat exhaustion – or if it sinks to abnormally low levels – hypothermia. The former condition is a problem of tropical countries and in some industries, and hypothermia is the cause of death in infants and old people — as well as in cases of prolonged exposure to cold in the sea or on mountains. In these situations the homeostatic mechanisms have been overstrained and have broken down.

Heat is generated by the metabolism of food and by muscular activity. Even at rest 40 calories per sq. metre of body surface an hour are produced and the usual condition is that excess heat must be lost in order to maintain the heat balance. The amount to be lost — or alternatively to be retained — depends upon the temperature, humidity, and cooling power of the external environment.

It must be understood that there are two levels of body temperature. The 'core' temperature of the organic systems and the deeper layers of the body differs from the surface temperature. The core temperature must not sink below 35 °C and fluctuations in the surface temperature reflect the action of the temperature regulating mechanism as a whole. Variation in mouth temperature on either side of 37 °C is a normal observation when the temperatures of a number of people are recorded.

The control of body temperature is effected by the shunting of blood from the body core to the surface or in the reverse direction. Nervous control is initiated by a group of nerve cells in the brain stem and nerve impulses flowing through the nerve network that surrounds the blood vessels either open up blood vessels or constrict them in such a way that the blood-flow is increased or diminished. When it is necessary to lose heat the blood-flow in the vessels of the skin is increased. The skin becomes warm and may be flushed, and the sweat glands are active. Heat is lost by radiation, convection, and evaporation of sweat — and also to a small extent through expired air. We can now see how an 'error' is corrected at the cost of making another 'error'. If sweating is excessive in order to lose heat, then the body loses also water and salt. The level of water and salt in the blood and in tissue fluids must also be maintained at a constant level. In order to retain water the kidney excretes less urine which is more highly concentrated than normal. Drinking to relieve thirst assists in the replenishment of water. Conversely, if the core temperature is in danger of falling because of cold external conditions, blood-flow in the skin is shut down, sweating ceases so that the body retains water. In this case the kidneys excrete a larger quantity of dilute urine. These fluctuations in kidney output are a matter of common experience and they bring to our consciousness the principles of homeostasis.

Organic System-Integration

We see now that, in addition to the circulation of the blood, the skin, lungs, and kidney are also involved in temperature regulation. Their functions are interdependent in this situation as though they were 'commanded' by the nervous system to make a contribution to the body's needs above that of oxygen transport and excretion of waste-products.

All human beings are equipped with homeostatic systems which make automatic adjustments to the usual states encountered in daily living. As in the case of temperature regulation, there are personal responsibilities for ensuring that the homeostatic mechanisms are not overstrained. This is important in the choice of suitable clothing, nutrition, activity, the control of external temperatures and ventilation to promote the maximum cooling power of the air. It is now recognized that survival from immersion in the water depends as much on protective clothing which can delay heat loss as on a life-jacket to keep one afloat. Cold injury in infants and old people calls for the maintenance of a relatively high room temperature. In the case of old people good nutrition and some physical activity are also important.

Hormonal Homeostatic Systems

The introduction of the oral contraceptive brings to our notice the existence of hormonal homeostatic mechanisms. The hormones are chemicals produced by the endocrine glands. The pituitary gland at the base of the skull is the master gland and its secretions initiate the production of hormones in other glands in the system — thyroid, adrenals (partial), part of the pancreas (insulin), and certain cells of the ovaries and testicles. Hormones were originally described as 'chemical messengers' because they pass to target organs via the bloodstream and cause changes in the functions of these organs.

A perfect example of homeostasis is the maintenance of the level of oestrogen in the blood. The pituitary gland initiates the cycle by secreting 'follicle stimulating hormone' (FSH) which, reaching the ovary via its blood supply, causes a single egg cell in the ovary's stock to ripen. During the ripening process the ovum produces its own hormone — oestrogen — which passes into the bloodstream to the uterus which is then stimulated to develop its lining in anticipation of the ovum's becoming fertilized.

When the level of oestrogen in the blood is high, the pituitary stops secretion of FSH but when ovulation is complete the level of oestrogen drops. The pituitary gland thus receives a 'feedback' and more FSH is produced leading to a further ovulation and the cycle restarts. The contraceptive pill containing oestrogen (and progesterone) enables the oestrogen blood-level to be maintained so that the pituitary gland receives no feedback stimulus which is necessary in order to secrete more FSH. This is an instance where biological technique enables us to interfere with a homeostatic situation to replace the normal fluctuation in blood-levels.

The primary source of well-being is homeostasis. Civilization has always depended upon this principle, e.g. the movement of populations away from the Equator to cold climates called for an adoption of clothing and artificial heating.

Nutrition

Food makes a direct contribution to well-being by the satisfaction of appetite and the supply of energy. This is a short-term contribution and for the maintenance of well-being food must also supply nutrients which repair the natural wear and tear of tissues and, in the case of children, the materials of growth. Nutrients are required for blood-formation and food must contain mineral salts for this purpose as well as for the general functions of the body. Vitamins occurring naturally in food provide protection against infection and the maintenance of connective tissues and membranes as well as for blood-formation and the preservation of the normal clotting power of the blood.

All the necessary food groups — proteins, carbohydrates, fats, minerals, and vitamins can be obtained from a variety of foods. The best safeguard against malnutrition is the use of a balanced diet in which the widest range of foodstuffs is included. Societies where diet is limited, e.g. to rice or other grains, are in danger if the supply of their staple food is threatened. In some national diets the protective foods and minerals are supplied by 'side dishes' which are erroneously regarded as luxuries or 'frills'. In sophisticated industrialized societies able to spend money on imports to supplement home-produced foods, there is a wide choice and no single article of diet can be considered as of paramount importance — it is the dietary pattern made up from the various foods chosen that matters.

Nutrition Education

A practical approach to nutrition education is to complete a questionnaire as to which foods were consumed on a given day and then to analyse the responses in dietary terms. For example we can ask — 'List all the meals, snacks and drinks you consumed yesterday. Did they contain at least one helping of meat; fish; egg; poultry; green, yellow, or red vegetable; fruit; cereal; and milk?'

The questionnaire could then be developed to enquire what further foods were consumed, e.g. bread, potatoes, sweets, puddings, jam, sweet fruit drinks, or substitute 'fruit-type' drinks. The dietary pattern for a week should indicate whether in fact a balanced diet representing all required nutrients is being taken.

Osman [3] in the USA has elaborated this method with high school students by requiring a record of six days intake of the various food groups including what he calls 'empty calories'.

Table 1. Student record of food intake

	Day 1	Day 2	Day 3	Day 4	Day 5	Day 6	Total	Average
Milk Group	√√	√√	√	√√√√	√		√√	12	2
Meat Group	√	√√√√		√√			√√	10	1.6
*Fruit and	√	√	√				√	4	.66
**Vegetable	√√	√		√√	√√	√√√	√	2	.33
Group		√ √						17	1.84/2.8
Bread and									
Cereal Group	√√	√√√√	√√		√√	√√√√	√√√√	20	3.3
Empty									
Calories	√√√	√√√√√√·√√√	√√	√√	√		√√	19	3.16

*Source of ascorbic acid.
**Dark green or yellow vegetable.
Source: Osman, J. D. (1972). 'Nutrition Education: Too Much, Too Little, or Too Bad?' *Journal of School Health* (USA).42(10):592–6.

Students were also asked to assign a rank order to certain items of diet as follows:

Table 2. Student rank order of certain food items

1. Rank as most nutritious (total nutrients)
   Instant breakfast with water
   Salted peanuts
   Pizza with pepperoni
   Orange drink with a B-complex vitamin pill

2. Rank food with most calories first
   Medium-sized baked potato
   9 potato chips
   Extra large apple
   10 celery stalks

3. Rank drink with most calories first
   8 oz. of beer
   8 oz. of whole milk
   8 oz. of skim milk
   8 oz. of cola drink

4. Rank as most reliable source of weight control information
   Dietician
   'Fat' Doctor
   Magazine ad
   Pharmacists

Source: Osman, J. D. (1972). 'Nutrition Education: Too Much, Too Little, or Too Bad?' *Journal of School Health* (USA). **42**(10): 592–6.

Food and weight control TV commercials are taped and played back to the class who are asked to evaluate the reliability and accuracy of the nutritional information.

Nutrition education at the public level must be meaningful in terms of familiar foods rather than food groups on a functional basis. Bender [4] states: 'No-one — not even the professional nutritionist — looks at the supermarket shelves with a view to buying his weekly raion of proteins and vitamins, rather he or she decides what will make a satisfying and attractive meal'.

The survey to which Bender was referring showed that few people know where to look for their nutrients — nutrition education should aim at enlarging people's experience and this has been only one of the benefits of the opportunities now available for foreign travel.

In scientific terms we all need daily abot 70 grams of protein (balanced as regarding its amino acid content), fourteen different vitamins, thirteen mineral salts, and 3000 calories in order to maintain well-being. 3000 calories are too generous for middle-aged sedentary people and, on the other hand, there are groups in the population at nutritional risk — babies and nursing mothers, the elderly, 'food faddists', and zealous but uninformed weight-reducers.

Bender rightly defends fish and chips from uninformed attack. He says that we can, and many do, live very well without raw carrots and liver but fish and chips provide good nutrition. We might add this — if nothing but fish and chips were eaten deprivation of other nutrients contained in vegetables, fruit, etc., would occur. But this only serves to emphasize the importance of variety.

Meaning of a Balanced Diet

The term 'balanced diet' is used without much understanding of its real meaning. MacDonald demonstrates the significance of balance in the diet in an article on sugar. [5] He points out that the nutritional priority of the body is energy. Man has hunger for energy only, there being no specific hunger for protein, fat, or even salt. If a diet is taken which is inadequate as regards energy but which contains proteins, then the protein would be used as an energy source and would not be available for growth and repair of tissues for which its amino acid content makes it unique. The addition of carbohydrate would mean that less of the protein would be diverted to energy. Despite the dangers of excessive consumption of refined sugar, in the light of MacDonald's comments, a completely carbohydrate-free diet would also be undesirable. There is a warning here for weight-reducers.

Deprivation of energy foods will result in excessive fatigue which will in turn diminish social and work performance and interfere with well-being. Deprivation of protein will lead to wasting of muscles and this will be increased by failure to take exercise. Muscle fibres are renewed and increase in number as a result of use. Uninformed slimming may produce results completely different from those desired.

Feeding Patterns

Human feeding patterns display an infinite variety as regards frequency of meals, timing, and the way in which it is prepared, cooked, and served. Social custom and convenience play a major part in this variation but so long as there is no gross violation of physiological processes this is not significant. Fatigue will be experienced when the level of blood-sugar is low, and in exacting ocupations and when driving long journeys frequent small meals are preferable to large meals at long intervals.

Maintenance of Blood-Glucose Levels

MacDonald illustrates yet another homeostatic mechanism which enables a constant response to metabolic demands, although eating is episodic.

He points out arrangements must be made to cope with times of excess and depletion during a twenty-four hour period. When the level of glucose in the blood rises after a meal, the pancreas increases its insulin output which results in the conversion of glucose to glycogen and fat which is temporarily stored. When the blood-glucose level is low, insulin output is reduced, glycogen in the liver is reconverted to glucose and deposit fats are broken down into fatty acids. The latter are then broken down in the liver and muscles with the release of energy.

Budgeting Priorities

Man's feeding patterns therefore seem to be adjusted to his metabolism but as in other homeostatic mechanisms they must not be overstrained and regular meals are desirable for the maintenance of uniform energy levels throughout the day. The subjective test of whether a diet is adequate is the experience of a uniform energy through the waking hours, satisfaction of appetite and steady weight. Food has a high priority for the maintenance of well-being and it is unsound economics to divert income from food to other needs. In the UK housing has always been a serious competitor and this was first observed by McGonigle, MOH of Stockton-on-Tees, in the 1930s. The high rents of new council houses and the expenditure on fares to work were shown to have an effect on the nutrition of children. Today the same events may be observed owing to the high cost of owner-occupied housing which can absorb more than 30% of income.

The Circadian Rhythm

The traditional agricultural pattern of living was work and other activity during the hours of daylight and sleep during the hours of darkness. A rest day every seventh day, a blessing bequeathed to civilization by Judaism, Christianity, and Islam, introduced a social element with a rhythm that was predictable and satisfied expectations. The deadlines were those of the seasons and apart from natural disasters like floods, emergencies did not arise. Human living was geared to the inherent rhythm of our terrestrial environment, but with the advent of industry and the development of technology economic necessity made it necessary to break away from natural limitations or activity. Deadlines became determined by economic and political considerations and the use of artificial lighting denied the truth of the Biblical statement that when night comes no man can work. Many of the Victorian epics of engineering were completed in a race against the clock — the building of the 'Great Eastern', for example, on which work went on at night by the light of flares.

Industrial Experience

It was in the early years of the First World War that it was found that technology could not triumph over biology. Increased hours of working in munitions factories resulted in decreased production and the advice of physiologists and psychologists was applied to a more biologically orientated management policy. The history of subsequent reforms in working conditions leading to the five-day week and standard forty-hour week can be studied in works on this subject. For the purposes of health education it is the recognition that there is a 'biological clock' which regulates individual activities and where influence can be measured even in such details as metabolic rates. The term given to this phenomenon is 'circadian rhythm'. This means that human activity and well-being follow roughly 'circa dies', a twenty-four hour period. Trans-continental air travel has drawn attention to this problem in the light of its effects on the health of travellers and on the performance of air-crew.

A predictable rhythm confers a sense of well-being. Temporary but not too frequent departures — such as spells on night duty, properly organized shift-working, and the occasional social indulgences can be tolerated.

Coming to Terms with the Biological Rhythm

If the circadian rhythm is deliberately and persistently violated then well-being and performance will be affected. The threats in modern civilization are the rigid measurement of industrial efficiency by cost-accounting and the restless energy of the few impatient people who control the lives of others. Some have drawn attention to the economic fact that roads are in use for only about half of the twenty-four hour period and they have suggested that full cost-benefit could be obtained by insisting on their use throughout the whole twenty-four hours. Suggestions have also been made for shift-working of schools to keep in pace with the shift-working of industry and to ensure completely economic use of the buildings. Such matters invoke value-judgments but they offer possibilities for fruitful discussion by senior pupils who will soon participate in democratic processes. So far as the individual is able to control his own circadian rhythm, he should be aware of its importance to well-being. The physiological fact is that activity is followed by fatigue from which recovery ensues after rest. There is no escaping this truth and it has to be taken into account even in space-travel — that most artificially adapted environment to which man has ever been exposed.

Personal Satisfaction

Well-being is not complete without a range of personal satisfactions which can be derived from daily living. Some of them are sensory — things seen, heard, smelt, and touched. Movement itself imparts a sensual pleasure and one of the great deprivations of imprisonment is the deprivation of movement. The skin, being developed from the same outer layer of the embryo as the brain and the nervous system, is a barometer of our emotions and satisfactions. We derive pleasure from cleanliness of the skin and of the clothing in contact with it, as we do on summer holidays from the contact of sea, sun, and wind. Personal hygiene is a matter of physical satisfaction as well as a matter of duty towards those around us.

Emotional satisfactions are dependent on a number of different factors that will be examined in detail in subsequent chapters. In part they depend upon skills in creating and maintaining human relationships and in part on our environment. A hostile environment grudging of recognition of personal worth and offering no aesthetic stimulus will make it more difficult to achieve emotional satisfactions. A sense of purpose in life and some challenge also contribute to the achievement of emotional satisfaction. When this is achieved minor physical disorders, which are no more than the normal body pressures reaching consciousness, disappear.

The Oxygen-Transport System

The oxygen-transport system of the body is fundamental to bodily comfort and performance, including mental alertness. This means that the heart and blood vessels and the lungs must be capable of peak performance during moments of demand, and of instantaneous adaptation to new environmental circumstances, either internal or external. We have already seen that we cannot dwell long upon the internal environment without considering the external environment. This has been obvious when considering the question of temperature regulation.

The basic life-process is oxidation which involves the consumption of oxygen with the production of energy, carbon dioxide, and water. The oxygen-transport system, using red blood cells as a vehicle, obtains oxygen from the atmosphere and transports it to the tissues where it is taken up by the cells, consumed, and carbon dioxide and water produced. The reverse process is now necessary, the carbon dioxide must be removed from the tissues and returned to the external environment. Carbon dioxide formed in the tissues is carried in the blood to the lungs in the form of carbinohaemoglobin and as bicarbonate, mainly in the red blood cells but also in the plasma. On arrival in the lungs, CO_2 and water are released. The respiratory centre is sensitive to the concentration of CO_2 in the blood and when it is high then the depth and rate of respiration are increased. Evolution has resulted in the four-chambered heart (the left and right sides are separate) which produces the figure of eight circulation required for this complicated process. The heart provides the pumping force to get blood from the lungs to the tissues. The veins provide the pumping force to get the blood back from the tissues to the heart, where it can be re-circulated.

The venous pumps or 'third' heart as they are sometimes called are generally neglected by most people. The pumping action of the veins which is essential to a brisk and efficient circulation is maintained by the action of muscles. When blood collects in any part of the body, it tends to produce a sensation of heaviness and sluggishness. This is partly responsible for the sensations following heavy meals and is inevitable when first waking and rising in the morning after blood has been pooled in the abdomen and in the head and neck during the recumbent position. The sluggish sensations on awaking and rising are quickly dispelled after a few minutes of muscular activity and this does not necessarily mean vigorous activity. The act of stretching and of gradually beginning to move about sends blood from the veins back to the heart and the circulation then begins to become brisker.

The oxygen-transport system is the most adaptable system in the body. During sleep and inactivity, it operates at a minimum level, but at a given notice, it can rise to a peak performance. Its efficiency is maintained only by effort. Like all organic systems in the body, it improves from use and disuse results in a falling off of performance. Most important of all, there must be reserves to call upon and these are important not only in young people for sudden calls of physical activity, but are important later in life too when the capacity to adapt to changing conditions diminishes. Physical education pays a good deal of attention to the building-up of reserves of heart and lungs, and it also trains the nervous system which is in control at all times, so that rapid changes in adaptation to changing environment can occur.

Athletic training actually enlarges the size of the oxygen-transport system and the athlete experiences a greater degree of well-being because his heart does not have to beat so fast, or his lungs expand and contract so quickly in order to produce the oxygen required for violent physical exertion.

Children should be made aware that well-being and the maintenance of reserves will depend on their taking appropriate exercise throughout the remainder of their lives. The significance of the venous pumps should be explained and here we see how the homeostatic mechanisms extend to the muscular system which in turn is under nervous control. Greater efficiency is achieved when people can achieve and maintain a good muscular tone and posture.

Effects of Tobacco

Apart from the lack of exercise and the neglect of posture which can lead to shallow breathing, perhaps the worst attack on the well-being of the oxygen-transport system results from smoking tobacco. Tobacco contains such a package of substances, that would be considered to be drugs in another context, that it is certain that if it had been discovered in the twentieth century no government would have permitted its use. Nicotine has a direct effect on the heart and blood vessels, as well as on the brain. The heart beats more quickly due to increased adrenalin production which is quite inappropriate since the heartbeat should normally respond to oxygen demands of the muscles alone. The blood vessels of the skin contract which in turn causes a rise of blood-pressure as well as a sensation of cold. The irritant gases and droplets in the tobacco smoke paralyse the cilia lining the bronchial tubes so that the automatic cleansing mechanism, which so conveniently removes debris of all kinds from the lungs and delivers it at the back of the throat, is paralysed. The breathing tubes also tend to contract so that the air-way is diminished. Breathing becomes more difficult, and this can be shown when people are asked to breathe into a spirometer which can measure the amount of air that can be expired from the chest.

We see therefore that tobacco embarrasses the oxygen-transport system in two ways. First, by artificially producing a rapid heartbeat but without producing a greater volume of blood per stroke, by raising the blood-pressure which is further embarrassing to the circulation, and by impeding the entrance of air into the lungs from which the oxygen can be removed by the circulation. In addition carbon monoxide is absorbed and is taken up by the red blood cells. As carbon monoxide forms a stable compound with haemoglobin some of the red blood cells are put out of action as regards their oxygen-carrying capacity.

We can now consider how the social environment enters into the picture as regards the oxygen-transport system of the body. Lack of amenities can discourage young people on leaving school from continuing the sports and athletics in which they acquired some skill. This is a matter for community responsibility. Personal failure to make constructive use of leisure may also result in a chronic physical inactivity which will create a problem in middle age and later in life. There may be too much preoccupation with economic and domestic problems and failures of planning in personal life.

Over-eating followed by the inevitable over-weight could disincline people for exercise and indeed they may run a distinct risk if they do attempt much exercise without weight reduction. Over-eating may have an emotional basis, but it is a hazard for those who are materially successful in whom it is part of a group pattern of behaviour. The same applies to smoking and the incentives to smoke are closely linked with feelings of prestige within a group, although later the smoking of tobacco can become part of an addiction. Anxiety may underlie both over-eating and smoking, but the solution to anxiety lies in its adequate constructive handling by the individual, a technique of living which should be taught as early in life as possible.

We have considered so far only a few of the many factors which have a bearing upon well-being. However, these suffice to show how hollow and superficial may be the traditional advice to people to take plenty of exercise, not to over-eat, and to abstain from smoking. Motivation for behaviour, and this includes not doing things as well as doing things, are derived from the primitive personal needs for success and recognition, but are modified considerably by a life-experience, lack of knowledge and skill, and the pressures in the social and economic environment.

An understanding of the principles of homeostasis should give everyone a greater confidence in his body as a going concern. But the matter should not stop there; it should also be understood that the thresholds of tolerance to homeostatic adaptation should be recognized and that something should be done to preserve the body's mechanisms against the strain of overcompensation-adaptation.

Adaptation is responsible for evolutionary change, as well as being, paradoxically, its own end-product. Darwin and the nineteenth century biologists taught the lesson that species must adapt in order to survive, but as no new visibly different kind of human being has emerged, it has not been easy to apply this lesson to ourselves. There is a growing body of thought now that many diseases and disorders in our community are the result of failure to adapt to circumstances which we have as a human race imposed upon ourselves. This has not been a question of one species competing for space with another, it is a question of one species unthinkingly creating a change in the internal and external environment for which the body has not sufficient powers of adaptation.

An example is the result of the consumption of refined sugar. Cleave has pointed out that the refining of sugar is only just over a hundred years old, so that the introduction of this article into the human diet, in evolutionary terms, happened yesterday. [6] Unrefined sugars require a lengthy process of digestion, being broken down gradually first by the saliva and then gastric and intestinal juices into glucose. Glucose is released in very small spurts into the circulation and the pancreas, producing insulin to metabolize glucose, can cope with this. When refined sugar is taken, on the other hand, larger doses of glucose flood the circulation almost instantaneously, and it seems plausible to believe that in many cases the pancreas cannot cope with this exceptional demand. In some people this may produce diabetes, and in other people the consumption of refined sugars is believed to be responsible for varicose veins, coronary artery disease, and intestinal disorders.

More recently attention has been drawn also to the results of consuming a diet in which there is little or no roughage. [7] Comparative studies conducted in communities where a coarse unrefined diet is taken, compared with Western European and American communities, shows that diseases of the large bowel and possibly even cancer can be related to the taking of a diet which does not produce sufficient stimulation for the musculature of the bowel to do its work.

Constipation and its attendant discomfort was once believed erroneously to be the cause of the absorption of toxic substances into the blood. There is no evidence for this, but there is evidence that constipation resulting from a feeble muscular contraction of the bowel and consequent engorgement and distension is responsible for disorders which may even require surgical treatment. For centuries, people have treated constipation by stimulating the bowel with violent purgatives. These were taken in ignorance of the fact that the bowel has muscles under nervous control which work automatically, perfectly well, when treated properly. This means consuming sufficient fluid and sufficient indigestible bulky roughage to produce the necessary stimulation. To attempt to stimulate a weakened muscle with purgatives is merely aggravating the condition and is adding to the danger of a development of cancer and other disorders.

When looking after our internal environment, we must be conscious of the forces of evolution and be wary of the introduction of new articles of diet, or new modes of living which may not result in an appropriate adaptive response. At the same time we should look to the outside social environment with its various pressures which may be demanding too much of the powers of adaptation.

QUESTIONS

1. What budgetary priorities in personal expenditure are required in order to maintain health and efficiency? Refer to the situation of an unmarried teacher in his or her first post.

2. In what ways is a person responsible for his own well-being?

REFERENCES

1. Bernard, Claude (1874). *Phénomènes de la vie*. Paris.
2. Cannon, W. B. (1963). *The Wisdom of the Body*. New York:Norton.
3. Osman, J. D. (1972). 'Nutrition Education: Too Much, Too Little, or Too Bad?' *Journal of School Health*(USA). 42(10):592–6.
4. Bender, A. (1969). *A Nutritional Evaluation: Food, Facts, and Figures*. Report of a National Survey. London: Margarine and Shortening Manufacturers' Association.
5. Macdonald, I. (1973). 'The Sugar in the Diet'. *British Nutrition Foundation Bulletin* No.8.
6. Campbell, G. D., Cleave, T. L., and Painter, N. S. (1967). *Diabetes, Coronary Thrombosis, and the Saccharine Disease*. Bristol: Wright.
7. Burkitt, D. P. (1971). 'Cancer and the Way we live'. Chapter 9 in G. Bennette (ed.) *Cancer Priorities*. London: British Cancer Council.

FURTHER READING

Conroy, T. T. W. L. and Mills, J. W. (1970). *Human Circadian Rhythms*. London: Churchill.
Dalzell-Ward, A. J. (1967). 'Physical Activity and Health'. Chapter in J. E. Kane, (ed.) *Readings in Physical Education*. London: Physical Education Association.
World Health Organization (1969). *Optimum Physical Performance Capacities in Adults*. Technical Report Series No. 436. London: HMSO.

FILMS

Title	Colour B/W	Running time	Distributor	Date
Body Defences against Disease	B/W	11 mins.	N.A.V.A.L.*	1949
External Respiration	Colour	14 mins.	N.A.V.A.L.	1952
The Nervous System in Man	Colour	18 mins.	N.A.V.A.L.	1968
The Fight against Bacteria	Colour	15 mins.	N.A.V.A.L.	1963
Immunisation	B/W	10 mins.	N.A.V.A.L.	1947
Nothing to Eat but Food	Colour	18 mins.	Free from Unilever Films	1962
Foods and Nutrition	B/W	11 mins.	N.A.V.A.L.	1949
Exploring Your Growth	Colour	11 mins.	N.A.V.A.L.	1965
A Question of Immunity	Colour	13 mins	Concord	1971
You – the Living Machine (USA)	Colour	8 mins.	Cancer Information Centre	1965
How the Body uses Energy	B/W	15 mins.	McGraw Hill	1966
Circulation and the Heart		17 mins.	Education Foundation for Visual Aids	1968
An Introduction to Nutrition (British)	Colour	10 mins	Rank Film Library**	1962
Cold can kill	Colour	33 mins	Ministry of Defence (Navy) Principal Supply and Transport Office, Section 7B/0572. HM Dockyard Portsmouth	1973
Pounds, Slimming and Sense	Colour	20 mins.	Guild Sound and Vision Ltd.	1969

*National Audio-Visual Aids Library, Paxton Place, Gipsy Road, London SE27
**Now Guild Sound and Vision Ltd., 85–129 Dundle Road, Peterborough PE2 9PY.

CHAPTER 3

Importance of the early years

We might consider the new born infant as the prototype of the healthy human being, assuming that the child is free of congenital defects and has escaped injury during the process of birth. Although it is true that many of the functions are still under-developed at this age, all the basic mechanisms for homeostasis are there and for the first six months of life the child even acquires from his mother an immunity to certain infections.

Growth and Development

The process of growth and development depends upon hormonal activity initiated by a growth hormone secreted by the pituitary gland which controls growth from birth to adolescence. [1,2,3] Other endocrine glands that are involved are the thyroid, adrenals, the endocrine portion of the pancreas (producing insulin) and certain cells of the testis and ovary. The velocity of growth is highest in the intra-uterine stage of development. There is an increase of size from the microscopic proportions of the embedded fertilized ovum to a baby of eight or nine pounds in nine months.

From birth the velocity of growth slows until it is complete with the fusion of the epiphyses of the long bones at about nineteen years and the final fusion of the epiphysis of the collar bone at about twenty-five. At puberty however there is a relatively rapid development of the testis and ovary leading to the development of secondary sex characteristics and the preparation for fertility.

Tanner has analysed the biological features of human growth as revealed by contemporary researches. There is a subtle relationship between hormonal activity and external factors. Once again homeostatic mechanisms are involved. Growth hormone is secreted in response to stimuli of which a drop in the level of sugar in the blood and a rise in the level of certain amino acids are examples. Exercise and emotion are associated with fluctuations in the level of growth hormone production.

The Growth Hormone

The homeostatic principle is represented by the existence of a 'feedback' circuit linking the entire endocrine complex. Changes in one gland are followed by compensatory changes in other glands. Tanner describes how pituitary activity itself is initiated by hormones produced in that basal part of the brain known as the hypothalamus. The hypothalamus has for long been known as the site of nerve-centres concerned with emotions such as aggression and fear and modern researches in neurophysiology have identified this region as an important traffic junction for circuits linking the higher cerebral centres concerned with thought and motivation with those subserving body functions. Now in addition it may be said that the *fons et origo* of all hormones originates in the hypothalamus. The pituitary gland is linked with this structure by a stalk supplied with nerve fibres as well as blood vessels. Thus events occurring in the higher cerebral centres are conveyed both by nerve impulses and chemically to the pituitary gland which then exercises general control over the members of the endocrine system.

The hormones secreted by the hypothalamus are said by Tanner to be 'switched on' by chemical stimuli resulting from alterations in the level of hormones in the blood stream. The cells in the hypothalamus which are sensitive to alterations in blood hormone levels are 'set' either to respond to a high or a low level of hormone. Before puberty the cells are 'set' so that a low level of oestrogen in the blood does not stimulate the production of FSH by the pituitary (see above). Thus ovulation and menstruation do not occur in the girl before puberty although the ovaries are complete with their stock of egg cells that will suffice throughout the reproductive life. After puberty the cells in the hypothalamus are then 'set' so that they are sensitive to higher levels of oestrogen. Then a fall in oestrogen level is followed by stimulation of the pituitary to produce FSH. Ovulation and menstruation can then occur.

Relevance to Child Care

These biological facts are meaningful in terms of the kind of care that children need in order that they should grow to their maximum potential and thrive. Widdowson observed in German nurseries after the Second World War that in a case where there was a very severe matron who was continually nagging and rebuking the children they failed to maintain their expected growth curve. [4] Severe psychological stress has been reported as being responsible for dwarfism presumably due to the 'switching off' of the growth hormone. These studies provide firm evidence that man is indivisible and they make plausible the observation that psychosomatic illness with physical changes is possible. Future researches in psychosomatic medicine will show the importance of the emotional environment in the causation of some organic diseases.

During the process of growth and development the home, social, and educational environment stimulates the development of behaviour, physical, intellectual, and emotional performance, and social functions that will characterize a human being in the twentieth century.

The Prototype of Health

There is no better point to commence study of the dependence upon environment and external factors for the promotion of health than the consideration of pregnancy itself. Before birth when the child is developing in the uterus, what happens to the mother is very important for his development. On the physical plane, if the mother suffers from virus infections during the third month of pregnancy and in particular, rubella, or if she takes certain drugs, then there is a likelihood that malformation of organs and limbs may occur. Both father and mother make an equal contribution of genes carrying physical and intellectual and possibly emotional characteristics. The human race exhibits a great degree of variation, more so than any other animal species. This is due to the gene mixture which occurs at random, and randomization is increased by freedom of choice of partners which is enjoyed in the Western world and to an increasing degree now in other parts of the world. [5] Such features as colour of the eyes and hair, shape of the body i.e. somatotype, are determined genetically, as also are intelligence and the susceptibility to certain disorders and infections. We must qualify this statement as it affects intelligence. The old controversy between 'nature' and 'nurture' has recently been revived by the contemporary debate between certain psychologists who would assign the maximum importance to genetic factors and the environmentalists — often as extreme in their views — who would place greater weight on environmental factors in the development of intelligence.

Smoking during pregnancy is now known to be a cause of low birth weight, which may not necessarily be a disadvantage, and also of an increase in the perinatal mortality rate i.e. stillbirth or death of the child within the first month of life. There is evidence also that children whose mothers have smoked during pregnancy tend to read later. Here we have perhaps the first clear-cut demonstration of the relationship between the maternal environment during development in the uterus and future educability.

The mother's emotions during pregnancy and labour are also important to the child's development. Because the mind and body are indivisible, the effects of emotional disturbance during pregnancy are shown in a physical way. The fact that a number of mothers could not tolerate their pregnancies without the use of tranquillizers to allay anxieties and fears is the primary cause of the disasters attributed to thalidomide. This is an extreme case, but if pregnancy cannot be accepted and experienced as a natural event, free from any undue discomfort, save, perhaps, inconvenience, then this is likely to have an effect upon labour, which may be difficult and prolonged and in which there is a greater likelihood of injury to the child's head. Cerebral palsy is one of the extreme examples of the effects of birth injury in which there is actual damage to the brain. In recent years there has been interest also in what is called minimal brain damage, which may be due either to something happening to the mother during pregnancy, such as infection, or to minor head injury during the process of birth.

The process of birth itself is influenced by the mother's emotions which are in turn influenced by those of the father. Both parents should be pleased when they learn of the pregnancy, be prepared to share the duties of care of the expectant mother, and the responsibilities of the birth, if the child is to be really welcomed into the world. A pregnancy may be inconvenient, however, and at the present day, it is likely to interfere with studies as well as the family economy. It has always been an economic burden, despite the provisions of the welfare state. It may interfere with career prospects, or it may be resented by one or other of the partners for some deeper reason.

Birth commences by the relaxation of the involuntary muscular ring that guards the exit to the uterus. This is called the cervix, and like all involuntary muscles, is under the influence of the emotions. If the cervix does not relax and stretch up to allow the passage of the baby's head, then labour will be delayed; there will be a recourse to anaesthesia, perhaps deep anaesthesia, and the use of instruments to assist the birth. The baby will be affected by the anaesthetics and starting breathing immediately after birth may be difficult. The mother will be either unconscious or so drowsy that she will not take an immediate interest in the child, and the husband will be anxious about his wife's survival. These are factors which have an effect upon the child's subsequent health and development.

Fate of 1,000 Children

If we study the survival rates of a cohort of a thousand children born in one year at the present time in England and Wales, we find that twenty-nine will not survive the first year of life. Of these, twelve will have been stillborn, and of the remaining seventeen, half will die in the first month of life. The general infant mortality rate, which is the number of children dying in the first year of life per 1,000 live births, is now only seventeen. This is not the lowest rate in the world as a whole and northern European countries do a bit better, the infant mortality rates being as low as 11 per 1,000 live births recorded in Scandinavian countries and in Holland. In Northern Ireland and in Scotland, the figures are 22 and 21 respectively, compared with the figure of 17 for England and Wales. In the USSR, the figure is 24 deaths per 1,000 live births in the first year, and in Yugoslavia as much as 56.

We can immediately see a geographical variation, which has nothing to do with climate, but which reflects social conditions. There is also a historical factor, for example, as recently as 1951, the general infant mortality rate was 29.8 per 1,000 live births, and if stillbirths and deaths under one month are isolated, that is the perinatal mortality rate, it was 38.2. At the beginning of the century, the general figure was round about 150.

To be born healthy therefore is not entirely a matter of luck, but much is also due to the quality of the society in which conception, pregnancy, labour, and care during the first year of life take place. The lowering of mortality rates in countries of Western Europe has been achieved partly by improved general education of the public, which in turn has led to industrial and technological development thus increasing the gross national product of the community. This has produced surpluses which can then be used by governments and voluntary agencies to provide services to cater for the special needs of expectant mothers, mothers in labour, and children during the first year of life.

The quality of family life is also a factor, and it is notable that the infant mortality rate amongst illegitimate children is higher than that of children born in wedlock. The reduction in family size and social changes which have encouraged husbands to share domestic duties and to take an interest in their wives' pregnancies and labour and in the care of the small child have also played their part. Health education carried on mainly by health visitors in welfare centres and in individual homes has raised the standard of child care.

Medical advances also must claim some of the credit for this improvement in the survival of infants during the first year of life. Antenatal care is usually undertaken early in pregnancy and during this period of supervision of her health the expectant mother has an opportunity for health education. Tests are done early in pregnancy to eliminate the possibility of the mother suffering from syphilis or gonorrhoea, so that congenital syphilis is becoming increasingly rare and infection of the child during labour which used to be an accident of maternal gonorrhoea is also almost unknown. The discovery of the rhesus factor has made it possible to prevent stillbirth or abnormalities as a result of rhesus incompatibility, a situation in which the mother becomes immunized against her own child.

Another threat to the child's development while in the uterus is toxaemia of pregnancy. This is detected by regular routine urine tests, and also measurements of blood-pressure, and if the condition is present, then it can be treated, and in most cases the baby survives to be born alive. Improvements in blood transfusion technique and the provision of blood-banks has made it possible for mothers suffering from severe haemorrhages in labour to be resuscitated. In the same way, exchange blood transfusion can be practised in the case where infants, despite all precautions, are suffering from a rhesus incompatibility factor.

Preparation of the mother during pregnancy to understand the nature of labour and to participate actively in it has reduced the need for deep anaesthesia and for instrumental interference. There are some mothers indeed who can go right through labour with only minimal discomfort and although claims are made that this has been made possible by psychological and emotional preparation, it is probable that these women enjoy a greater degree of security of personality than the majority.

When the child is born, the parents now have available a wide range of equipment specially designed for small children. This extends from clothing to toys and includes food preparations for use during weaning, always a vulnerable time for the baby. The industries which service the needs of mothers and small children have also made their contribution, and in addition to distributing their products, a good deal of health education is often included as some of them employ qualified health visitors who have concentrated on child care education.

The child is an emotional being even before birth, and from birth onwards he will require the kind of care which includes the demonstration of affection by physical contact in the first place. It is significant that the skin is developed from the same outer layer of the embryo from which the brain and nervous system develop. Throughout the whole of life the skin and the mind are closely linked. Not only can disorders of the mind affect the skin adversely, but conversely pleasurable stimulation of the skin imparts a sense of well-being. It is particularly important in the case of a small infant whose only communication channels are through physical contact.

The child requires stimulation verbally also, and stimulation by experience. As he grows stronger and physical skills develop, he has a need for movement and play and for responding to physical challenges.

For the first six months of life, the child will enjoy an immunity to various infections acquired from his mother. This unfortunately does not extend to immunity to the common cold and bronchitis and during the first few months of life, the baby is very vulnerable to infection brought in by people outside the family. From six months onwards, however, he requires protection by artificial immunization and the present schedule is extensive. It includes protection against diphtheria, whooping cough and tetanus which can be combined in single injections, and against poliomyelitis — the vaccine for which is administered by mouth on a lump of sugar. Early in the first year, he will require protection against measles by vaccination. Vaccination against smallpox was discontinued in 1971 as a routine.

This basic immunity requires reinforcement on entering school by the administration of booster doses. Later on in childhood, it is advisable that girls should be protected against rubella between the ages of eleven and fourteen and the purpose of this is the protection of their own children when they eventually become pregnant. Between thirteen and fifteen protection against tuberculosis is given by the administration of B.C.G. vaccine. Therefore the greatest medical contribution has been in the preventive field by the gradual elimination from communities in Western Europe and in the United States of dangerous killing diseases which exacted a terrible toll of child life in the nineteenth century.

Table 3. Schedule of vaccination and immunization

Age	Vaccine
During the first year of life.	Diph/Tet/Pert/* and oral polio vaccine. 1st dose. Diph/Tet/Pert/ and oral polio vaccine. 2nd dose. Diph/Tet/Pert/ and oral polio vaccine. 3rd dose.
During the second year of life	Measles Vaccine.
At 5 years of age or school entry.	Diph/Tet/toxoid and oral polio vaccine, or inactivated polio vaccine.
Between 10 and 13 years of age.	B.C.G. Vaccine (for tuberculin negative children).
All girls aged 11—13 years.	Rubella Vaccine.
At 15—19 years of age or on leaving school.	Polio Vaccine (oral or inactivated) and tetanus toxoid.

*Combined injection: protects against diphtheria, tetanus, and whooping cough. 'Pertussis' is the name of the organism causing whooping cough.

Protection against diphtheria and tetanus is by toxoids which immunize against the toxin produced by the organisms. The other infections are prevented by vaccines which stimulate antibody formation against the actual organisms.

Source: Department of Health and Social Security. (1972). *Immunization against Infectious Diseases.*

Reproduced by permission of the Comptroller, HMSO.

EDUCATION FOR PARENTHOOD

Another important preventive measure has been the provision of health education for parents. The modern parent requires to know facts regarding child development, physical, emotional and social needs of the child, prevention of illness, care of the sick child, protection from common danger and the promotion of the greatest possible potential development of the intellect by education. Not only must facts be known, but there must be skills in applying them, and these skills are not only physical or manual. The difficult problem of toilet-training for example can only be undertaken by parents who understand that during the first year of life the nerve pathways controlling the voluntary action of the bowels are as yet undeveloped. They must also be aware of the emotional damage done to children by associating defecation and the passage of urine with goodness or badness. Later on, they will need to be able to distinguish between temper tantrums and emotional disturbance that requires professional advice. They must be aware that the human being needs stimulation and challenge in order that the functions develop and are maintained.

In addition to these basic facts, modern parents have to know about the social and medical services now available to assist them in the care of their children. Many benefits either financial or of services are not taken up because people are unaware of them, or because they are daunted by the prospect of filling in forms or other formalities. To be a complete and efficient parent in the twentieth century, however, it is essential to understand the social services of the welfare state in whichever country one lives.

This is where we may now relate health education to a successful birth and survival of the child which is the beginning of a healthy life. The general principles that emerge from the study of the personal, social and economic environment that contributes towards the birth of healthy children must be regarded as a prototype of a health-contributing environment throughout the rest of life. The emphasis and the slant changes, but the general principles remain.

QUESTIONS

1. Indicate briefly some of the practices you would include in a health education programme in (a) an infants' school, and (b) a junior school.

2. Why is 'play' so important for normal development?

3. Why is it necessary that a teacher should have a reasonable understanding of the process of maturation of children in the age range that he/she is teaching?

4. What advice would you give to a parent of a five-year-old when the former complains that her child has 'dirty habits' (plays with its genitals) and asks questions about the origin of babies?

5. In what ways may illegitimate children be disadvantaged?

6. How may health education and antenatal care influence a child's future educability?

7. Do the provisions of the welfare state diminish the responsibility of parents?

REFERENCES

1. Tanner, J. M. (1970). 'Postnatal Growth'. Chapter in R. G. Mitchell (ed.) *Child Life and Health*. London: Churchill.
2. Tanner, J. M. (1961). *Education and Physical Growth*. London: University of London Press.
3. Tanner, J. M. (1969). *Growth at Adolescence*. 2nd. ed. Oxford: Blackwell.
4. Widdowson, E. M. (1951). 'Mental Contentment and Physical Growth'. *Lancet* 1:1316–18.
5. Winchester, A. M. (1971). *Human Genetics*. Ohio: Charles E. Merrill.

FURTHER READING

BBC (1968). *Formative Years*. London: BBC Publications.

Illingworth, R. S. (1968). 'The Normal Child'. *Studies in Child Development* No.2 (National Children's Bureau). 4th.ed. London:Churchill. (The Bureau publishes a series of monographs on child development and its relationship to the standards of child care.)

Isaacs, Susan (1968). *Children and Parents: Their Problems and Difficulties*. London: Routledge and Kegan Paul.

Kellmer-Pringle, M. L., Davie, R. and Hancock, L. E. (eds.) (1969). *Directory of Voluntary Organizations concerned with Children*. (National Children's Bureau). London:Longmans. (It is as much a guide to the needs of children as a source of addresses and information.)

Ratcliffe, T. A. (1967). *The Development of the Personality*. London: Allen and Unwin.

Winnicott, D. W. (1957). *The Child and the Family*. London: Tavistock Pubns.

FILMS

Title	Colour B/W	Running time	Distributor	Date
Biography before Birth	B/W	18 mins.	N.A.V.A.L.	1952
The First Days of Life	Colour	22 mins.	N.A.V.A.L.	1971
Barnet (The Child)	Colour	48 mins.	N.A.V.A.L.	1969
To Janet a Son	Colour	18½ mins.	Free from Farley's Ltd., Golymead Road, Colnbrook, Bucks.	1961
Preparation for Parenthood	B/W	17 mins.	N.A.V.A.L.	1952
Childhood — The Right of Every Child	B/W	30 mins.	Concord	1968
Terrible Twos and Trusting Threes	Colour	22 mins.	Concord	1950
The Frustrating Fours and Fascinating Fives	Colour	22 mins.	Concord	1952
Sociable Six to Noisy Nine	Colour	21 mins.	Concord	1956
The World of Three	B/W	28 mins.	Concord	1966
Seven Up	B/W	35 mins.	Concord	1964
Immunization	B/W	10 mins.	N.A.V.A.L.	1949
Fair Families (by Margaret Mead)	B/W	60 mins.	Concord	1959
Moving Off In the Beginning From Hand to Mouth	B/W	20 mins.	Concord	1969—71
Early Mother—Baby Relationships	B/W	10 mins.	Concord	1967
Human Hereditary (American, for secondary schools)	Colour	14 mins.	N.A.V.A.L. Boulton Hawker Films, Ltd., Hadleigh, Ipswich, Suffolk.	1960
The Science of Man, series 3: Egg to Adult (on sexual reproduction) (10 films)	B/W	30 mins. each	BBC Television Enterprises	1964
Child Development (*four parts, filmstrip*) 1. Birth to Two Years 2. Development of Love Sentiment 3. Emotional Development to Adolescence 4. Development 1—3 years			Camera Talks Ltd.	
Human Development (*filmstrip*)			Camera Talks Ltd.	
Learning about People (*12 short strips*)			Encyclopaedia Britannica	
Fear and Horror	B/W	13 mins.	Guild Sound and Vision	

CHAPTER 4

The community's health

In preparation for adult responsibility, it is important that all school-leavers have a sound idea of the health patterns in the community and can identify and interpret their significance. They should be encouraged to speculate on what further improvements can be achieved, but also on the ways in which present standards can be maintained and what factors in society can threaten them. It should be clearly understood that the pattern of health and disease in every community is the result of a complex of factors which includes personal and group behaviour, economic standards, geographical location, balance of ecology, education, and standards of living as well as medical treatment. With the use of modern medical techniques even after disastrous wars, modern states can regain the level of public health which obtain in peace-time. We do not have to look far afield in the E.E.C. for witness of this in our own time. The decline of public health is due not only to the casualties caused by military operations, but even more important, the breakdown of health and social services and environmental control, all of which have to be maintained at a peak of efficiency to keep disease at bay and to preserve the quality of life.

Annual Medical Audit

In the United Kingdom there is an annual medical audit of the nation's health in the form of the annual report of the Chief Medical Officer, Department of Health and Social Security. Since 1972 the Secretary of State for Wales has presented a report to Parliament which contains (amongst other matters) information concerning the Health and Personal Social Services and Housing and Environmental Services. The Chief Medical Officers of the Scottish Home and Health Department and the Ministry of Health and Social Affairs of Northern Ireland respectively also publish annual reports. To obtain a complete picture of the United Kingdom, all four reports should be read, particularly as there are distinct differences in the various regions of the United Kingdom.

In addition to these documents, the health of the schoolchild is dealt with separately in a report published every two years by the Chief Medical Officer of the Department of Education and Science. There is an increasing availability of sources of information about health, disease, mortality, and causes of disease at the present day. The statistical basis of all of these depends upon the work of the Registrar-General whose Department, the Office of Population Censuses and Surveys, collects and analyses information on all aspects of demography, including the causes of death and produces special reports on the causes of certain illnesses. There have been special studies to analyse records kept by family doctors which throw a new light on the incidence of the less serious illnesses and their nature. The reports of the Office of Health Economics, a privately financed institute, provide us with yet another source of information from which we can draw a picture of the nation's health.

Favoured Age-Groups

One of the first things that the school-leaver will discover is that his own age-group enjoys the highest standard of health and lowest mortality rate of any group in the community. In fact the death rate of the age-group from five to thirty-four in the United Kingdom is the lowest in Europe. The countries of the E.E.C. show a fairly similar picture and the lowest general death rates are seen in the Scandinavian countries. A male infant in the United Kingdom born between 1969 and 1971 will on the average survive to the age of 69.2 years. A female infant born in the same period will on average survive to the age of 75. These figures are somewhat misleadingly called 'expectation of life', but in reality they are figures showing the average age at death, which varies according to the age (i.e. under five or between five and thirty-four) at which the expectation is calculated. These survival rates do not seem much superior to the Biblical three score years and ten which was apparently the norm in those times in the pastoral countries of the Middle East. The greatest improvement in survival has been in the earlier years of life with the reduction of the infant mortality rate and subsequently the reduction of mortality during the school years.

There are variations in mortality experience even within the United Kingdom. Whereas the figures for expectation of life in England and Wales and in Northern Ireland are practically indentical they are lower in the case of Scotland, where a male infant born in 1968 will enjoy an average survival rate to the age of 67.3 years, and a female infant to the age of 74.4 years. The variations in Europe in terms of expectation of life are relatively slight with the exception of the Scandinavian countries referred to. When one looks at the picture in the *Third World*, however, there are profound differences. This is due to the persistence of severe infectious diseases such as diphtheria and tuberculosis which threaten infant and child life, to lack of development of environmental control as it affects the protection of water supplies and the disposal of waste, coupled with the lack of development of social and medical services for the adult population. There are also problems of malnutrition and in many communities severe parasitic infestation e.g. hookworm or bilharzia. Rheumatic fever which has undergone a 'massive decline' in prevalence in Western Europe is a problem in the U.A.R. and Caribbean. Fortunately, the resources of the World Health Organization are devoted to public health programmes in these countries.

Retreat of Major Infectious Diseases

If we consider progress in public health in the last three decades in Western Europe, the most important feature is the retreat of killing infectious diseases. In particular, tuberculosis has declined considerably and is now most likely to occur in middle-aged men and we do not see the bovine type of tuberculosis which used to cause so much damage to bones and joints in children. Immunization in childhood has caused the disappearance of diphtheria and polio-myelitis, and a great reduction in the incidence of whooping cough and measles. Smallpox, having been controlled for nearly two hundred years by vaccination, now does not occur unless imported from other countries, and the practice of routine vaccination against smallpox in infancy has been discontinued.

The conquest of tuberculosis has been due to several factors: improvement in social conditions and the isolation of infectious people from the vulnerable community; the introduction of antibiotics and chemotherapy and of course the immunization of school children by B.C.G. This does not mean to say that there is no longer any anxiety about tuberculosis in this country, but the total deaths due to this cause in 1971 were only 1,329 and the notifications of new cases of the disease totalled 11,137. Case-finding and persuasion to accept treatment have been important factors in the reduction of this disease, and at one time mass-miniature radiography units worked continuously in all parts of the country offering free chest X-Rays to the general public, and also to personnel in factories and offices. The recent wave of immigrants from countries where tuberculosis is still a serious health problem has made it necessary for health authorities to give special attention to the detection of tuberculosis in this group.

A new dimension in the use of immunization has been the recent

Figure 1.   A comparison of the incidence of mortality due to tuberculosis in 1930, and lung cancer in 1968

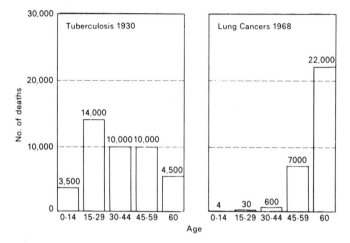

Source: Office of Health Economics. (1972). *Medicine and Society.*
Note: A dramatic illustration of the exchange of one health problem for another after an interval of forty years. Note the shift towards older age-groups.

introduction of vaccination against rubella, which is offered to schoolgirls aged 10—11. In this case the purpose of the immunization is to prevent the occurrence of rubella in pregnancy and thus to prevent congenital malformation in future children.

Unfortunately, the picture is marred by the continual occurrence of epidemics of influenza and because of the frequent change in the character of the virus causing the epidemic, it is very difficult to prepare vaccines that would be useful on a mass basis. However, people in certain occupations, such as doctors, mid-wives, ambulance drivers and those who are particularly vulnerable to infection can be protected by vaccination against this disease.

Sexually Transmitted Diseases

There is one infectious disease, however, which having declined considerably in the years 1950 to 1956 in the United Kingdom now shows a sharp rise in incidence. In the Annual Report for 1971, the Chief Medical Officer, D.H.S.S., said that this infection (gonorrhoea) is still uncontrolled. The highest incidence is in the age group 20—24, but 400 girls under the age of 16 contracted this infection in that year, and 129 boys. The report went on to say, 'the increasing incidence of gonorrhoea in young people remains the greatest cause for concern. It is sometimes suggested that increasing use of the contraceptive pill is a factor, but it is well known that many girls take the risk of pregnancy and indeed the incidence of births and legal termination of pregnancy at these ages has risen.'

Gonorrhoea is not the only one of the sexually transmitted diseases which represents a major public health problem. We are particularly fortunate in the United Kingdom that the incidence of syphilis has not increased and the number of new cases diagnosed each year is very low compared with other countries. Nevertheless, there are over 1,000 early infections each year. Other genital infections transmitted by sexual intercourse are non-specific urethritis which accounted for a total of 72,420 cases of which 59,023 were in men and 13,397 in women in 1971. There is also infection with non-bacterial organisms of which trichomoniasis accounted for 17,407 female cases and 1,300 male cases in 1971, and an infection by a yeast-like organism, candidosis, which accounted for a total of 24,420 cases, 2,881 in males and 21,539 in females.

The list of identifiable sexually transmitted infections is growing, and some of them can have serious consequences. For example, the virus of herpes simplex, which causes the familiar cold sore around the lips in the course of a common cold, can also cause a genital infection. In 1971, 3,671 cases were diagnosed at special clinics.

Figure 2   Number of cases of gonorrhoea dealt with for the first time in England and Wales from 1940

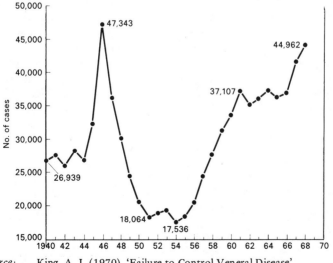

Source: King, A. J. (1970). 'Failure to Control Venereal Disease'. *Brit. Med. J.* **21.**

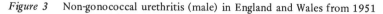

Figure 3   Non-gonococcal urethritis (male) in England and Wales from 1951

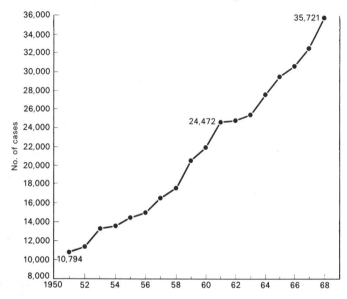

Source: King, A. J. (1970). 'Failure to Control Venereal Disease'.
Brit. Med. J. 21.

The possibility that infection with this virus could be associated with the occurrence of carcinoma of the cervix in women later in life is supported by a considerable amount of evidence gathered from the study of large samples of populations in the United States.

For this group of sexually transmitted infections, there is at present no effective method of prevention, save the regulation of personal behaviour. At best, the spread of this disease can be controlled if those who have run the risk by casual sexual contact go immediately to a special clinic for diagnosis and treatment, and if they abstain from having sexual intercourse until they are pronounced clear of infection. Despite extensive researches, no vaccine has yet been produced, although there is a possibility that a vaccine effective against syphilis may be available before long. In the case of gonorrhoea, the biological conditions, which are essential for the production of a vaccine, seem to be absent. The fact that an attack of gonorrhoea does not confer immunity against further attacks is not now considered to rule out the effectiveness of a vaccine.

With regard to the other genital infections mentioned, there is no possibility of a vaccine being available. High standards of personal hygiene, the restricting of intercourse to one partner, whether in marriage or out of marriage, and the development of emotional maturity in sexual matters remain the best preventive measures against this group of infections. It is unique in that personal behaviour is the determining factor.

Intestinal Infections

Infections which spread from the intestine also remain a problem, although in the United Kingdom the highly efficient systems of sewage-disposal combined with protected water supplies and the great rise in standards of personal hygiene during the last three decades have helped to keep these infections at a minimum. Diseases, such as typhoid fever, however, can easily be imported into this country now that so many people travel to parts of Europe where the diseases are still endemic. Travellers are advised to have protective inoculations against typhoid fever before travelling to these countries, but from time to time, cases of typhoid fever are imported and the numbers fluctuate annually from 150 plus. It has been established that only 6% of the people who suffer from typhoid fever in any particular year and who contracted the infection abroad had received inoculations against typhoid before starting their travels.

Infections spread by food occur each year. Ice-cream is sometimes a vehicle in the spread of para-typhoid fever, and about 7,000 cases of food poisoning caused by germs entering the food during production, preparation, storage, or serving occur each year. It is suspected that the numbers are under-reported. Food poisoning is a particular problem in large-scale catering including the school meals service, but the strict application of the Food Hygiene Regulations and the training of catering staff in the principles of safe food-handling should restrict the incidence of food poisoning to the occasional accident.

Dysentery is a problem in schools and a number of outbreaks occur each year in day nurseries or infant schools. The prevention of the spread of dysentery is a matter for strict personal and environmental hygiene. This is one case where the teaching of personal health habits, such as washing the hands after going to the lavatory, regular bathing and the wearing of clean underclothing and the maintenance of scrupulous cleanliness in w.c.s has a direct application to the prevention of disease.

Prevention of Respiratory Infections

There remains the problem of the transmission of infection by droplets from the nose and throat. Although scarlet fever is now very rare, tonsillitis is still very common, and as it is not a notifiable disease, the exact numbers are not known. It is however a common illness amongst school teachers who are exposed more than other adults to large numbers of children at close quarters. The common cold and its complications such as bronchitis represent hazards to the school teacher's health. Research suggests that apart from the spread by direct droplet infection from the nose and throat during talking, sneezing or coughing, there is also the spread of germs through dust and fluff from clothing. Here is an instance where the traditional hygienic principles applied to the environment of the classroom can have a direct effect upon the prevention of disease. Adequate ventilation will dilute the concentration of droplet nuclei in the air, whether these be due to spray from the nose and throat, or dust and fluff from clothing. Ventilation, oiling of floors and other wooden surfaces, and the avoidance of dry sweeping to prevent dispersal of dust are all useful preventive measures.

When we consider the infectious diseases as part of the general national health picture, we can summarize the position as follows. The major killng diseases, which used to take a particular toll of child life, have retreated as a result of immunization, improved standards of hygiene, personal, domestic, and communal, and the higher degree of education and awareness about the dangers of these infections. Control of movements at international frontiers and the requirements for vaccination and inoculation in the case of travel to certain countries are also important factors. These measures have had no effect on influenza, the common cold, and other upper-respiratory infections, or on the sexually transmitted diseases. Preventive measures are not 100% effective in the case of intestinal infections, or food infections. In some cases, personal

Table 4. Mortality: Principal causes, England 1971

Cause	Deaths	Rate per million	SMR (1968 = 100)	%
Tuberculosis of the respiratory system	846	18.4	63	0.16
Tuberculosis, other forms	484	10.5	81	0.09
Diphtheria	1	0.02	–	–
Whooping cough	23	0.5	188	0.004
Streptococcal sore throat and scarlet fever	6	0.1	119	0.001
Meningococcal infection	116	2.5	117	0.02
Acute poliomyelitis	3	0.1	–*	
Smallpox	–	–	–	
Measles	24	0.5	53	0.005
Syphilis and sequelae	121	2.6	68	0.02
All other infective and parasitic diseases	1,459	31.7	91	0.27

Table 4. (*continued*)

Cause	Deaths	Rate per million	SMR (1968 = 100)	%	
Malignant neoplasms					
Buccal cavity and pharynx	1,494	32.4	95	0.28	⎫
Oesophagus	2,825	61.3	103	0.53	
Stomach	11,531	250.2	95	2.17	
Intestine and rectum	15,111	327.9	98	2.84	
Larynx	673	14.6	106	0.13	
Trachea, bronchus and lung	29,291	635.5	104	5.50	⎬ 20.7
Breast	10,603	230.1	108	1.99	
Uterus	3,607	78.3	96	0.68	
Prostate	3,812	82.7	99	0.72	
Leukaemia	2,847	61.8	95	0.53	⎭
Other malignant neoplasms	28,505	618.5	105	5.35	
Diabetes mellitus	4,561	99.0	103	0.86	
Hypertensive disease	8,534	185.2	82	1.60	
Ischaemic heart disease	133,765	902.3	101	25.12	
Other forms of heart disease	33,653	730.2	89	6.32	
Cerebrovascular disease	74,842	1,623.8	97	14.06	
Influenza	650	14.1	14	0.12	
Pneumonia	37,629	816.4	94	7.07	
Bronchitis, emphysema and asthma	26,557	576.2	84	4.99	
Peptic ulcer	3,636	78.9	89	0.68	
Nephritis and nephrosis	2,249	48.8	97	0.42	
Hyperplasia of prostate	1,108	24.0	75	0.21	
Complications of pregnancy, childbirth and the puerperium	129	2.8	67	0.02	
Congenital anomalies	4,234	91.9	99	0.80	
All other diseases	66,305	1,438.6	98	12.45	
Motor vehicle accidents	6,624	143.7	109	1.24	
All other accidents	9,370	203.3	97	1.76	
Suicide and self-inflicted injury	3,739	81.1	86	0.70	
All other external causes	1,491	32.3	100	0.28	
All causes	532,445	11,552.3	96		

*SMR → infinity: because no deaths from acute poliomyelitis in base year 1968.
Source: Department of Health and Social Security. (1971). *On the State of the Public Health.* Annual Report of the Chief Medical Officer.
Reproduced by permission of the Comptroller, HMSO.

behaviour and the application of hygienic knowledge could reduce the incidence of these infections considerably. An indication of the need for education on so basic a matter as personal cleanliness is the prevalence of infestation by head lice and the itch mite — the cause of scabies. In the period 1969—70 well over 200,000 school children were found on inspection to be infested with one or other of these parasites. The irritation, rashes and secondary infection resulting is not dangerous but a serious interference with personal well-being. Pubic lice are also transmitted during sexual contact and are an additional hazard of sexual promiscuity. In some countries infestation with body lice is a serious matter as these insects are the vectors of typhus fever. Here is a direct relevance to health education. Not only has there been success in preventing the major infectious diseases, but the sequels to these infections have also either disappeared or declined considerably e.g. bone and joint tuberculosis resulting in deformity.

Health in Europe

The low mortality rates prevailing in the countries of the Western European community are due then to a number of factors. First there is the retreat of the serious infectious diseases; secondly there is the fact that expectant mothers and women in labour and newly-born children are given very much better medical and social care than in former times, and thirdly, there has been a natural decline of certain diseases like scarlet fever which used to be a cause of mortality and of chronic disabilities in the younger age-groups. Over all, there is the influence of social betterment.

From the point of view of health education, individual responsibility here lies principally in obtaining prompt medical care early in pregnancy and in co-operating with doctors, health visitors, social workers, and other advisers on the care of the child in early infancy. Immunization against the major infectious diseases is also a personal responsibility, principally, of course, of parents. It must be realized also that improvements in personal, domestic, and environmental hygiene and the works of the public health inspector have also played an important part in reducing the incidence of major infections. There is therefore an individual duty to keep oneself and one's clothing clean and to be careful about the disposal of excreta, to protect food and drink from infection, and to co-operate generally with the public authorities who have a responsibility for environmental control. In some respects, bye-laws made by local authorities require the compliance of the individual citizen in his household. Enforcement of these bye-laws by legal process is seldom necessary because of the raised standards of education which have been responsible for a greater awareness of personal responsibility for hygiene of the environment.

Table 5. Health indices in various countries

Country	Standardized Mortality Ratios*			Expectation of life (years) at age 1 year		
	Year	Males	Females	Years	Males	Females
Australia	1969	104	102	1960–62	68.5	74.5
Austria	1969	110	116	1969	67.5	73.9
Belgium	1968	104	112	1959–63	68.4	73.9
Bulgaria	1969	94	119	1965–67	70.3	73.8
Canada	1969	90	91	1965–67	69.5	75.7
Czechoslovakia	1968	109	116	1966	68.2	74.1
Denmark	1968	82	96	1967–68	71.0	75.4
Eire	1969	99	119	1960–62	69.3	72.7
Finland	1968	123	123	1961–65	65.8	72.8
France	1968	95	91	1968	68.3	75.6
Germany—East	1968	110	127	1965–66	69.5	74.2
Federal Republic	1968	114	128	1966–68	68.3	74.1
Greece	1969	77	97	1960–62	70.5	73.5
Hungary	1969	105	122	1964	69.1	73.5
Iceland	1969	77	91	1961–65	71.2	76.3
Israel	1969	88	117	1969	70.1	73.5
Italy	1968	96	104	1960–62	69.4	74.1
Japan	1968	95	106	1968	69.3	74.3
Netherlands	1969	82	92	1968	71.0	76.3
New Zealand	1968	102	106	1960–62	69.2	74.2
Norway	1968	80	89	1956–60	71.9	75.9
Poland	1969	106	109	1965–66	69.0	74.4
Portugal	1969	114	129	1959–62	65.8	70.9
Roumania	1969	113	140	1964–67	68.9	72.5
Spain	1960	101	117	1960	69.2	73.3
Sweden	1968	78	94	1967	71.9	76.4
Switzerland	1969	63	133	1958–63	69.4	74.5
UK—England and Wales	1970	100	100	1967–69	69.1	75.1
Northern Ireland	1970	105	113	1967–69	69.2	74.3
Scotland	1970	112	115	1967–69	67.7	73.6
USA	1968	103	102	1968	67.3	74.4
USSR	:	:	:	:	:	:
Yugoslavia	1968	109	133	1966–67	68.2	72.4

*Using 1970 England and Wales death rate.
: Not available.

Source: Department of Health and Social Security. (1971). *On the State of the Public Health.* Annual Report of the Chief Medical Officer.
Reproduced by permission of the Comptroller, HMSO.

The Contribution of Medicine

The overall mortality figure for the countries of Western Europe, however, is misleading and cannot be used in any way to assess their level of health. From the point of view of people living in the developing countries of the *Third World*, the mortality rates of Europe might be an indication of an extremely healthy state. This is not so. First the mortality rates have shifted towards the older age-groups of the population, and secondly, premature mortality in the younger age-groups is prevented by the more effective treatment of dangerous organic diseases which still occur. An idea of the extent of this illness can be obtained from the figures available for the average daily number of beds occupied in hospitals in England and Wales during a representative year. This is about 379,000 and the figure of 70% is quoted for all hospital beds occupied by patients who are mentally ill, mentally handicapped or over sixty-five. The remainder are occupied by patients who are acutely ill, requiring surgery or complicated medical treatment, and under modern conditions, the average stay is not very long.

We have a situation therefore of highly-developed technological medicine being applied to the health problems of relatively few people. There is an increasing tendency to avoid admission to hospital if this is possible, and increasing interest in detection of the early stages of disease which may require early relatively minor treatment.

The practice of medicine and surgery is newsworthy, and the public is well informed via the television, radio, press, and magazines. Technical achievements, such as organ transplants, are now taken largely for granted, but there is little consideration as to the alternative methods that might have been employed to avoid the patient having come to need such treatment. All these technical advances in medicine have been made possible by the growth of industries and research in a number of allied disciplines, chemistry, physics, biology, and engineering, including the very important electronics industry. Many procedures which are accepted by the public as commonplace would not have been possible without the development of polythene tubing for example. Automation has made its appearance in medical techniques, and it is now possible to have a completely automated laboratory which can handle enormous numbers of specimens of blood, urine, and other tissue fluids, and which can provide a printed-out result at the end of the process.

A television programme which recalled one working day in a London teaching hospital fifty years ago showed graphically how much progress has been made in so short a time. At that time the role of hospitals, from the patient's point of view, was mainly to provide temporary shelter and nursing care, and from the point of view of medical science, to provide the opportunities for the observation of disease, its classification, and research into its causation.

In 1922, the middle-aged woman with pernicious anaemia could only receive reassurance and comfort, and medicines which might help her symptoms. The young man with a bacterial infection of his heart, a sequel incidentally to rheumatic fever which now is extremely rare in this country, would only get progressively worse and his death was inevitable, as indeed was that of the woman with pernicious anaemia. The young man with tuberculosis could not go to a sanitorium because he was staying at home to look after the children while his wife went out to work to support the family. The old woman at the end of her life after six months relative luxury in the hospital wards was cured of her fractured hip, and was transported to a workhouse where her clothes were taken away from her; she was made to wear uniform and set to work. The major operation shown in the programme was performed without the cover of blood transfusion and the patient eventually died after several hours from the effects of severe haemorrhage.

The Need for Social Services

Not only did this programme show how relatively crude and undeveloped was the state of medical practice at the time (and here it must be understood that this is not a criticism), but it also indicated the lack of social care for patients after discharge from hospital. The major feature of the National Health Service in this country has been the integration of social care and rehabilitation as supportive of medical treatment. Once again, we see how questions of health and disease are indivisible from questions of social and economic factors.

Major medical advances in the last fifty years have been in the field of blood-transfusion, chemotherapy, anaesthesia, the introduction of insulin to preserve the life of the diabetic, and the development of the group of drugs called corticosteroids which reinforce the natural action of the adrenal gland and are invaluable in all branches of medicine and surgery. These advances would not have been possible without a vigorous and progressive pharmaceutical industry which has itself engaged in the research which has reinforced work conducted in university laboratories. These industries have supported the medical profession in such a way that lives now can be saved in conditions which were not so long ago accepted as hopeless.

Preventive Medicine

It must not be thought that this brief description of medical advances is in any way a matter for self-satisfaction on the part of the countries of Western Europe. Progress must be maintained in preventive medicine, and whereas we have already seen the disappearance of the fever hospital and the separate hospitals for children, save in one or two specialized cases, we should also look forward to the era when hospital wards can be progressively closed as the need for treating such desperate conditions will gradually have diminished.

At the present time, accidents, which account for a considerable amount of admission to hospital and necessitate emergency surgery and often long periods of rehabilitation, should be tackled on a preventive basis. Accidents are directly related to human behaviour, even though environmental conditions such as the state of roads, and vehicles, or imperfect design in domestic dwellings are relevant. When we say that the mortality rates of the five to thirty-four-year-old age-group in the United Kingdom are the lowest in Europe, it must be recognized that this record is marred by the mortality and the invalidism which results from avoidable accidents.

If the figures for mortality are no guide to the health of a nation, similarly figures for hospital admissions which affect a minority of the population are also misleading. There are a number of conditions for which estimates are available, which indicate that the nation is by no means healthy. It has been said, for example, that ill health is the norm in this country at the present time.

The Cancers

Cancers of various sites are important causes of admission to hospital where they are treated by radiotherapy or surgery. In general the outlook for people with this type of disease is more hopeful than formerly. There is an interest in prevention of cancer, for example, in industry by avoiding contact with certain chemicals; the control of cancer of the cervix of the uterus by cervical cytology and its possible prevention by attention to personal hygiene in sexual intercourse; and the prevention of lung cancer, which accounts for many times the number of deaths that occur in road accidents each year. Lung cancer remains the one type of cancer which shows no tendency to improve, and which is now affecting women significantly as well as men. The figures for lung cancer are a monument to the disregard for personal health and safety of a population which has been informed for nearly twenty years of the association between cigarette smoking and this disease.

Dental Health

There are other causes of ill health, however, which come within the purview of health education, and which should be of interest to the school-leaver. We have been said to have the 'worst teeth in the world' in England and about thirty million fillings in permanent teeth are carried out each year by dentists in England and Wales. A good deal of this dental health affects children, although it has been reported in 1972 that the figures for the dental health of school children show a slight improvement compared with previous years. The incidence of dental decay could be halved at least if fluoridation of water supplies was introduced in areas in which there is less than one part per million of fluoride.

Abortions

126,000 abortions were performed in England and Wales in a representative year under the provisions of the Abortion Act. This shows that people have not adopted a responsible attitude to conception and that they are not prepared to use contraceptive methods, even though these have been increasingly available for many years. In addition to the abortions, there are a number of illegitimate births about 70,000 a year of whom a high proportion are children who will need to be taken into care and who will be deprived of the benefits of a normal home life.

Alcohol and Drugs

It is estimated that there are about 300,000 alcoholics in England and Wales and this does not include the numbers of people in whom heavy drinking prevents their working from time to time. Alcoholism is also related to home accidents, violence, and sexual misbehaviour. Estimates of people who are taking drugs without medical authority vary considerably and are not easy to obtain. With regard to the taking of dangerous drugs, there are about 3,000 addicts to heroin known to the Home Office and receiving treatment in official treatment centres. Recent figures have shown a slight decrease of new cases over the years. Figures for the smoking of cannabis are impossible to obtain as only the occasional prosecution brings cases to light. It has been estimated that about 100,000 individuals in the community are taking amphetamines without medical authority.

Mental Illness

As regards mental illness, we know the numbers of people suffering from mental disorder as diagnosed or certified by psychiatrists. The figure is about 350,000 and it has been calculated that in a representative year, over 30 million working days were lost in the United Kingdom through mental disorder. These figures do not take into account the mental illness revealed by inadequacy of personality, causing poor social and work performance, aggression and violence, and conflict in homes, in neighbourhoods and in industry as a result of emotional insecurity. When we turn to figures recording the numbers of people who consult their general practitioners we find that at least one third of them do so for illnesses which although presenting themselves in a physical way have a decidedly psychological background.

Heart Disease

Premature deaths occur in the middle age-group, mainly from diseases from the heart and blood vessels, and research so far indicates several possible causes, most of which could be tackled by health education. The problem of over-weight and too little exercise is the obvious one, but it is dangerous to oversimplify this matter as it is possible that there is a genetic element operating in the case of people who develop high blood-pressure and allied disorders at a fairly early age. A recent interesting observation is the relationship between the softness of water supplies, and the occurrence of diseases of the heart and circulation. These diseases tend to occur more frequently in soft water areas, but these are also geographically separate from the hard water areas, so that this observation may merely conceal other causes related to geography and social characteristics of the region.

An Unhealthy Society

When we turn to the figures for consulting family doctors, it is clear that we could not describe our society as healthy at all. To quote a publication of the Office of Health Economics, it is suggested that now that the probability of early death has been so greatly reduced, and many of the more serious and disabling illnesses have been brought under control, individuals have apparently started to regard more seriously their minor diseases and discomforts. [1]

These are reflected in the statistics for claims for sickness benefit and sickness absence from industry. It is paradoxical that, in a community with a low general mortality rate and with such ample provision of medical-care services and a high ratio of doctors to population, demands for medical care should continue to increase. It is now recognized that symptoms for which people consult their doctors may be an expression of discontent or anxiety at work or in the home. The relevance to health education is that there is still little idea in the general public mind of the relationship between the emotions and physical processes.

Symptoms which appear to be entirely physical are very often produced by anxiety, tension, conflict, and general insecurity. Doctors are now obliged, therefore, to make a social diagnosis, and

Table 6. Sickness Benefit: New spells (a) and days (b) of certified incapacity, analysed by cause of incapacity, Great Britain, 1969--70

Cause	New spells (a)		Days (b)	
	Males	Females	Males	Females
	Thousands		Millions	
All causes	8,065	2,532	267.0	75.0
All causes except influenza	6,404	2,109	246.4	70.0
Infective and parasitic diseases	559	201	10.2	3.6
Tuberculosis of respiratory system	6	1	2.8	0.8
Neoplasms	15	5	1.2	0.4
Endocrine, nutritional and metabolic diseases	32	7	3.0	1.1
Diseases of blood and blood-forming organs	17	30	0.9	1.0
Mental disorders	202	99	20.7	9.9
Diseases of nervous system and sense organs	210	60	16.2	4.4
Diseases of circulatory system	238	37	37.5	5.8
Hypertensive disease	36	10	6.1	1.5
Ischaemic heart disease	69	3	15.8	1.0
Diseases of respiratory system	3,703	1,124	76.8	15.8
Influenza	1,660	422	20.7	5.0
Bronchitis excluding acute bronchitis	693	129	33.1	4.0
Emphysema	5	—	1.4	0.1
Diseases of digestive system	580	141	17.0	3.6
Diseases of genito-urinary system	92	135	3.3	3.4
Complications of pregnancy, childbirth and puerperium		106		5.0
Diseases of skin and subcutaneous tissue	218	64	4.7	1.3
Diseases of musculoskeletal system and connective tissue	642	113	26.0	6.8
Arthritis and rheumatism except rheumatic fever	413	73	17.4	4.8
Congenital anomalies	3	1	0.3	0.2
Symptoms and ill-defined conditions	653	268	24.7	8.8
Accidents, poisonings and violence	898	143	24.6	3.8

(a) Spells commencing in period.
(b) Days in spells current at some time in period.
Source: Department of Health and Social Security. (1971). *On the State of the Public Health*. Annual Report of the Chief Medical Officer.
   Reproduced by permission of the Comptroller, HMSO.

in the National Health Service, in its present structure, much more attention is now given to social needs and social care than in former times.

Claims for sickness benefit appear to affect all age-groups in the population, and in this case, younger people do not show the abundant health one might expect when looking at mortality statistics alone. Respiratory disease is a fairly common cause for sickness absence, and this runs right through the age-groups with bronchitis being an important cause of sickness absence and disability in the middle years of life. Bronchitis is aggravated by smoking, although it is probable that most middle-aged people with bronchitis had damaged chests early in childhood and one of the results of immunization against whooping cough and measles may well be to reduce the incidence of this disease in future generations.

Studies of the health of university students have rather surprisingly shown also that a substantial number of them are by no means healthy. They suffer from a number of minor ailments, and once again psychological maladjustment comes high on the list, very often mingled with sex problems. It is also surprising to find that they are even deficient in standards of personal hygiene in many cases, and this may be revealed when they consult the university physician for sexual problems. [2,3]

It is this group of disorders, which do not lead to major hospital treatment that constitute the greatest justification for health education. A feature of the new National Health Service is that health education has been included in the structure 'by name' for the first time. Health education, which used to be confined mainly to the activities of the Public Health Service and was related only to mothers and children is now available for the whole population, and in the hospital and family doctor areas of medical care, as well as the preventive areas.

Cultivating the Right Attitudes to Health

The health education of the schoolchild to prepare him for this adult world in which sickness is so prevalent, and yet much of it preventable, must concentrate on cultivating the right attitudes to health, that is, the need to preserve the body as an active efficient going-concern, and to know the kind of care and use which maintains it in this happy state. In addition, those leaving the school for the adult world should be aware of the way in which the National Health Service can give them personal support in the maintenance of their health and the facilities it can offer, should they fall ill.

Table 7. Birth rates and infant mortality rates in various countries

Country	Perinatal mortality rate per 1,000 live births (1969)	Infant mortality rate per 1,000 live births (1970)	Sum of late fetal death and infant mortality rates per 1,000 live births (1969)	Live birth rate per 1,000 population (1970)
Australia	23.1**	17.9	29.6**	20.5
Austria	27.3	25.9	35.9	15.1
Belgium	25.0†	21.7*	33.9†	14.7
Bulgaria	17.8	27.3	39.1	16.3
Canada	22.5	19.3*	29.3	17.5*
Czechoslovakia	20.7†	22.1	30.2	15.8
Denmark	19.1†	14.8*	23.4	14.4
Eire	26.1	19.2	34.8	21.8
Finland	19.9†	12.5	23.3	13.7
France	22.5†	15.1	34.7†	16.7
Germany — East	23.5†	20.0*	31.0	13.9
Federal Republic	26.7†	23.5	34.0	13.3
Greece	29.5	31.8*	46.3	17.4*
Hungary	33.2	35.7	45.6	14.7
Iceland	18.6	11.7*	22.9	20.7*
Israel	22.3	23.6	34.6	27.0
Italy	34.0†	29.2	46.6	16.8
Japan	24.5†	15.3*	32.5†	18.9
Netherlands	19.8	12.7	24.3	18.4
New Zealand	20.9+	16.7	26.9	22.1
Norway	19.9†	13.7†	24.9†	16.2
Poland	24.2	33.1	44.7	16.7
Portugal	41.6	58.0	81.9	18.0
Roumania	27.6	49.5	69.9	21.1
Spain	:	27.8	48.3	19.8
Sweden	18.9**	13.1†	22.4**	13.6
Switzerland	21.7+	15.4*	24.8	15.9
UK — England and Wales	23.7	17.9	31.3	16.2
Northern Ireland	29.2	22.7	39.9	21.1
Scotland	25.6	21.1*	35.3	16.8
USA	27.1†	19.8	34.3†	18.2
USSR	:	24.4	:	17.5
Yugoslavia	26.3†	56.3	65.1	17.6

+ 1966   ** 1967   † 1968   * 1969.
: Not available.

Source: Department of Health and Social Security (1971). *On the State of the Public Health.* Annual Report of the Chief Medical Officer.
Reproduced by permission of the Comptroller, HMSO.

National Expenditure on Medical Care

The National Health Service of the United Kingdom is an enormous enterprise, bigger than British Rail, and rivalling great commercial empires like Shell in sheer size, and in capital investment, and revenue expenditure. It is therefore a large employer, and every teacher will have through his hands children who will eventually take up some kind of employment in the National Health Service. At present, the community in the United Kingdom invests some 6% of the gross national product in health care. This is not the top of the league. As we might expect the United States, Canada and Sweden exceed this, and even France invests a slightly higher proportion. Nevertheless, the higher investment in other countries is not necessarily matched by a superior health picture.

In order of rank of *expenditure* on health service, Canada comes first with 9.66% of the G.N.P., followed by the USA (8.22%), Sweden (7.12%), France (6.56%), and the UK (6.02%). [4] When the rank order is decided by a statistical index combining death rates, perinatal, and maternal death rates, Sweden is first with the lowest rates, followed by Canada, the UK and USA (tied), and finally, France.

These figures for expenditure are not strictly comparable since the systems of medical care range from almost total private enterprise to a mainly nationalized service. However, the mortality rates can be compared as the figures have been standardized for this purpose. They serve to reinforce the evidence that a community's health depends on factors other than medical treatment.

QUESTIONS

1. Compare the causes of illness and mortality in the nineteenth century with those operating at the present day.

2. What is the contribution of medical science and technology to public health?

3. What are the immediate needs in the *Third World* in order to raise the standard of health of its populations?

4. There is a great reservoir of information in the Biennial Report of the Chief Medical Officer of the Department of Education and Science. Give a few examples of how you would make some selected topics or statistics acceptable to a pupil.

5. The health of the community is continually at risk. Give an account of a model lesson you would take to illustrate two selected threats to the community's health (14-year-old pupils).

6. How can we best get children to realize that they have a part to play in the community's health?

7. Upon whom does the responsibility of the community's health rest most heavily? Give some examples of how this responsibility is honoured.

REFERENCES

1. Office of Health Economics. (1972). *Medicine and Society*. London.
2. Gunn, A. (1970). *The Privileged Adolescent: An Outline of the Physical and Mental Problems of the Student Society*. Aylesbury: Medical and Technical Publishing.
3. Still, R. (1973). 'Student Problems'. *Hlth. Educ. J.* 32(2):36.
4. Kings Fund Centre. (1971). *Do we spend enough on Health Care?* London.

FURTHER READING

Brockington, C. (1968). *The Health of the Community.*. London: Churchill.
Caplan, G. (1969). *An Approach to Community Mental Health*. London: Tavistock Pubns.
Christie, A. B. (1968). *Infectious Diseases*. London: Faber and Faber.
Cymru: Wales. Annual Report presented to Parliament by the Secretary of State for Wales. (This Report is in Welsh and English.)
Department of Education and Science. *The Health of the School Child*. Report of the Chief Medical Officer. London: HMSO.
Department of Health and Social Security. *Annual Report of the Chief Medical Officer*. London: HMSO. (Can be obtained in most libraries.)
Leff, Sonya (1970). *You, Your Health and Your Community*. London: Heinemann. (A guide to personal and communal health problems throughout the world for sixth-form students and teachers.)
Office of Population Censuses and Surveys. *Weekly statistical returns, annual surveys and occasional supplements on special subjects*.
World Health Organization. *Annual Report of the Director-General, and many reports and monographs*. (Information regarding these from UK Committee for WHO, London School of Hygiene and Tropical Medicine. WHO publications can be purchased from HMSO.)

FILMS AND FILMSTRIPS

Title	Colour B/W	Running time	Distributor	Date
Clean Air			Camera Talks Ltd.	
Food Hygiene			Camera Talks Ltd.	
Insect Pests			Camera Talks Ltd.	
Refuse Collection			Camera Talks Ltd.	
Safeguarding Our Meat			Camera Talks Ltd.	
The House Fly			Educational Productions	
Prevention of T.B.			Camera Talks Ltd.	

FILMS AND FILMSTRIPS (*Continued*)

Title	Colour B/W	Running time	Distributor	Date
Food Poisoning			Ealing Public Health Dept.	
Food Free from Germs			Camera Talks Ltd.	
Don't Spoil our World (*filmstrip*)	Colour		Concord	1973
From the Cradle to the Grave (3 parts) 1. Deals with Education 2. Deals with Housing 3. Deals with Health	B/W	20 mins. each	Concord	1973
Health Services			Camera Talks Ltd.	
Public Health Inspector			Camera Talks Ltd.	
The Mental Health Service			Camera Talks Ltd.	
School Health Services			Camera Talks Ltd.	
By Whose Hand	Colour	16 mins.	Central Film Library	1962
Health of a City	B/W	26 mins.	Films of Scotland, Film House, 3 Randolph Crescent, Edinburgh EH3 7TH	1965
Modern Pied Piper of Hamlin	Colour	21 mins.	Rentokil Library, 16 Dover Street London W1	
Island of Coal			National Coal Board	

CHAPTER 5

Health consequences of behaviour

Although the body has a natural tendency to healthiness, it is impossible to lead an active and productive life without being subjected to a number of factors which may stress the body's defences to the point where disorder or disease occurs. We have seen that a number of these have been effectively controlled by the community by the application of medical and social techniques. Much of the progress that has been made in this field of health has called only for the co-operation of the individual who usually has had complete faith in the advice offered him. Knowledge of environmental causes of ill health is extending with each advance in medical research, and although at the present time there appear to be many human disorders which are inborn, for example, metabolic disorders like diabetes, and those cancers for which we do not at present know the cause, every fresh discovery suggests that there are hidden factors in the environment which, once revealed, will then give us further opportunity for the prevention of disease.

Determinism and Existentialism

We might call these, to coin a term, the *determinist* causes of ill health. There are in addition *existentialist* causes which reside in the autonomous individual who has free will and liberty to create his own environment and to control it, or to ignore it according to his needs at the time. It will be remembered from the previous chapter that the paradox in Western Europe is that although the mortality figures are the lowest in the world and although the early part of life is almost free from serious illness, in the working population, even from the immediate post-school years until retirement, there is a considerable burden of ill health which causes absence from work and requires medical treatment. It is in this area of ill health that the social scientist has become interested in recent years, and the concept has grown up of illness which is a direct result of behaviour. Other factors such as the intervention of bacteria, or changes in physiological adjustment as a result of deprivation or disuse, are factors in the middle of the chain as it were, and not at its beginning.

Four Main Springs of Ill Health

It is often said nowadays that the main purpose of health education is to change behaviour. We know how choice of certain kinds of behaviour sets in train a series of events which leads to one of the following four main springs of ill health: *neglect, disuse, misuse*, or *abuse*. These four words have a strong emotional content and imply value-judgments, but this is not the intention. They are useful terms to use technically in that they represent the four ways in which the individual can destroy the health with which he is naturally endowed.

The literature on behaviour in relation to health practices is extensive and studies are being conducted in all parts of the world in every type of community from the most primitive, where taboos and superstitions colour the social environment, which may be inimical to health, to the most sophisticated and affluent indus-trialized societies. Behaviour can be quantified by surveys which enquire into the attitudes of groups of people towards their health and to health practices. The responses can be analysed according to age, sex, social class, occupation, or any other parameter which we care to introduce. By the application of statistical methods of sampling, the plotting of frequency distributions, and the calcu-lation of limits of probability and significance, we have a fair picture of the way in which different groups in the community are likely to behave either in relation to the preservation of their health or into taking action if their health appears to be threatened.

The Gap Between Perception and Application

Studies of this kind first drew attention to the gap between the perception of a message and its practical application. This is the basic problem of practical health education. It should not imply, as some do, that information is no longer important and that we should take steps to influence behaviour. In an open society which preserves personal liberty, this will not work.

The quantification of behaviour is aimed primarily at identifying social pressures and is therefore an environmental study. We also have to take into account *existentialist* aspects of health behaviour. These are not so easily quantifiable, although personality inven-tories and group personality projection tests have been used in some surveys in order to identify what is called a personality profile. It has been done for example in studies of sexual behaviour and smoking. Smoking, in fact, has offered the widest field for this type of enquiry so far. It is impossible however to separate quantifiable human behaviour from basic psychology and the study of the emotions.

Setting aside moral considerations, all behaviour is concerned with the obtaining of satisfactions and the preservation of emotional security. Here again, it is very difficult to separate the two, and in the case of the infant, they are indivisible. The infantile satisfactions of food, sleep, and close bodily contact with the mother represent a complete fusion of both motivations. Infantile behaviour is the prototype of human behaviour which becomes modified as growth of development and socialization proceeds.

Social Satisfactions

Heimler has classified social satisfactions into five main categories, financial, work, family, sexual, and the chosen group. [1] He has been able to show how an average score distributed through these five social satisfactions can be regarded as an index of mental health, there being often a compensation in one type of satisfaction for a deficiency in another. In addition there are the normal sensual satisfactions associated with eating, drinking, and general bodily comfort. Satisfaction gained from physical movement and activity is partly sensual and partly emotional and it also has a social component.

It would be impossible to enumerate all the various personal satisfactions that constitute the goals of every individual in the community. Suffice it to say that they differ very little from one society to another; what differs is the value-system of the society in which one lives and the degree to which personal security can be achieved. It is little use having complete financial satisfaction if one is not accepted by any group, or if there is a continual threat to one's financial gains. Similarly sexual satisfaction, perhaps the most general desire at the present day, can be diminished by economic and social deprivation and will certainly be marred by contracting venereal disease or producing an unwanted pregnancy. In Lord Chesterfield's words, 'The posture is ridiculous, the pleasure momentary and the price damnable.' In order that satisfactions we attempt to achieve can endure, it is necessary also to achieve emotional security.

The relevance to health education is that there are many occasions in a person's life when he is dissuaded from taking appropriate action to protect his health because he feels threatened by other factors which then assume a greater importance. In many cases the threat is imaginary, and is the product of an inadequate personality, so that mental health education, which means helping the child to develop an adequate personality, must be closely identified with the behavioural aspects of health and disease.

Forgoing Immediate Satisfactions

Because it takes a long time for the body to suffer as a result of *neglect, disuse, misuse*, or *abuse*, and because a number of people get by and survive to the average expectation of life, young people are disinclined to accept the idea that they should deprive themselves of any immediate satisfaction in order to protect their health. Nevertheless if the school has an important part to play in education for citizenship, then health education is no different in any respect from other subjects in the curriculum where the child is encouraged to take a long view and an attempt is made to help him to develop into a co-operative, productive, and useful citizen.

Calculated Risks

One result of the attempts to quantify human behaviour has been that it is now possible to calculate risks to health as a result of certain kinds of behaviour. It must be recognized that it is impossible to live at all without incurring some risk, but that the probabilities of a risk occurring to an individual vary greatly, according to the nature of the risk, and according to his mode of life. In communicating information about health, it is necessary to include the calculated risks that people will run, and it is then left for them to make a decision.

Health education therefore may eventually concentrate on training people to run calculated risks where the demands of their occupation or mode of life require this. It is certainly the case in the prevention of accidents where the positive approach which aims at producing a higher degree of skill will reduce the risks, rather than preventing people from taking advantage of transport and equipment which is essential to modern living.

Help from Statistics

To understand the theory of probability, it is necessary to have a smattering of statistical theory, and there is a good case for including the teaching of statistics in mathematics courses in all schools. We have found that the general public fails to comprehend a message regarding health, because the message is itself based upon statistics. This is true of fluoridation as of smoking; it is certainly true of the use and non-use of the various contraceptive methods, and with a little mathematical ingenuity, it could soon be true regarding the hazards of contracting gonorrhoea or syphilis. The contribution of mathematics to health education is relevant because in the modern world people need to be numerate as well as literate.

A good example is the calculated risk of contracting lung cancer as a result of smoking ten to twenty cigarettes a day for a period of ten or more years. In the heavy smoker, it is 1 in 8; in the moderate smoker, it is 1 in 25; in the non-smoker, it is 1 in 300. Lord Platt, at the time President of the Royal College of Physicians, is quoted as having said that if airlines advertised their accident rates in such terms, intending passengers would have no hesitation in the choices they made. Here, we offer the public the choice of running a 1 in 300 risk of contracting lung cancer, as opposed to a 1 in 8 risk. Those who are accustomed to investing in football pools, or in various forms of betting, are very sensible of the need for information about calculated risk. It can be the same in the field of health.

The Seat-Belt Problem

However, emotional factors intervene. An example is the reluctance of the majority of motorists to wear seat-belts. Statistically it is possible to calculate the risk of serious facial or head injury as a result of being flung violently forward in journeys only a short distance from home, and at relatively low speeds. Propaganda about this subject has had very little effect, but it must be realized that no propaganda has ever been necessary to require passengers in aircraft to adjust seat-belts on take-off, before landing, and at other times during the flight when directed to do so.

The calculated risk of injury from the non-adjustment of a seat-belt in an aircraft is considerably less than that of driving a car without a seat-belt. It is not sufficient to point to the authoritarian environment in an aircraft where a passenger would not be allowed to travel if he failed to adjust his seat-belt before take-off. There is no resentment at being asked to adjust a seat-belt in an aircraft, and there is no resentment at being asked to refrain from smoking. In an attempt to analyse the two situations, it is possible that the satisfaction of personal prestige is completely different.

It is the older and experienced motorists who are most reluctant to adjust the seat-belt. They have had a long accident-free motoring life, are proud of their personal skills, and believe that these confer an immunity upon them. With regard to front seat passengers, they may be influenced by the skill and experience of the driver, which of course can be annulled at any time by a sudden incident. In some cases, for example, a puncture or a collapse of a front wheel has brought a car speeding on a motorway to an abrupt halt, and no other driver has been involved. It is notable that younger motorists and passengers are more likely to adjust seat-belts, and in fact demand that they should use them if they are travelling in a strange car. In air travel however, the adjusting of the seat-belt has always been the standard ritual, and advertising has promoted the 'jet set' image. This is in accord with Festinger's theory of 'cognitive dissonance' i.e. that behaviour conditions attitude. There is no reflection upon the passenger's skill and it is recognized by passengers who take an active interest in flying that the purpose of the seat-belt is not only to prevent personal injury, but to prevent passengers wandering about the aircraft at times when the flight crew are occupied with maintaining its trim.

Capacity to Make Adjustments

In less dramatic threats to health and life, the capacity of the body to make temporary and long-term adjustments to various misuse and abuse is the temporary ally of the individual who is not interested in his health, or who disregards advice given him. It must also be recognized that there are episodes during life in which there has to be a complete disregard of the need to preserve one's health. Even the inmates of concentration camps, who have been able to survive the various privations to which they have been subjected, have been able to lead healthy and active lives after rehabilitation. There are also moments of urgency where care for others, or the need to take action to prevent disaster means that risks must be taken, even *uncalculated* risks. This reflects the flexible aspect of the human condition, and it is understandable that the older type of health education which appears to be overcautious and to aim at preventing people doing things that they wanted to do has not appealed very much to young people.

The key to an understanding of this problem lies in the study of the need for satisfaction and emotional security. Qualitatively, any satisfaction produces the same degree of emotional and physical well-being. This means that satisfactions which carry a health hazard can be eliminated and substitute satisfactions put in their place. For example, the satisfaction from eating heavily of large quantities of rich food, which cause a rise in the blood cholesterol and predisposition to arterial disease, can be weighed against the satisfaction of feeling light and alert and free of the abdominal discomforts and clumsiness which accompanies overweight.

Personal Recognition of Motivation

Group discussion methods applied to weight reduction take advantage of the psychological phenomenon that one can substitute one satisfaction for another and that once the substitute satisfaction has been incorporated into our life-style, it also then becomes a habit. Techniques of health education in a person-to-person situation aim at helping people to recognize their own motivations and to change their attitude and behaviour in the light of this recognition. Heavy smokers have confessed, for example, that as a result of discussing smoking habits, or of writing down the situations when they felt compelled to smoke, they have been able to cut down smoking, and in some cases, to give it up altogether.

Coincidence of Factors

Areas of behaviour which are directly related to health are necessarily restricted within our present limited definition. Behaviour which *a priori* would appear to be a threat to health does not necessarily do so. There must be a coincidence of factors, factors related to the behaviour itself and the factors related to health, before a direct effect can occur. All people go through life striving to achieve satisfactions and attempting to maintain a sense of emotional security. From time to time accidentally, they 'collide' with a situation where there is a threat to health. In this situation, the choice of behaviour may increase the risk which is already calculable. There are situations where the imposition of change in one's life may threaten the familiar satisfactions, or may even cause an alteration in biological rythm, for example changes in working conditions or hours and the resulting conflict which arises from attempts to maintain satisfactions and to retrieve emotional security may cause an undue stress. Although it is commonplace nowadays to say that people must be educated to accept change, a moral problem also arises for the community as there are often too many changes for change's sake without consultation. Here we find an environmental factor virtually out of the control of the individual.

Dental Hygiene

Concrete examples of the way in which behaviour affects health can be found in the problems which are now tending to dominate health education in schools. Reference has already been made in a previous chapter to the low standard of dental health in the population of the United Kingdom. It is unfortunate that dental enamel is the only tissue in the body, with the exception of parts of the nervous system, which cannot regenerate after damage. Damage occurs only rarely through violence, and almost consistently in a large number of children it is due to erosion of the enamel by acids which form in the mouth as a result of fermentation of carbohydrate. This process is aggravated by stagnation, and dental decay tends to occur at specific tooth surfaces where the stagnation of food is most likely.

Some individuals are fortunate enough to have a dental enamel which is more resistant to the effect of acid. Microscopical studies suggest that this is due to a higher degree of development of the dental enamel during the period of growth. It is known that the consumption of water containing one part per million of fluoride from birth onwards encourages the full development of enamel so that the teeth become more resistant. This fact has been known for over thirty years and for an almost equivalent length of time many communities in North America have adjusted the fluoride content of their water supply to one part per million, where this has been deficient.

This general community measure results in the reduction of dental decay in children from between 50% and 60% and this has been demonstrated in the United Kingdom in the trials conducted in Kilmarnock in Scotland, in the Island of Anglesey, and in Watford in Hertfordshire. Other measures which will prevent dental decay consist of oral hygiene which means cleansing the mouth adequately after meals, and the avoidance of eating sticky carbohydrates in between meals. The consumption of refined sugar harms the teeth. Toothbrushing itself is now believed to have a more beneficial effect on the health of the gums, rather than the teeth themselves; nevertheless, it is preventive of disease affecting the soft tissues which in turn can cause serious disability, pain, and cosmetic defects. Regular dental care is also part of the package of personal care which is required in order to maintain dental health.

Individual and Community Responsibility

These are the basic scientific facts, but their application depends entirely upon people's attitude to dental health and their willingness to take the trouble to give their mouths this little extra attention which is required. Responsibility is split squarely between community and individuals. The community at large so far does not accept that fluoridation of water supplies is desirable. This is despite the demonstration of its effectiveness in reducing dental decay and its complete safety in every respect. Although legislation permitting local authorities to adjust the fluoride level of their water supplies to one part per million has been on the statute book for over ten years, few authorities have taken advantage of it. There has in fact been an organized opposition to fluoridation and although this is the interest of only a minority, it has been sufficiently powerful to influence the opinion of those responsible for enacting legislation, if not of the public at large.

This pressure-group offers opposition to fluoridation as a public policy. The grounds on which opposition is based include effectiveness, safety, and ethics, a frequent complaint being that fluoridation is an example of mass medication. Any evidence adduced on strictly scientific grounds in support of such opposition can be refuted but in any case the issue of fluoridation has passed from the educational to the political arena.

When the attitudes towards fluoridation of one representative sample of the public were studied it was seen that the general public is by no means committed to the view-point of the anti-fluoridation lobby. Beal and Dickson, who studied a sample of 367 mothers with five-year-old children living in the West Midlands area, found that two-thirds of them had heard of fluoridation and one-third actively favoured fluoridation as a public health policy. Only 8% were against fluoridation. [2] These authors point out — and this is important in view of the fact that the opponents of fluoridation concentrate on local councillors as their target — that the elected representatives know very little about the opinions of those who elect them.

The school community also bears some responsibility, and here the organization of school meals, the choice of menus, and the provision of water for drinking, which itself has a cleansing effect, are all important. The school tuck shop has been under continual criticism by dentists and medical officers of health because it concentrates on the selling of sweets and sweet biscuits. Attempts to get tuck shops to sell or even give away apples or carrots have not been successful. [3] The arguments in favour of school tuck shops are entirely economic, it being pointed out that the proceeds from these shops provide funds for various amenities which are not provided by the local education authority.

Life-Style

The responsibility of the individual for dental health consists of the practice of personal oral hygiene to avoid stagnation of food, the avoiding of eating food at any time when immediate cleansing of the mouth is impossible — eating food in bed before going to sleep for example — the choice of non-sticky carbohydrate foods as opposed to sticky ones, and the acceptance of the need for regular dental inspection and early treatment if required. There are groups in the community who accept these measures as part of their normal life-style. The importance of life-style to health cannot be exaggerated. Groups who do not accept the general life-style referred to will regard the measures of oral hygiene as being 'middle class' and will consider that they are not for them. Overall lies the general attitude that the preservation of the natural teeth is *not* a matter of high priority and that dentists can extract decayed teeth and supply substitutes very easily. There is more concern that there should be enough dentists and facilities for treatment than that preventive measures should be instituted.

In the case of school children, it has already been mentioned that there is some sign of improvement in the level of dental health, but it has yet to return to the high level which was observed by school medical officers and dentists in the years immediately following the end of the Second World War. Sweet rationing and the preference of children in that generation for savoury snacks, rather than sweets or biscuits, were responsible. The home therefore also bears a responsibility for the maintenance of dental health, not only in training children to observe the habits of oral hygiene, but in providing suitable food at times and in a form where stagnation in the mouth is less likely to occur. In attempting to analyse behaviour in relation to dental health, one can identify the need for satisfaction, i.e. the satisfaction of carbohydrate foods, the satisfaction of group behaviour where all children are accustomed to buying sweets and to eating them during the day, and the satisfaction derived from familiar habits, such as for example, taking biscuits up to bed before going to sleep, or being rewarded by sweets or biscuits for hurt feelings. With regard to the choice of food, emotional security which is linked with feeding-patterns is a powerful influence.

Sexually Transmitted Diseases

Other examples of the link between behaviour and health concern the problems of venereal disease, unauthorized taking of drugs, smoking, and alcoholism. It is now preferable to talk about sexually transmitted infections, and these are acquired as a result of accidental contact sexually with an infected person. If two people have intercourse only with each other and have been completely exclusive, they will not acquire these infections. The risk of acquiring them however is increased as soon as people have intercourse with more than one partner, and is at its maximum when people are promiscuous. It may be truly said therefore that sexually transmitted infections are caused by the choice of a particular behaviour-pattern. It is an oversimplification to suggest that the innate human sex drive is itself responsible.

Studies carried out during the last twelve years have indicated that in the age-group fifteen to nineteen, only about one-third of the boys, and less than one-third of the girls have had sexual intercourse. [4] In older age-groups, there are similar findings. We can detect a difference between the promiscuous and the non-promiscuous. The non-promiscuous include people who have intercourse outside marriage, but who confine this to one partner. The motives for sexual promiscuity appear to be a split between sexuality and the capacity for affection. In the mature individual, there is a blending of sexuality and affection, so that the sexual act is associated with a personal relationship which carries a mutual acceptance of responsibility. [5]

Nature of Sexual Promiscuity

We cannot claim therefore that sexual promiscuity is encouraged by a lack of information about sexually transmitted diseases. It is true that surveys have found that there is a need for accurate information, but this lack of information is shared by the non-promiscuous. In the human subject, the regulator of sexual behaviour is emotional. Sexual activity can be repressed, and this probably still occurs despite the impact of Freud. It can be channelled into an alternative outlet — this used to be called 'sublimation', and the phenomenon is observed in animals as displacement activity — or it can be identified only with a special personal relationship. Value-judgments exert an influence.

Studies of the promiscuous have suggested that they have attitudes to society, to older people, and to institutions which tend to be rebellious, and they reject moral values in respect of sexual behaviour as they reject other value-systems. [6] In such people, sexual promiscuity may be part of a protest. Perhaps the most bizarre example of protest was that described by a venereologist at an international conference who had evidence that many young drop-outs from society refused treatment for gonorrhoea as part of their general protest against society.

The problem of sexually transmitted infections involves the whole community as it is necessary to control the spread of infection, and here again we find that behaviour-patterns are important. For example, a patient who has contracted gonorrhoea or syphilis should co-operate with the physician and social workers at the clinic so that the contact from whom he caught the infection can be traced and persuaded to come in for treatment. The attitude of the patient will be the determining factor. If the patient recognizes the need of the community to control the spread of these infections, then he or she will co-operate.

Physiology of the Sex Instinct

The nature of the sexual drive is such that stimulation of the appropriate nerve-centres by ideas evoked by sights, sounds, or communicated thoughts set in train a series of physiological changes leading to the engorgement of the genital organs and preparation for the sexual act. The younger people are, the more urgent the need for expression and relief of this tension. It follows therefore that the community must bear a responsibility for the unwitting or even deliberate stimulation through the mass media publications, advertising, and other aspects of the contemporary social scene which are sexually titillating. The community must also accept the need for open discussion of sexually transmitted infections and the

erns of behaviour which increase the risk of contracting them.
chools must accept responsibility for including a sound pro-
mme of sex education in the health education curriculum,
dealing with biological matters before puberty, and with matters of
personal responsibility by discussion after puberty. Throughout, the
importance of human relationships and personal responsibility must
be stressed. This will be an encouragement to emotional maturity,
rather than mere factual instruction. The individual must be aware
of the existence of an unidentifiable group of infected men and
women who make up the reservoir of infection in the community.
The individual must also recognize the personal responsibility to
co-operate with those whose duty it is to control the spread of
these infections.

The Contraceptive Pill

With the introduction of the contraceptive pill and its prescription
to unmarried girls, new health and ethical problems have now
arisen. There is evidence that the increased use of the contraceptive
pill is associated with an increase in sexually transmitted infections. [7] The reason appears to be the obvious one that when the
male partner uses a condom there is a physical barrier which does
confer a certain protective effect, although not a complete one. If
an unmarried girl taking the pill leads a promiscuous life, she is
therefore not only likely to contract gonorrhoea herself, but to pass
it on to her friends.

An interesting situation may arise where, as a result of taking the
pill, serious side-effects occur in a small proportion of women who
require hospital treatment. Such treatment will not be given in a
venereal diseases clinic, but in a general ward associated with all the
sympathy and social support that is customary on such occasions.
The promiscuous girl who contracts gonorrhoea, on the other hand,
will not advertise the fact to her relatives and friends, and will not
expect them to turn up with gifts of flowers and fruit and 'get-well'
cards. The sexual motivation of both girls may not differ.

The satisfaction involved in sexual behaviour involves more than
physical pleasure. If the satisfaction is identified with a human
relationship, then a dangerous pattern of behaviour will not emerge.
The need for emotional security is very prominent. Sexual
promiscuity is frequently a result of group behaviour when people
who desire to be accepted are obliged to conform. There is evidence
that most girls are under pressure today to accept sexual intercourse
as the inevitable consequence of a chance acquaintance. Their need
for emotional security may persuade them to consent and it is this
rather than the need for physical satisfaction that appears to be
operative.

Drug Abuse

The problem of the unauthorized taking of drugs
small one, although any tendency for it to incre
looked upon with some alarm by the communi
people today will claim that they have had contact
are taking drugs, or who have offered them drugs, and we ...
accept that the opportunities for the unauthorized use of drugs
exist. It is self-evident that the personality of the drug-taker and his
motivations, needs, and drives are different from those who, having
the opportunity, are not tempted. One authority has suggested that
both normal and emotionally disturbed young people are fascinated
by the idea of drugs because the drugs offer them very special
meanings. He suggests that they are a direct source of pleasure; they
are a vehicle for acting out adolescent rebellion; they can be part of
a challenge to virility and the key to an admission to a privileged
group; and finally they represent a voyage into uncharted territory. [8]

Reasons for Drug-Taking

Studies of the reason why young people take drugs will support
these ideas. There are those who take them in order to be
over-active and to resist fatigue, or to be especially brilliant at social
gatherings. There are those who take other kinds of drugs in order
to escape from the too painful reality which they cannot face.
There are those who take drugs, and this applies particularly to
cannabis, because it is part of group behaviour, and it is identified
with admired models, e.g. the frequency with which the pop music
industry is associated with cannabis. Cannabis also offers the escape
into uncharted territory but the supreme trip into this particular
field is offered by LSD.

There are harmful physical, emotional, and intellectual effects
from all unauthorized drug-taking. An essential difference between
taking a drug prescribed for a specific illness by a doctor is that the
latter accepts full responsibility for all effects of the drug, the doses
are controlled, the supply is limited, and the taking of the drug is
confined to the short period when it is necessary to influence the
cause of the illness. The unauthorized taking of drugs purely to
alter mood has neither the merit that it is curing illness, nor the
safety-margin conferred by strict medical control.

Coping with Stress

Apart from the immediate and long-term physical effects, the
taking of drugs to alter mood provides an illusionary support and it
has the grave disadvantage that the person taking the drugs is

prived of the emotional and intellectual exercise involved in confronting his problems. All human beings face situations of stress and they learn to survive by direct confrontation. It is possible that, in the case of young people who take drugs, their own parents have deprived them of this opportunity of confrontation with the reality of their problems by over-protection, and this has resulted in rebellion. In some cases, depression is so strong that drugs may offer the prospect of destroying one's own ego. As this is part of a current ideology, it is plausible that a confused youngster might think that taking drugs had a certain merit.

Role of Parent and Teacher

The role of the parent and teacher in this problem is to concentrate rather on observations of behaviour and behaviour-change than on attempts to diagnose drug-taking in itself. There must also be a search for causes for frustration or dissatisfaction, and a home and school environment must be contrived which allows legitimate self-expression and the healthy development of the ego. We see therefore that the problem is not simply one of the chemical actions of various substances on the nervous system and on subsequent behaviour, but rather of the behavioural disorders which led up to the taking of drugs.

Smoking

When we come to the subject of smoking, we find that the literature describing reasons why people start to smoke is enormous. Some of the studies involve complicated behavioural theory, but Bynner's study of schoolboys who smoke suggests that a powerful motivation for taking up the habit is that it is associated with toughness. [9] One of the conclusions drawn up by Bynner is that health education designed to stop boys taking up smoking, or to persuade them to stop, should attempt to explain ways in which boys can be tough or appear tough without the necessity to smoke. On the other hand, this stereotype of toughness has been derived from the adult world, and in particular from advertising of cigarettes and tobacco products and it does reflect the values of society outside the school. The prohibition of television advertising of cigarettes should have had a positive effect in diminishing this image of toughness, which comes over much more effectively from the medium of television than in any other form of advertising. Interest has been shown also in eliminating smoking from television drama and in deliberately inserting non-smoking episodes where people deliberately refuse cigarettes.

The association in the schoolboy's mind of cigarette smoking with toughness and the desirability of that attribute illustrates another behavioural concept which recognizes that people tend to identify with admired models whom they wish to emulate, but refuse to identify with models who do not appeal to them. It is therefore possible to attach one's liking or prejudice in respect of a person to an inanimate object or to a particular habit. The oft heard criticism that health education seems to attempt to implant middle-class habits in working-class children is perhaps a non-personalized example of this tendency.

Behavioural Science

Behavioural scientists have introduced two technical terms, dissonance and consonance, to describe personal attitudes reflecting conflict or dislike in association with personal health behaviour and those which reflect the feeling of being satisfied and at ease with one's behaviour. From the point of view of health education, groups of people falling into the dissonant category are more important. In studies of adult smoking behaviour, smokers have been divided into consonant smokers and dissonant smokers. [10] The consonant smokers are aware of the hazards to health, but have no conflict about them and are able to give up smoking with little difficulty. The dissonant smokers on the other hand are aware of the hazards they run, are fearful, and would like to give up the habit, but are unable to do so. To label the dissonant group as being addictive is an oversimplification. There is a decidedly addictive aspect of the use of tobacco and perhaps nearly half of smokers are addicted to some degree. However it is the dissonance and the conflict which makes it impossible for this group to apply the knowledge they have about the hazards of smoking to their own personal behaviour.

Smoking and School Children

Much of the study of smoking behaviour and attitudes pertains to the adult sector of society. With regard to school children, many parameters have been measured in relation to smoking habits, and it has been found that educational attainments, relationships with parents and other elders, smoking habits of parents and of friends, and the desire for group conformity are all involved. The reasons for smoking in the case of schoolgirls are more obscure, and it is remarkable that in all studies that have been carried out in many countries there is a sharp difference between boys and girls when it comes to association of smoking with educational attainment. In the case of boys, those of lower educational attainments and little or no prospect of qualification for higher education are most likely to smoke. In the case of girls, the position is almost reversed and girls of 'O' and 'A' level calibre who are going on to higher education seem more likely to smoke than in the case of boys of the same age. This may be related to the relatively greater maturity of girls compared with boys in the same age-group. There is evidence in studies conducted in the United States and in New Zealand that smoking may be part of a general protest against the older generation. It is claimed in one study, for example, that when New Zealand and the United States are compared, the greater degree of authoritarianism amongst New Zealand parents is likely to be conducive to their children smoking. [11] In the case of the United States, among those with parents who are said to be more permissive in their attitudes, smoking is less attractive as a gesture of protest, as presumably it will not be challenged or corrected, and it is possible that in these circumstances, adolescents might decide to experiment with drugs as an alternative.

These studies of the behavioural aspects of the smoking of tobacco both in children and in adults are relevant to the method of health education employed in order to prevent children and adolescents from taking up the habit. It can be said at the present time we have not yet found the ideal method, although so far studies of anti-smoking programmes in schools have indicated that the didactic authoritarian approach has been more effective in converting smokers into non-smokers than other approaches which have endeavoured to take into account more modern and sophisticated methods of health education, including group discussion. Where the head teachers have taken part in these programmes, there appears to have been a greater degree of success than where the programmes have been left to outside visitors such as doctors or school nurses.

When the smoking habit is well ingrained, and there may be addiction to nicotine, various minor personal satisfactions are contributory to continuance of the habit. It must be remembered that the smoking gives pleasure, and therefore all attempts at stopping people smoking by referring to the habit as filthy, disgusting, or unpleasant are likely to fail. These are arguments that appeal to the non-smoker, but research has shown they only arouse antagonism and aggression in established smokers, most of whom are in fact well behaved and careful to avoid giving offence to others. It is unfortunate that this pleasure can only be obtained at great risk to health for the reasons outlined in a previous chapter.

The Smoking Ritual

Tobacco as it is at present cured and processed for the making of cigarettes is a highly toxic substance, and apart from the damage done to the smoker, there is evidence that non-smokers in their immediate vicinity may also be harmed, e.g. by irritation of nose and throat, and absorption of carbon monoxide. The act of smoking gives pleasure for a variety of reasons, apart from the aroma and taste of the tobacco and the momentary stimulation that nicotine produces. The equipment for cigarette smoking is attractive, e.g. cigarette cases and lighters, some of which may be in silver or gold, and which give pleasure in handling as part of the ritual that accompanies the selection of a cigarette and lighting up. When we are dealing with the established smoker, who will usually need help in an anti-smoking clinic, insight into the importance of these marginal pleasures in the smoking ritual must be achieved and substitute pleasures must be sought. What we have learned from the behavioural studies of smoking is that one cannot approach all smokers in the same way. There are varieties of smoker and the variations in the habit frequently reflect variations in attitude and behaviour and separate approaches have to be contrived for each type.

Alcohol

Our understanding of the excessive consumption of alcohol and of alcoholism itself, which must be classed as a disease, has also been illuminated in recent years by behavioural studies. Although some of the motivations for drinking are similar to those of smoking tobacco, for example in young people the feeling that this is the initiation into the adult world or a symbol of toughness, there the parallel ceases. It would not be too strong a statement to say that tobacco cannot be used safely by anybody. On the other hand, the majority of adults of normal personality and stability can consume alcohol in amounts which do not reach toxic levels. There is a minority however who abuse alcohol and become ill after episodes of anti-social behaviour, gradual failure at work-performance, and domestic strife. The numbers of men and women in the United Kingdom community who suffer from alcoholism is estimated to be between 200,000 and 300,000. There is now concern at the fact that boys and girls are beginning to drink much earlier. In the 1930s, the average age of seventeen to nineteen years was quoted as the time in which boys had their first drink. In an inner London Borough, it has been found that some boys are drinking at the age of 12.8 years, and girls at 12.3 years. [12] This is despite the stringent licensing precautions which make it an offence to serve young people under the age of eighteen years with alcoholic liquors on licensed premises. Alcoholics Anonymous, the voluntary organization which helps alcoholics to overcome the habit, estimates that 4% of alcoholics in Britain are in their teens or very early twenties.

Social factors are obviously important here. Young people have a greater amount of money to spend; girls tend to associate with boys old enough to be served legally at licensed premises, and who can obtain alcoholic drinks for them; and there is a great increase of teenage parties in which alcoholic drinks are provided legally in private homes. This indicates that the subject of alcohol, its use, and abuse, and the problem of alcoholism should be included in school health programmes.

Education for Responsible Drinking

The intention should be to educate for responsible drinking in order to prevent abnormal drinking amongst young people. The social and group pressures and the behavioural motivations leading to abnormal drinking should be understood. If we return to our behavioural model which combines the motivation to obtain satisfaction with that to maintain emotional security, the satisfactions derived from being accepted by a heavily drinking group will soon be offset by the exclusion from other groups which may have a greater value from the long-term point of view of the individual's emotional and social development. Problem-drinking is more likely to occur in cultures where there is a tendency to moral condemnation of the use of alcohol than in cultures that accept alcohol as a normal commodity to use and where young people are introduced to drinking in the family circle. It follows that any attempt at moral education in this field is more likely to produce a reaction which can lead to problem-drinking.

Problem Drinkers

Psychiatric studies of boys who have become problem-drinkers reveal a history of conflict during childhood, and particularly a conflict involving a clash between a desire for dependency and a desire for independence. Where the conflict has been with fathers, there has been an attempt to follow a stereotype of masculine behaviour, aided by the consumption of alcohol. The prevention of problem-drinking in this group of young people is more in the therapeutic than the educational field, but the school can help by detecting early signs of neurotic behaviour which require psychiatric help through the school health service. There is always the danger however that a normal well-adjusted boy or girl may be attracted to a group of problem-drinkers.

Role Identification and Advertising

Throughout all these behavioural studies relating to specific problems of public health and health education, the importance of role identification is emphasized. Individual human beings all assume a role according to age, occupation, and social status. There is a tendency for such role identification to be stereotyped, and this stereotype is deliberately encouraged by advertising. Both in the case of tobacco and with alcohol, advertisers deliberately link consumption of these products with a stereotype masculinity for men and a sexually attractive sterotype for women. When young boy-smokers say that smoking is identified with toughness, they are merely referring to an image which perhaps they little understand. Toughness here means toughness of the film and television man of action dominating others by his physical strength and readiness to use it in self-defence or defence of others. The stereotype of toughness which is associated also with the underworld appeals to those boys who are in conflict with their parents and other elders and wish to make their gesture against society in a totally different way from that adopted by politically aligned young demonstrators or drop-out groups.

The need for role identification and the compulsion to play one's role appropriately is a necessary condition of man as a social animal. Thus all teachers have a recognizable role, as do doctors, lawyers, and other professional occupational groups which are characterized by self-imposed codes of behaviour. In addition to these occupational roles, there are also roles appropriate to parents, to the middle-aged, and the elderly. The compulsion to play the appropriate role has a direct effect upon health behaviour and in the field of mental health the too slavish adherence to a stereotype of age-group, for example, may result in conflict and tension.

Peer Groups and Reference Groups

The adolescent age-group has identified a role of its own of reaction against the adult world and protest. The significant difference here is that the adolescent age-group is its own reference group. In human society, two groups are recognized which are responsible for a regulation of behaviour. The first is the peer membership group, and the second is the reference group. Where a peer group is also its own reference group, it may behave in a way that is totally indifferent to the needs of society as a whole. In a healthy society, a reference group stands outside the membership group and regulates its behaviour.

The work of behavioural science in the field of public health has resulted in the identification of varying roles that people adopt when their health is threatened or when they become ill.

Health Roles and Sickness Roles

For example, when a person believes himself to be healthy then he may still undertake activity for the purpose of preventing disease or of detecting disease in its early stages. This can be called health behaviour. When a person feels himself to be ill, he may then undertake activities to identify the cause for his illness and to discover a suitable remedy. This can be called illness behaviour. Finally, if a person is sick, he then adops a special sick role, i.e. the role of dependence upon professional advisers, of the temporary cessation of his normal activities, withdrawal from his normal social and work groups, and co-operation with his professional advisers in the matter of treatment. [13]

Health education is closely concerned with these three aspects of behaviour in health and illness. The assumption of the sick role is one which will cause great anxiety and concern with most responsible adults, not on account of the dangers of their illness, but rather from the withdrawal from their normal activities and associations. Even the removal of the economic threat implied by illness and the loss of earnings by social welfare legislation such as that obtaining in the countries of the E.E.C. has not diminished the anxiety felt at the assumption of the sick role. Interest in this aspect has led to studies showing how people tend to avoid seeking medical advice, or submitting to treatment, even when they are conscious of symptoms of ill health.

The relevance to health education in schools lies in the responsibility to implant responsible attitudes towards the personal solution of health problems. It will be seen that even in the younger age-groups of employed persons in the postschool years, the sick role is frequently assumed. The differences revealed in the claims for sickness benefit for the same illnesses by the two sexes indicate that men and women differ in their attitudes to the sick role. This may well have an adverse effect upon the future health of men and this may well be reflected in the greater instance of claims for sickness benefit for diseases like bronchitis in the middle-aged male, compared with the middle-aged female.

Whereas we naturally do not wish the sickness role to obtrude into school health education, and we hope that attention to primary health behaviour will eventually reduce the amount of sickness, it has to be borne in mind, and it is a suitable subject for discussion by older pupils. Such discussion should go far beyond fields of social conscience to save the community loss in productive work and the cost in the treatment of sickness. It is the avoidance of emotional upset caused by the necessity to assume the sickness role, which should be an additional incentive to preserve health and normal activity as far as is possible.

Relevance to Health Education Method

Behavioural studies are also relevant to the methods to be used in health education. It has been recognized for more than a quarter of a century that the mere imparting of information is not enough to change health behaviour in most cases. This means that methods of communication and teaching must include ways of influencing motivation of attitude and that these must be included in all health education procedures. The use of films offers the greatest opportunity for influencing motivation, and this places a premium on the more sophisticated sociological type of film as compared with the conventional documentary. The use of thematic films referred to later in this book has been an important advance in the methodology of health education. In general, it can be said that when an individual has insight into his own motivation then it becomes easier to change behaviour. Although insight is acquired more easily in a group situation, for those who are determined to change their behaviour in the interests of their health, individual effort is also rewarding. This has been shown in the case both of weight reduction and of giving up smoking. The practice of making a note of the situation in which there is a temptation to smoke is one of the therapeutic measures for people to undertake themselves.

QUESTIONS

1. In a multi-cultural society, how can the health educator teach practices that have a 'class' image?

2. Discuss the phenomenon of role identification in relation to health behaviour.

3. Smoking and the drinking of alcoholic beverages are both said to be socially acceptable. What effect has this situation on the teaching of the dangers of such practices?

4. How do you account for the fact that so many 'old wives tales' persist? Do any of them have a real scientific value? Why is it sometimes difficult to get people to reject them?

5. Very few, if any, pupils in secondary schools have not heard about sexually transmitted diseases. How would you attempt to get this problem into perspective including the associated problem of promiscuity?

6. If you are a smoker and/or drinker of alcoholic beverages, how can you reconcile this behaviour with your teaching on the danger of these activities?

7. 'Contraception or Abortion.' Discuss this statement and give a brief account of the currently accepted types of contraceptives. Quote any 'old wives tales' you may have heard in this connection. Why is the 'withdrawal' technique so unreliable?

8. Under what circumstances do you consider that 'Cleanliness is next to Godliness'? Quote examples showing when such practice is very difficult. Does it always really matter? Give examples.

9. Have you any comments to make on the consequences of parents preparing their babies for 'Baby Shows', 'Bonniest Babies Contests', etc.?

REFERENCES

1. Davies, N. and Heimler, E. (1967). 'An Experiment in the Assessment of Social Function'. *Med. Officer.* **117**:31—2.
2. Beal, J. F. and Dickson, S. (1973). 'The Attitudes of West Midlands Mothers to Water Fluoridation'. *Publ. Hlth. J.* **87**:75—80.
3. Young, M. (1971). 'Nibbling', *Hlth. Educ. J.* **10**:62.
4. Schofield, M. G. (1965). *The Sexual Behaviour of Young People.* London: Longmans.
5. Wittkower, E. D. and Cowan, J. (1944). 'Some Psychological Aspects of Sexual Promiscuity'. *Journal of Psychosomatic Medicine.* **6**:287.
6. Schofield, M. G. *op. cit.*
7. Juhlin, L. and Liden, S. 'Influence of Contraceptive Oestrogen Pills on Sexual Behaviour and the Spread of Gonorrhoea'. *Brit. J. Ven. Dis.* **45**(4):421.
8. Boyd, P. (1972). 'Adolescents, Drug Abuse, and Addiction'. *Brit. Med. J.* **4**:540—43.
9. Bynner, J. M. (1969). *The Young Smoker.* London: HMSO.
10. McKennell, A. C. and Thomas, R. K. (1967). *Adults' and Adolescents' Smoking Habits and Attitudes.* Government Social Survey Report, SS 353B. London: HMSO.
11. Newman, I. M., Irwin, R., Ang, J. and Smith, J. M. C. (1971). 'Adolescent Cigarette Smoking in Two Societies'. *Int. J. Hlth. Educ.* **14**(3):114—20.
12. Searle-Jordan, V. T. (1970). *The Social Drinking Scene.* (Foreword by Dr A. D. C. S. Cameron.) London: London Borough of Hammersmith Health Education Service.
13. Robinson, D. (1971). *The Process of Becoming Ill.* London: Routledge and Kegan Paul.

FURTHER READING ON FLUORIDATION

Cannell, W. A. (1960). *Medical and Dental Aspects of Fluoridation.* London: Lewis.

Committee on Research into Fluoridation. (1969). *Fluoridation Studies in the United Kingdom and the Results achieved after Eleven Years.* Reports on Public Health and Medical Subjects No.122. London: HMSO.

Gamson, W. A. (1961). 'Social Science Aspects of Fluoridation: A Summary of Research'. *Hlth. Educ. J.* **19**:159—69.

Gamson, W. A. (1968). 'Social Science Aspects of Fluoridation: A Supplement', *Hlth. Educ. J.* **23**—**24**:135—43.

Murray, J. (1973). 'A History of Water Fluoridation.' *Brit. Dental J.* **134**(6):247—50; see also **134**(7):299 — 302.

The Oral Hygiene Service. (1970). *Symposium on the Role of Fluoride in Preventive Dentistry.* Revised edition. London.

FILMS

Title	Colour B/W	Running time	Distributor	Date
About Abortion	Colour	22 mins.	Concord	1970
Caught for a Baby	B/W	25 mins.	Concord	1970
Beyond Conception	Colour	25 mins.	Concord	1968
The Day before Tomorrow	Colour	30 mins.	Concord	1971
Save This One	Colour	25 mins.	Concord	1972
Every 30 Seconds (VD)	Colour	17 mins.	N.A.V.A.L.	1973
Prevent It	Colour	11 mins.	N.A.V.A.L.	1972
A Half Million Teenagers	Colour	16 mins.	N.A.V.A.L.	1970
Her Name was Ellie His Name was Lyle	B/W	40 mins.	N.A.V.A.L.	1967
The Game	B/W	30 mins.	Concord	1966
Sex Can be a Problem	B/W	45 mins.	Concord	1972
The Merry-go-Round	B/W	23 mins.	Concord	1966
Unmarried Mothers (Granada Television)	B/W	50 mins.	Concord	1968
My Parents Don't Understand Me	B/W	30 mins.	Concord	1966
Crutch for All Seasons	Colour	20 mins.	British Temperance Society	1969
Gale is Dead	B/W	50 mins.	Concord	1970
V.D. − Out of Control?	B/W	30 mins.	Concord	1971
One Way Ticket	Colour	23 mins.	Guild Sound and Vision, South Staffordshire Medical Centre, New Cross Hosp., WV10 OPQ	1971
The Mindbenders	Colour	25 mins.	Concord	
Population & Pollution	Colour	18 mins.	Concord	1970
A Matter of Attitudes	B/W	30 mins.	Concord	1968
Smoking & Health − Report to Youth	Colour	13 mins.	N.A.V.A.L.	1969
Dying for a Smoke	Colour	10 mins.	Central Film Library	1967
The Drag	Colour	9 mins.	Concord	1967
Let's Discuss Smoking	B/W	16 mins.	Concord	1964
Smoking & Lung Cancer	B/W	28 mins.	Concord	1965
Smoking Machine	Colour	16 mins.	Central Film Library	1964
Black Sheep	B/W	16 mins.	Tenovus Cancer Information Centre, 111 Cathedral Road, Cardiff	1965
Cancer by the Carton	Colour	27 mins.	Tenovus Cancer Information Centre	1965
Is Smoking Worth It?	Colour	16 mins.	Tenovus Cancer Information Centre	1962

F I L M S (*continued*)

Title	Colour B/W	Running time	Distributor	Date
Up in Smoke	Colour	23 mins.	British Temperance Society (U.S.A.)	
Spotlight on Smoking			Scottish Central Film Library	
Time Pulls the Trigger	Colour	23 mins.	Tenovus Cancer Information Centre	1961
Traitor Within	Colour	9 mins.	Tenovus Cancer Information Centre	
Who? Me?	Colour	20 mins.	Tenovus Cancer Information Centre	1965

CHAPTER 6

Areas of community responsibility

Human communities have always accepted responsibility for the care of the sick and relief of poverty. This is the basic principle from which have developed elaborate systems of medical care and social security which characterize most countries in the modern world. Action has always been taken by a minority of the members of the community motivated either by religious or humanist feelings and in the long evolutionary chain that stretches from the early Christian era to the contemporary National Health Service and Social Security Agencies, members of religious orders have given way to responsibly minded landowners who in turn have given way to philanthropists and then successively to statesmen in the nineteenth century and politicians in the twentieth century. In the nineteenth and twentieth centuries there has been the development of an indispensable infra-structure of administrators. Despite the taking over by governments of welfare tasks formerly borne by voluntary agencies, the voluntary principle has survived and can be seen even in countries of the Eastern European bloc, where the Red Cross and its Muslim counterpart, the Red Crescent Society, complement the work of state health services.

Economic and Political Structure of Communities

The term community is loosely applied by modern commentators frequently with some undertone of idealism or ideology. From a purely descriptive point of view, the term community can be applied to any group of human beings who exist in a state of inter-dependence and so the basic principle of community life is necessarily economic. This does not eliminate the importance of human relationships and human emotions which include compassion and the concern for the welfare of others. This should be at its height in the family as a community, but even in the family, there is an economic inter-dependence. At the present time there is a growing realization that the enjoyment of amenities involves the principle of interdependence and this is at the heart of the present movement towards conservation. Such a simple view of the structure of the community would have held good in medieval times in Europe and was characteristic of the welfare situation before the dissolution of the monasteries in England in the reign of Henry VIII. Since that time, the structures of communities have been more varied, and there has also been a gradual evolutionary tendency towards the realization of a world community. The League of Nations was an early, valiant attempt at this, but the United Nations has had more real powers, and in one of its technical agencies, the World Health Organization, we have the realization of the acceptance by the world of community responsibility for the health of its members. The United Nations can be cited as the supreme example of a politically structured community, supported by a technical and administrative infra-structure and making use of scientific research, advances, and techniques of administration in order to apply these advances to the practical problems of health.

The European Economic Community is a political structure with a strong administrative element, and is based upon the principle of economic interdependence. There is as yet however no uniform system of welfare services in the representative countries of the Community each of which has developed its own system according to its historical and social evolution. At the present stage of world development, it is impossible to translate any national health service into another country, as each service represents the aspirations of the people concerned expressed through their elected representatives in parliament, and these aspirations in turn reflect national character and national history.

Thus in the United Kingdom, the dissolution of the monasteries was a disaster as regards the voluntary care of the sick and the relief of the poor, but the traditional characteristics of English feudalism included the willing acceptance of responsibility, even of the duty, on the part of the landed aristocracy to care for their tenants and workers. It is possible to discern the faint remnants of this kind of feudalism, even in modern legislation, but it must be remembered that the transition from private charity to community organization in order to help people to be as self-reliant as possible and to prevent breakdown of health or of personal economy was effected at the end of the nineteenth century by voluntary agencies and by individual philanthropists.

Emergence of the Insurance Principle

The insurance principle for the provision of health care was discovered by working-class movements in England in the nineteenth century, resulting in the foundation of industrial insurance and industrial sickness schemes. Whereas in Germany in the 1880s, a National Health Insurance Scheme based upon compulsory insurance was established by Bismarck as an act of administration, it was not until 1911 that Lloyd George introduced the National Health Insurance Act which, using the principle of compulsory insurance, provided a very limited form of medical care for wage-earners up to certain limits, but not including their families.

Health Services and Political Reform

We can consider the term community at three levels. First there is the apparatus of the modern state, which in the countries of the E.E.C. and in the United States is based upon representative democracy. Again it is a minority of the community who assume responsibility, but this responsibility is assigned to them by the majority of the members who then accept government by consent. It is significant that, when the progress towards universal franchise is traced from the first reform bills at the beginning of the nineteenth century, we find that interest in health and welfare problems of vulnerable members of the community, i.e. women and young children and elderly people, increases as the extent of franchise increases.

Action was concerned with environmental control of infectious diseases and this included the provision of hospitals. Hospital accommodation was also provided at public expense for the insane. General hospital accommodation was provided for the needy by the same Boards of Guardians who controlled the workhouses. Voluntary hospitals which made their appearance in the eighteenth century were set up in all major centres of population. It was not until the beginning of the twentieth century that the efforts of voluntary agencies concerned with maternal and child welfare began to attract the attention of politicians, and the Midwives Act of 1902 was the first example of twentieth century health legislation in which the community accepted responsibility for the health care of some of its members. The history of education is very similar, and this is yet another justification for considering health and education together.

The community from the political and administrative aspects, then, has resulted in this country in the setting up of elaborate schemes of health and social security. From the beginning of the twentieth century, these have included promotion of health and prevention of disease in the individual as well as maintaining the control over the environment which was firmly established by the end of the nineteenth century. These developments will be considered in detail later in this chapter.

Consensus Politics

The influence of the mass media over personal lives has resulted in the creation of a community of the mind which forms public opinion which then influences political events. A fashionable phrase at the present time is 'consensus politics' and although this can be misused as in cases where this is justified by minority groups to defy existing acts of Parliament, it makes sense when it refers to the effect of a public opinion in which the silent majority makes its views and needs known through the medium of journalists, writers, television commentators, and the like. Consensus politics in this form has a profound effect upon the protection of the health of the community, but in turn it places a responsibility on the silent majority for making judgments on issues of social concern in the light of information and discussion. It is another situation in which we must stress the relevance to health education in schools.

Public opinion surveys conducted either on statistically random samples of the population by age-groups, or sex, or occupation, or by random enquiry simply of passers-by, reveal an increasing interest in community health problems and a sense of responsibility for their solution. In some respects, the results of such public opinion surveys reflect credit on the health education which has already been carried out in schools, and one sees this particularly when questions regarding sexual behaviour, venereal disease, unmarried mothers, abortion, and so on, are raised. It will be remembered that the first of the aims of health education suggested by WHO was to ensure that health is accepted by the community as a valued asset. We are slowly moving towards this, but not fast enough. There is still too much preoccupation with the delivery of medical care and with costly and dramatic procedures such as organ transplants, and too little with the general aim to raise the health of the community to the level at which many aspects of medical care today will be no longer necessary. Yet as long ago as 1946, the late Professor John Ryle, the first professor of social medicine in this country at the University of Oxford, could write, after having spent his own lifetime as a consultant physician in London, that we should look forward to the time when hospital wards would close, and we should no longer need the vast armies of medical nursing and auxiliary personnel at present required to staff a modern health service, and that governments should look to the basic requirements of people for the maintenance of good health. [1]

We might modify this statement a little and say that the people themselves should look to the supply of these requirements, and should then press their elected representatives to ensure that they are supplied. Unfortunately there has not been sufficient definition of the factors which promote health in individuals and groups. In some ways, we are behind the nineteenth century thoughts which grasped the fact that housing, sanitation, and pure water supplies were the basic requirements for healthy living. There are many groups in the population in all countries of the E.E.C. where most health problems would be solved immediately by adequate housing and a minimum standard of comfort and security. In most countries in the *Third World*, it is not doctors and nurses who are needed so much as regular employment, good housing, adequate nutrition, and freedom from fear. The world community is helping to a certain extent here insofar as the United Nation's technical agencies are much more concerned with these basic factors to promote health than with the translation of elaborate Western European and American systems for medical care to these countries.

The Mass Media and Consensus Politics

Community responsibility in this general amorphous concept of the community will extend to the total environment in which its members have to live. We have already made reference in the previous chapter on behavioural concepts of health to the importance of the emotional climate and the maintenance of a general moral tone of society. To blame the mass media entirely for any deterioration of moral tone is merely finding a scapegoat. Mass media in general follow the public consensus, and then go one step ahead of it.

Nothing could illustrate this more clearly than the present discussion on the topic of abortion. There is a general consensus that legalized abortion undertaken under the best medical conditions supplies a social need for a certain number of women and that they should not be denied this. Although this may be regarded as consensus, there are substantial minorities in the community who disagree. It is accepted, however, that there is nothing in the Abortion Act which forces people to have abortions, but too many commentators appear to think that doctors and nurses are also forced to undertake these operations to which they may have conscientious objections.

Perhaps this arouses very little sympathy outside the ranks of the medical and nursing professions, but of greater importance is the publicity given to informal and casual abortion procedures. They have even been referred to as 'lunchtime' abortions, in which it is suggested that women could simply take an hour or two off from work, have an abortion, and then go back to their occupation. (These comments do not refer to the day care of women who have an abortion early in pregnancy by the vacuum extraction method and who can leave the hospital the same day.) Such ideas ignore medical, psychological, and emotional considerations. Psychiatrists and social workers who have had the care of women who have elected for abortion have evidence of the psychological trauma that occurs before and after this operation. Profound depression can follow this experience and supportive treatment from the psychological point of view is as important as medical supervision to ensure that no complications have occurred.

A community which has had the advantages of a good broad general health education would have anticipated such complications of legislation which has been represented purely as an advance in the delivery of medical care.

Ethics and the Doctor-Patient Relationship

Ethical considerations in medical practice are now presenting considerable problems in all countries of the world, and here again it is the community which by consensus will influence events. It may now be accepted that the educational gulf between medical practitioners and their patients has narrowed considerably. This means that traditional authoritarianism of medicine and nursing is fast disappearing. Nevertheless, there is still the tendency by the community to accept a sick role of complete dependency upon their professional attendants and this arouses considerable problems in the field of clinical research. Clinical research is necessary for the advancement of medicine and it is accepted by the medical profession that no experiment should be conducted on patients without their being consulted beforehand and having given their consent with understanding. In the case of children, the responsibility for consent lies with the parents, but in this era of 'children's lib,' one wonders at what age the limit can be set. Unless patients and their relatives are well informed however and have had developed in them a capacity for deduction and judgment, consent may either be withheld unreasonably and without regard to community responsibility for the advancement of medicine, or on the other hand may be too readily given, thus laying open the way to a general abuse.

Participatory Democracy

We now have to consider the third aspect of the community and this can be described as participatory democracy. In Europe this is seen in a limited sense in the work of various voluntary organizations in which their constitution is itself democratic. A new aspect of participatory democracy in the United Kingdom and also in certain countries in Europe is a formation of citizens' groups or committees in order to defend some amenity, or to demand social justice. Because these concern minorities and local communities, such efforts frequently excite the derision or hostility of the wider community. We have seen this in the case of participatory democracy mobilized for the purpose of influencing the choice of site for the third London airport. We see this activity also in the field of education where issues regarding safety of children in approaching their schools, school meals, and the choice of secondary education are the main topics. Unfortunately most of these movements are doomed to failure because they are attacking an established administration which in turn derives its powers from the people through their elected representatives and government by consent. It is in the United States that we find community movements involving participatory democracy in the field of health care and for the promotion of health.

American Democracy and Medical Care

In order to understand the peculiar democracy of the United States, it is necessary to read de Tocqueville's work published in 1830 where the evolution of the republic from the former British colony is described. [2] The American principle that everyone should be able to stand on his own feet has to be supported from time to time by collective action. It has also been suggested that the absence of an aristocracy in the European sense has meant that groups of people have had to combine in order to provide services, amenity, and protection which is not available to them from a feudal system The situation in the United States today is complicated by the fact that the structure of the community depends upon national and ethnic characters. Because large groups of Europeans have emigrated to the United States and have maintained their national cultures, we find German communities, Italian communities, Scandinavian communities and so on. In some cities in the United States, for example Philadelphia, we find hospitals that have been paid for and built entirely by one community. Sociological studies of health care in the United States show that the stimulus for participatory democracy is very often the need for conformity. For example, [3] the upper income-groups will ensure that their children have regular dental treatment, immunization and health check-ups, simply because it is the correct thing for their social group. Lower income-groups, being unable to afford such things, will deny their importance, or in some cases will resort to unorthodox medical practitioners, such as osteopaths, chiropractice, nature cure experts and the like.

Voluntary Insurance

The system of health care itself in the United States is predominantly one of private enterprise, financed to a varying degree by voluntary insurance in the same way that the working-class institutions in nineteenth century England attempted to cover the cost of essential medical care. The cost of care in the United States from the point of view of direct contribution by the individual is the highest in the world. However, such a system satisfies the national aspiration to be self-reliant and forms a part of the national economy. It is a direct result of the history of social development in the United States but it has the disadvantage that lower income-groups are unable to afford the high premiums for health insurance and must accept a lower standard of medical care, and perhaps in some communities, virtually no *preventive* care at all.

The principle of participatory democracy also seems to fall down in that there is little or no representation of the consumer of medical care in the United States, where the medical profession enjoys power, authority, and status far higher than in any other country in the world. It must not be thought however that it is the power of the medical profession alone that holds back progress towards a national health service. Systems of medical care grow and evolve from the social development of the country.

The National Health Service

The British National Health Service represents the most comprehensive acceptance by the community for the care of the health of its members that could be found anywhere in the world. The coming into operation of the provisions of the National Health Service Reorganization Act in 1974 represents an advanced stage in the evolution of community health care by the application of politics and administration, which commenced early in the nineteenth century. The National Health Service Act of 1946 was based on the principle that ill health and poverty go hand in hand and the scheme put into operation by this Act was the work of a distinguished economist, Sir William (later Lord) Beveridge. The reorganization effected in 1974 on the other hand is the work of administrators and experts in management. This reflects the contemporary political and administrative preoccupation in what is called the delivery of the package of medical care. This has been necessitated by the increasing technological complexity involved in the diagnosis and the treatment of disease and its prevention which requires the large human and financial resources referred to in a previous chapter. The working of the National Health Service also depends upon a national insurance system and the 1946 Act was not implemented until 1948 in order to allow time for the implementation of the sister Act, the National Insurance Act of 1946. Like all measures designed to improve the public's health in the United Kingdom, there is also a strong link with a local government structure and one of the forerunners to the Act of 1974 was the decision to re-organize the local authorities which were established as administrative units of local government during the nineteenth century.

The 1946 National Health Service Act, being based primarily on economic considerations, achieved the aim of making medical care freely available to all who needed it without the necessity for payment at the time, based on an insurance principle supplemented by finance from taxation. In making the necessary provisions, however, the traditional boundaries between the three aspects of medical care — preventive or public health, hospital, and family doctor treatment — were preserved, and the three branches of the National Health Service were administered by separate authorities between 1948 and 1974.

Since 1948, however, more progressive ideas on the administration of medical care services have appeared, and it has been recognized that boundaries between curative and preventive medicine are artificial, and that the needs of the community will be better served by one authority to provide and administer all three branches of the service. Services for environmental control, i.e. sewage disposal, the provision and protection of water supplies, the maintenance of standards in the provision of safe food, both chemically and bacteriologically, housing, and the problems of noise abatement and protection of the community from radio-activity still remain the duties of the new local authorities, the metropolitan counties and the county councils. The all-purpose type of authority, the county borough, which was set up as an administrative unit in 1888, disappears and all functions connected with the National Health Service pass to regional health authorities and area health authorities with certain functions being sub-served by district councils. Representative democracy has been provided for by the inclusion of community health councils based on area health authorities. Half the members will be nominated by local authorities from their elected members and half will represent voluntary bodies.

A National Health Service Commissioner (Ombudsman) was appointed as the guardian of the public interest.

New Health Officials

This is a radical change in the administration of health services. It has meant the disappearance of the familiar medical officer of health and his replacement by administrative medical officers at regional and area level, and a new type of medically qualified health official, called the 'Community Physician'. What was formerly described as 'public health', now becomes 'community medicine' and this is in accordance with scientific and professional thinking of the last decade.

Teachers will be particularly interested in the school health service, and this continues as before as a service to the local education authority staffed by doctors and nurses, seconded from the area health authority. The close partnership between teachers and doctors which has been a feature of the school health service, which is in fact the senior of the community health services having been founded as long ago as 1907, will continue.

The new administrative arrangements recognize that a patient's needs may involve family doctor, hospitals, and preventive health services and that co-operation between the personnel of these three branches can be improved by their being employed by one single authority.

Social Services

The growing importance of social work in medical care is a feature of the last two decades. Since 1971 social service departments have been set up by local authorities under the direction of directors of social services who have been appointed by social services committees. This is under the provision of the Local Authority Social Services Act 1970 which came into operation on January 1 1971. This Act followed the recommendations of the Committee on Local Authority and Allied Personal Services (the Seebohm Committee). The effect of this Act has been to bring under one administrative department the social aspects of care and after-care and prevention of illness which were formerly provided under Part III of the National Health Service Act 1946 by the local health authority, and also the care of deprived children under the Children Act of 1948. The separation of the social work departments from the health departments has come in for a considerable amount of criticism particularly in regard to the care of the mentally sick in the community.

At the top of this pyramid of health and social services, the two aspects of health care are brought together in the form of the Department of Health and Social Security, although the responsible secretary of state's title is Secretary of State for Social Services. This Department succeeds the Ministry of Health which was set up relatively recently in 1919 and which had in turn succeeded the Local Government Board set up in 1871 which included in its responsibilities a supervision of the environmental control services administered by the local authorities.

In summary, the history of the health service in the United Kingdom is bound up with the history of local government itself, and is characterized by continual overhaul of the services with administrative reconstruction during successive epochs. It is possible to discern the direct effects of community consensus politics with these various phases of reorganization and reconstruction. Since its inception in 1948 the National Health Service has been a subject of debate in medical circles and in both Houses of Parliament. A new trend which must be accepted as a sign of healthy participatory democracy is the public debate often introducing severe criticisms of the service which is now carried on in the Press. A number of journalists specialize in health and social service matters and their penetrating criticisms are of value to a free society whose members should be well informed on all matters touching their personal lives. The consensus however is that the National Health Service itself is of inestimable value to the British community, even if some reforms are called for.

Nineteenth Century Precedents

At the beginning of the nineteenth century, public attention was alerted to the adverse sanitary conditions in the towns of England. This was the subject of the famous report by Edwin Chadwick, one of the Poor Law commissioners. The effect on public opinion of the severe cholera epidemics which continued even up to the 1860s also influenced the executive in their decisions. So imperfect was the protection of water supplies that it was possible even for the Prince Consort to contract typhoid fever and die of that disease. Reports by Chadwick and a medical colleague, Southwood-Smith, gave graphic accounts of the appalling conditions in working-class housing — many cases having been proven of families being drowned in sewage. Such reports can be regarded as health education of the community, and consensus politics resulted in the executive's taking action.

Nineteenth century health legislation is characterized by successive royal commissions followed by bills and acts of Parliament on housing and sanitation and the implementation of these acts by delegating duties and powers to local authorities.

Despite the harshness of the times there was a recognition of the association between industrial employment and ill health. The early acts controlling conditions of work in factories operated mainly in favour of women and children. Some of them applied only to the cotton and woollen industries where conditions were particularly bad. Nearly forty years before the first Education Act of 1870, the Factory Act of 1833 laid down that children aged 9–13 should attend school for two hours a day on six days a week. Limitation of hours of work and progressive control of toxic hazards, prevention of accidents, and improvement in factory hygiene proceeded during the nineteenth century. The twentieth century saw the development of industrial medicine and the extension of factory health services provided by employers. The Trades Union Congress appointed its own Medical Adviser. The setting up in 1972 of the Employment Medical Service of the Department of Employment was the first step towards a nationalized industrial health service. There is a veritable spate of legislation during the second half of the nineteenth century with remarkably speedy implementation, bearing in mind that the administrative techniques and the techniques of data collection and analysis depends entirely upon personal and human labour. The establishment of the General Register Office in 1836 with authority to conduct a decennial census of the population was the first administrative act which made it possible to produce health statistics which have been the guide for legislation and administration ever since. It is interesting to note that the General Register Office itself has undergone a change of title and that it is now referred to as the Office of Population and Census Surveys. From the mere collection of data, research taking advantage of modern data-processing equipment has speeded up the pace of change in organization and also has given clues to the causation and prevention of diseases.

Pioneer Voluntary Effort

The recognition that expectant and nursing mothers and very young children were particularly vulnerable members of the community started in train a similar process which led to the setting up of special services for medical care for these groups. Following the British tradition, voluntary effort preceded official action and, by 1901, it was possible for boroughs with the necessary financial resources to set up schemes for domiciliary midwifery and the supervision of the health of mothers and children. The history of the 1907 Education Act setting up the School Health Service has already been outlined and this was to be followed in 1918 by the first Maternal and Child Welfare Act which conferred powers on county councils and county boroughs to provide special services for mothers and children. These services, like those for school children, had a strong educational component from the beginning, and the history of health education in the United Kingdom is largely the history of the maternal and child welfare services and the trained nurses and health visitors who have worked in them.

Trend towards Unification

Thus, progress was piecemeal and involved the extravagance of an unnecessarily large number of separate administrative bodies until the first stage of unification was reached with the 1946 National Health Service Act.

Before that time in 1930, the British Medical Association had itself proposed a form of national health service based on economic needs. From the subsequent history of the National Health Service, it is clear that any service not firmly supported by the National Insurance scheme, supplemented by taxation, would have quickly become bankrupt. The flaw in Beveridge's thinking was that he genuinely believed that ill health would gradually disappear from the community as a result of the provision of free medical treatment. The costs of the National Health Service have escalated until they reach about 6% of the gross national product. The major benefit of the National Health Service between 1948 and the present day has been in the field of hospital treatment and specialist consultation which has been available in all parts of the country, whereas previously specialists were concentrated in the major cities and domiciliary visits were not possible, save to those who could pay the fees.

On the preventive side, the provision of immunization schemes, the growth of health education, and the social care of the needy have all resulted in improvements in the community health. The very low figures for mortality, reduction of maternal mortality to virtually nil, and the substantial reduction of infant mortality are largely the fruits of the work of the last twenty years. It must be remembered, however, that this has not been the result of medical care in the sense that Beveridge meant, but rather in the improvement of preventive services and of health education. Immunization schemes are to be regarded as a most important aspect of these, and they can be most easily evaluated.

Consensus Politics, Contraception, and Mental Health

The effect of consensus politics on the executive can be seen in two aspects of modern medical care, namely contraceptive services and the care of the mentally sick. In 1972, it was revealed that two elderly women had spent fifty years of their life in a mental deficiency institution, having been committed there at about the age of seventeen or eighteen because they had been unmarried mothers. Remarkably, they had been committed there by a magistrate on the application of their own parents who had not known how to handle their problems in any other way. At the age of sixty-eight it was found that neither of them was in fact mentally retarded.

In the same year, the National Health Service Reorganization Bill proposed that free contraceptive services should be available to all who wanted them. Previously to that, the Family Planning Act of 1969 had conferred powers on local health authorities to provide free services to all. No greater contrast in attitude could be imagined, particularly when we remember that these two unfortunate women were committed to what was virtually a medical prison as recently as 1920. Public opinion is now overwhelmingly in favour of the free availability of contraceptive advice and contraceptives. This is not only in order to prevent the births of unwanted babies and the distressing sequels which follow, but also to reduce the incidence of abortion which causes concern to many. It is also recognized that sexual intercourse has a function in human society and in relationships, apart from procreation.

In 1920 the 'birds and bees' era of sex education had been ushered in. This was based entirely upon the view that sexual intercourse has only one function — that of procreation. Later in the 1930s, there was a timid acceptance of the fact that certain women's health or even life might be threatened by repeated childbearing, so that contraceptive advice could be offered to married women who were suffering from ill health. The fact that sexual intercourse is a normal part of married life with a positive contribution to health and well-being was only reluctantly conceded. At the present day, public opinion which has been influenced undoubtedly by sex education and by the freer discussion of sexual matters in public has now persuaded the executive to take the necessary action. It must also be the first instance of health legislation where services are offered with the intention of directly promoting normal health, rather than preventing ill health itself.

Care of the Mentally Sick

The care of the mentally sick was once regarded entirely as a semi-penal system designed to remove lunatics from a community where they were a nuisance or a danger, and to incarcerate them by legal process. In certain States in the United States of America, this is still the case. Thus the mentally sick became the responsibility of the Board of Guardians. Even when harsh treatment of the mentally sick was abandoned (and the movement started simultaneously in this country and in France at the end of the eighteenth century), hospitals to receive the mentally sick were isolated as far as possible from the community, and there was an emphasis upon guardianship and custody, rather than treatment. It has been recognized in recent years, however, that the mentally sick will recover, and be rehabilitated more easily if they can continue to live in the community of which they are members. The Mental Health Act of 1959 is a direct example of health education carried on by the National Association for Mental Health. This was the beginning of a new era of the care of the mentally sick in which hospitals provided only one aspect of care -- that, perhaps, during acute episodes of illness. Local authorities were required to provide hostel accommodation for those who could not live at home, and the former isolation of mental hospitals from the community began to end.

Process of Change

In both cases we have cited, the process of change starts by a few innovators who may never see the results of their own work, but who are followed in time by those who implement the innovation. During the second phase, public education is carried on by the media of mass communication, stimulated by voluntary societies who are composed mainly of innovators. Politicians are invariably involved and eventually the executive of the party in power at Westminster prepares the necessary legislation conferring powers on administrative bodies to implement the reforms.

These are instances of where health education of the community makes sense in terms of the community's responsibility for the health of its members. Such health education must necessarily start at school by ensuring that all school-leavers know the facts regarding community health, such as we have outlined in this book. It must be reinforced however by the mass media, and this is the other side of the coin, since, whatever criticism may be levelled at the mass media, without their facilities, ideas would not circulate and become discussed and the need for reforms would not be appreciated. The advent of television which is a most penetrating form of the mass media, bringing into the home ideas which formerly could only be gained by going out to inconvenient public meetings, has obviously forced the pace of change in community attitudes.

Limits of Legal Compulsion

No discussion of community responsibility for health would be complete without the consideration of the value of legal compulsion to regulate health behaviour. It is interesting to observe that those with the most liberal ideas can become extremely enthusiastic when the question of legal compulsion for healthy behaviour arises. Basic and practical questions involved are: how far can you regulate people's behaviour by law, how can you enforce laws compelling them to do things, or not to do things, and whether by attempting such compulsion, evasion and crime will be encouraged? Young people frequently ask why the government has not abolished smoking, instead of merely drawing the public's attention to the dangers of smoking. Smoking can be prohibited, if not abolished, under certain circumstances, which people accept without question. To go back to our air travel analogy, no one objects to being stopped from smoking when approaching an aircraft or during taking off or landing; similarly, no one objects to the prohibition of smoking at petrol-filling stations. The abolition of smoking in public places is well received in most countries of the world and many department stores in big cities in the United Kingdom now require customers to refrain from smoking. In other situations, social custom and convention make smoking out of the question. For example, there may be couples who have smoked while dancing, but it is extremely unlikely, and certainly no one smokes in church. To attempt to abolish smoking by law, however, would result in an underground movement for the importation and the processing of tobacco and the distribution of its products. No country in the world, not even the most severely totalitarian, has attempted to abolish smoking. The unfortunate history of prohibition in the United States showed how worse evils could occur and that more serious consequences would arise from illicit drinking than if drinking was permitted and controlled by licensing regulations.

There have been two attempts to control personal behaviour in respect of venereal diseases. The Contagious Diseases Act of 1864 provided that women who were suspected of spreading infection could be arrested, brought before the justices, and compelled to submit to medical examination and, if found to be infected, could be compulsorily detained in hospital. Public opinion eventually recognized that this was unfair to women and as a result of the efforts of Josephine Butler, a pioneer in the movement to abolish organized prostitution, the Act was repealed in 1886. During the Second World War, Regulation 33B, a Defence Regulation, was introduced under which persons named as a source of infection by two or more patients could be compelled to appear before a magistrate and directed to undergo medical examination and treatment if they refused to come forward voluntarily. Although this regulation did not discriminate against women it was never popular with the doctors and social workers who were responsible for the control of venereal diseases. The risk of blackmail was considerable and it was believed that this regulation actually deterred patients from naming contacts.

The Public Health Act of 1936 contains provisions for the compulsory detention and treatment of a patient suffering from a dangerous contagious disease, e.g. smallpox, or open tuberculosis, where co-operation is refused. This power has been very rarely invoked save in exceptional situations such as the case of a man suffering from mild smallpox who refused to leave a hotel in which he was staying.

The procedure would be for the medical officer of health to obtain the necessary order from a magistrate and for his action to be confirmed by the Health Committee. It should be noted that powers for restraint of liberty are vested in the local authority, not in a medical man whose professional duty is to offer advice and to support his application for an order with medical evidence.

The difficulty about attempting to control personal behaviour that does not infringe the common law is enforcement. The problem is less in the case of statutory control of the production and distribution of food, drink, and other articles which carry a potential risk to health. In such a case there is an obligation or a contractual relationship, the business or undertaking is carried on under accepted legal sanctions, and local authorities have statutory powers to enforce the provisions of the various acts and regulations that provide for the control of the environment and of the supply of goods to the public. Legal control here is on a community basis and is for the common good. Thus we have effective laws regulating the food and drink trades, ensuring quality control, and the prevention of bacterial infection or chemical adulteration. Certain statutory 'nuisances' are defined and committal of such nuisances, if detected, is followed by prosecution. The Clean Air Act is mainly preventive in scope and is an example of legislation requiring people to do things for the public good rather than providing merely for penalties for non-compliance.

The public health inspector is the enforcement officer acting on behalf of the local authority but he does not measure the success of his work by the number of prosecutions he initiates. The public health inspector is a primary health educator in the area of environmental control and he relies mainly on the explanation and interpretation of the statutes to the tradesmen and manufacturers whose establishments come under his jurisdiction. In the field of food hygiene, for example, the public health inspector carries out health education campaigns and organizes courses of instruction for food handlers in which he undertakes the major part of the teaching and examining. This is obviously of greater importance in that such work is truly preventive whereas prosecution for an offence does not undo the harm that may have occurred to the health and safety of the public.

This aspect of community health education is important when new legislation is about to be introduced. For example, the Clean Air Act which exacts certain requirements of householders as well as industrialists came into operation smoothly because medical officers of health organized educational campaigns in which public health inspectors held meetings, set up exhibits etc., before the Act came into operation. To the extent then that personal behaviour is related to the community's health, sanitary law is effective and, if there are gaps, common law can be invoked. On the personal plane, however, particularly if liberty and enjoyment of amenities and convenience are involved, legal enforcement of health has serious limitations.

The difficulty about attempting to enforce certain codes of behaviour by law is the problem of enforcement. Already, in the field of environmental control, we have very effective laws regulating the production and distribution of food, quality control of drugs, labelling orders to prevent adulteration, the prevention of the pollution of the air by black smoke, and the sanitary disposal of waste material. In fact, powers conferred on local authorities for the protection of the environment are being extended as new hazards are indentified. An example is the Deposit of Poisonous Waste Act of 1972 under which prosecution may be brought against firms or individuals who jettison substances such as cyanide without regard to public safety.

APPENDIX ONE

The Structure of the National Health Service

The National Health Service (Reorganization) Act which came into force in April 1974 ended the administrative boundaries between curative and preventive medicine and provided one authority to cover all aspects of medical care. The coming into operation of the Act coincided with the reform of local government whereby metropolitan counties and counties were created each with district councils. London local government which had been reformed in 1965 was left unchanged. All personal health services are now the responsibility of the new health authorities, but social services remain the responsibility of the new local authorities. Environmental control is also the responsibility of the local authorities. The school health service is now staffed by doctors and nurses seconded from the area health authorities.

The overall responsibility for the National Health Service is vested in the Secretary of State for Social Services who is assisted by two Ministers of State, one for health and one for social services. These ministers are accountable to Parliament. There are fourteen regional health authorities each of which has at least one teaching hospital in its area. These RHAs are appointed by the Secretary of State and they are responsible for the regional planning of all services in the region.

The next tier comprises the area health authorities of which there are ninety-two and each is subdivided into a number of health districts up to a maximum of five. These form the next administrative tier. There are 150 health districts of population size of 200—500,000 and each contains at least one district hospital. Each area health authority comprises fifteen members representing medicine, community health services, and, where applicable, teaching hospitals. The chairman is appointed by the Secretary of State. The boundaries of area health authorities are coterminous with those of the new local authorities and in order to facilitate medical services to these authorities joint liaison councils have been appointed containing representatives of local authorities and area health authorities.

Community health councils have been appointed at area health authority level. These comprise thirty members, half of whom are nominated by the local authorities and half representing voluntary agencies. Their funds are provided by the area health authorities.

General practitioners retain their status as independent contractors under the aegis of family practice committees. The area health authority will plan health centres — these were provided for in the Act of 1946 — and will provide the premises and ancilliary staff for the general practitioners.

The Act has introduced a new principle of executive control. The medical officer of health disappears after a period of nearly 130 years during which he has been the guardian of the community's health. He reappears in the new role of community physician at area and district level and as a member of the management team which will undertake the day-to-day management of the service accountable to the area health authority. The district management team comprises six members, three of whom must be doctors including one each from the hospital and general practitioner services respectively, one nurse or midwife, and a treasurer and an administrator.

This structure applies to England and there are separate but similar schemes applicable to Wales, Scotland, and Northern Ireland. In these countries there are modifications necessary in the light of their political structure — each has its own central department for example — and also because of the population distribution.

APPENDIX TWO

Health and Welfare Legislation in Force in the UK

Note on legislation. There are three ways in which legal powers are conferred on public bodies for the purpose either of the sanitary control of the environment and regulation of public conduct, or for the provision of health and social services. There are general acts of Parliament, subordinate legislation — that is statutory instruments and orders made by a Secretary of State under the provision of an Act — and by-laws adopted by local authorities or other authorities clothed with statutory powers, for example, water and sewage undertakings. Such by-laws are confirmed by the appropriate Secretary of State. By-laws are mainly concerned with the compulsion to do something or the prohibition of doing something, and they come nearest — in the public health field to compulsion for health. However health and social welfare has a positive aim and prosecutions are relatively rare, reliance being placed on making the legal requirements known — e.g. posting a list of by-laws or distributing leaflets and posters — and expecting that the majority of people will comply.

Statutes for the provision of services

The National Health Reorganization Act 1973 (came into force in April 1974)
The Abortion Act 1967
The Local Government Social Services Act 1971
The Mental Health Act 1959

Statutes to enable public authorities to control the environment

The Public Health Act 1936 (and 1961)
This Act covers the following main aspects:
    Sanitation and buildings
    Nuisances and offensive trades
    Drinking water
    Prevention of pollution
    Prevention, notification and treatment of (infectious) disease
    Nursing homes

Baths and washhouses
Common lodging houses
Canal boats

The Offices, Shops and Railway Premises Act 1963. (This provides for inspection and enforcement of standards of accommodation, hygiene, lighting, etc.
The Food and Drugs Act 1955.
Food Hygiene Regulations 1960–62.
Clean Air Act 1956.
Radioactive Substances Act 1948 and 1960.
The Noise Abatement Act 1960.
The Home Safety Act 1961.
The Housing Act 1957 and 1961.
The Town and Country Planning Act 1962.
The Factory Act 1961 (successor to a long line of acts dating from 1819).
The Deposit of Waste Act 1972.
Note: regulations have been made under the provisions of these acts to cover all eventualities, and codes of practice have been drawn up for the guidance of those directly concerned, e.g. food production staff and food handlers, dairymen, etc.

Statutes and regulations concerned with the welfare of children.

The Children and Young Persons Acts — 1933, 1938, 1952–63.
Births and Deaths Registration Act 1953. (This provides *inter alia* for the compulsory registration of all live births as well as stillbirths.)
The Children's Act 1948 and 1958.
The Adoption Act 1958.
The Nurseries and Child Minder's Regulation Act 1948 and 1968.
The Education Acts 1944 and 1968.
School Health Services Regulations (made under the Act) 1959.
The acts and regulations quoted above apply generally to England and Wales. There is separate legislation in Scotland.

APPENDIX THREE

Landmarks in the Historical Development of Health and Social Services in the United Kingdom.

1836 *The Births and Registration Act.* Under the provisions of this statute the General Register Office was set up and the appointment of Registrar-General created.
1848 General Board of Health established.
1858 Transfer of functions from General Board of Health to the Privy Council.
1871 Local Government Board (with Medical Department) established.
1871 *Vaccination Act* (superseded Act of 1867). Appointment of public vaccinators and administrative officers — Vaccination Officers. Vaccination

against smallpox compulsory with exception of those who declared a conscientious objection. Compulsory vaccination came to an end in 1946 when the acts were repealed under the National Health Service Act.

1875   *The Public Health Act.*

1888   *Local Government Act.* Administrative counties and county boroughs created.

1894   *Local Government Act.* Urban and rural district councils created.

1902   *Midwives Act.*

1904   Report of Interdepartmental Committee on Physical Deterioration.

1907   School Medical Service established. Thus the Board of Education became a health authority.

1911   *The National Health Insurance Act.*

1913   Royal Commission on Venereal Diseases.

1917   *The Venereal Diseases Act.*

1918   *The Maternity and Child Welfare Act.*

1919   *The Ministry of Health Act.* Local Government Board abolished and Ministry of Health created.

1929   *Local Government Act.* Poor Law functions absorbed into general system administered by administrative counties and county boroughs. Local authorities now responsible for vaccination, collection of vital statistics, provision of institutions for care of physical and mental illness, and child life protection.

1946   *National Health Service Act.* First comprehensive health service available to all. Part III services (prevention, care and after-care, midwifery and health visiting services, ambulance services and home help service) administered by local health authorities, counties and county boroughs.

1948–58   *Children's Acts.* Existing duties for child life protection imposed on local authorities now extended to include the taking into care of those under the age of seventeen who are deprived of a normal home life and who are without parent or guardian.

1969   Department of Health and Social Security established, succeeding the Ministry of Health and bringing under one direction all services concerned with medical care and social services.

1971   *Local Government Social Service Act.* (came into operation January 1972) Social service departments set up by local authorities separately from health departments. The new departments took over certain Part III functions from health departments.

1972   *Local Government Reorganization Act.* Existing local authorities with their geographical boundaries abolished and replaced by counties, metropolitan counties with county districts.

1973   *National Health Service Reorganization Act.* All health services unified under one authority.

These landmarks demonstrate the essentially evolutionary and dynamic character of British political and public life in the field of human welfare. There is a continual re-examination of institutions and their reform based both on scientific methods, as in the case where legislation has followed Royal Commissions or other fact-finding operations, and partly empirical. For example the General Board of Health was set up because of the serious epidemics of cholera at the time. Compulsory vaccination was introduced after a major epidemic of smallpox. Revelations of social and health problems arising as a result of mobilization for war created a pressure of public opinion leading to the establishment of the school health service and to legislation regulating the treatment of venereal disease.

Throughout this history there has been a consistent assurance that the administrative machine and statistical services were ready to apply the new knowledge produced by research. This trend is shown today when the new Health Service was timed to come into operation at the same time as the reforms in local government.

It is interesting to note that whereas in the nineteenth century and early twentieth century there was a devolution of responsibility from the centre to local government, there is now a move in the opposite direction. There has also been a change in nomenclature of central departments and their ministers. In the nineteenth century there were 'Boards' with 'Presidents'. In the early twentieth century the Boards became Ministries with Ministers. In the late twentieth century we now have Departments with Secretaries of State having Ministers under them to discharge special functions and detail.

QUESTIONS

1. In what ways did nineteenth century politics show a greater appreciation of preventive medicine than is shown today?

2. Could legislation be devised to control the modern social environment in order to maintain health and prevent breakdown?

3. What is the relationship between the professional health worker and the community? Is there a lesson here for the teacher?

REFERENCES

1. Ryle, J. A. (1947). *Changing Disciplines*. Oxford:OUP.
2. de Tocqueville, A. (1835). *Democracy in America*. 1961 edition. Translated by Henry Reeve. Oxford: OUP.
3. Koos, E. L. (1954). *The Health of Regionville*. Ithaca, New York: Columbia University Press.

FURTHER READING

Abel-Smith, B. (1963). *Paying for Health Services: A Study of the Costs and Sources of Finance in Six Countries*. World Health Organization, Public Health Papers No.17. London: HMSO.
Brockington, C. F. (1955). *The People's Health*. London:Batchworth Press.
Brockington, C. F. (1958). *World Health*. (Pelican Medical Series). Harmondsworth: Penguin.
Hatch, S. (ed.) (1973) *Towards Participation in Local Services*. Fabian Tract 418. London:Fabian Society.
Paul, B. D. (ed.) (1955). *Health, Culture and Community:Case Studies of Public Reactions to Health Programs*. New York:Russell Sage Foundation.

Weston, T. (1972). *How is the Health Service?* London:Conservative Political Centre.

World Health Organization. (1973). *Interrelationships between Health Programmes and Socio-Economic Development.* Public Health Papers No.49. London:HMSO.

Public Health Law and the History of Health Services

Frazer, W. M. (1950). *A History of English Public Health.* London: Baillière, Tindall and Cox.

Roberts, L. and Shaw, C. H. (1966). *A Synopsis of Hygiene.* 12th ed. London:Churchill.

FILMS

Title	Colour B/W	Running time	Distributor	Date
Little Man, Big City	Colour	10 mins.	Concord	
Pity of it All	B/W	45 mins.	Concord	1966
River with a Problem	B/W	28 mins.	Concord	1961
Limits to Growth	Colour	60 mins.	Concord	1972
A Funny Thing Happened on the Way to the Garbage Dump	B/W	51 mins.	Concord	1970
First Mile Up	B/W	30 mins.	Concord	1961
Community Responsibilities — What's Your Opinion	B/W	10 mins.	Concord	1955
Community Care of the Mentally Sick	Colour	19 mins.	Concord	1966
Tomorrow's Children	Colour	17 mins.	Concord	1971
Somewhere to Play	B/W	15 mins.	Concord	1971
Do Something	B/W	17 mins.	Concord	1970
Two of a Kind	B/W	30 mins.	Concord	1967
The Earth and Mankind (*Six films*)	B/W	30 mins. each	Concord	1961
Accidents	B/W	25 mins.	Concord	1966
Born Losers	B/W	25 mins.	Concord	1969
Cathy Come Home	B/W	70 mins.	Concord	
A Completely Different Way of Life	B/W	50 mins.	Concord	1971
David and Hazel	B/W	30 mins.	Concord	1964
Conformity	B/W	45 mins.	Concord	1967
Flowers on a One Way Street	B/W	60 mins.	Concord	1967
Last Bus	B/W	30 mins.	Concord	1969
Suspects All		20 mins.	Guild Sound and Vision Ltd.	

CHAPTER 7

Areas of personal responsibility

Although all modern states offer an elaborate system of medical care and protection of health, such official systems cannot cover every eventuality. In the final analysis we are all independent and autonomous users of our physical, emotional, and intellectual equipment and we are in command of the environment in which we spend most of our lives, i.e. the home. Everyone is responsible for other people in some way, either through parenthood, occupation (as in the case of teachers and youth leaders, as well as industrial managers), and in voluntary organizations which provide the social needs for the different age-groups in the community. In order to carry out these personal responsibilities both for our own individual well-being and health and also for that of others, it is necessary to understand the nature of man and his ecology, as well as the various hazards that can threaten well-being, health, or life itself.

Evaluation of a Summer Camp

An understanding of the way in which responsibility depends upon knowledge and experience can be obtained by considering the formal evaluation of the results of a camping expedition. When a teacher returns his charges to their families on the conclusion of a camping trip, no doubt his first criterion of success is the degree to which all the children are satisfied with their experience and have actually undergone a visible improvement in physical, emotional, and social well-being compared with the time at which they set out.

To achieve such a result, however, means that certain negative criteria will have to be applied in the check-list which could be used in assessing results. This list would read as follows:

1. All children have returned and none were left behind in hospital.
2. There were no serious accidents.
3. At no time during the camp did any child suffer from diarrhoea and vomiting.

4. There was no serious aggression or friction amongst the children or between the group of children and residents in the camping area.
5. There were no cases of snake-bite or attacks by farm animals.
6. No child refused his food.
7. No child was excluded by the other members of the group, bullied, or made to feel unhappy, or homesick.

On the positive side, the check-list would show that the camp site was left clean and tidy, that all litter was disposed of satisfactorily, and that no food was left lying about to attract flies or vermin. It might also be of interest to include the fact that the children had learned something new about the area in which they were camping.

The Camping Life-Style

To the experienced camper, none of the things mentioned above would appear to be unusual or new in concept. This is because the whole situation adds up to what can be called a life-style which is appropriate for camping. To experienced campers, this life-style is so instinctive that they do not bother to analyse it, but they make use of their experience in order to plan a camping trip in such a way that the calculated hazards will be reduced to a minimum. The teacher leading a camping trip enjoys the advantage of having authority conferred upon him by consent of parents and children and of being able to exert discipline and restraint when he considers it necessary. For him the life-style of camping resembles the Mosaic law. The rules of personal conduct and environmental control laid down by Moses have been shown to be effective for the prevention of tapeworm infestation, bacterial toxin food poisoning from bovine carcasses, and the prevention of the spread of gonorrhoea, to mention only a few examples. It may be regarded either as an extraordinary feat of serendipity, or a practical example of divine inspiration. Teachers of divinity might make use of this story for an interesting intellectual exercise.

Principles of Field Hygiene

When we consider the preparations that a teacher must make for camping, on the other hand, we see that far from this being a matter of instinctive life-style or serendipity, a camp is organized on lines that fit in exactly with the principles of human physiology and ecology. Credit should be given to the Royal Army Medical Corps for the discovery of the principles of field hygiene both in camp and on lines of communication, and their application in situations where improvisation is required. The contribution of military hygiene to military success is well accepted and it has always taken into account physical and emotional well-being as well as barriers to the communication of serious infectious diseases, particularly those affecting the intestines.

The teacher subconsciously applies the same principles when instructing his pupils about their conduct during the camp in the interests of their safety and health, and also in giving them lists of equipment that they should provide for themselves personally. He is exercising his imagination by examining the calculated risks (which he does not have to communicate to his pupils since this might unnecessarily alarm them or their parents) both to physical health and to other people's emotional security and enjoyment of living. It is therefore our personal responsibility to handle anxiety effectively in a constructive way, and not to communicate one's own insecurity to others so that they break down. This is a skill that comes from experience and the guidance of parents, teachers, and other elders. It is, fortunately, a skill that can be acquired at any age and an understanding of human relations and group dynamics is an essential part of mental health education.

All the foregoing are components of well-being and, in addition, there are certain practical skills required of the individual in order to protect health or to secure prompt professional attention to departures from health. These include the prevention of infection, and in the camping example, cited above, food-hygiene was involved. [1,2] In addition there is the prevention of infection by prompt isolation in the case of the common cold or tonsillitis or influenza in addition to the precaution taken by a full immunization programme. The prevention of accidents depends upon an orderly organization of the home environment and calls for an awareness of situations in which human judgment will fail and be likely to cause an accident. Here the human being can be regarded as the host of an accident and his environment presents a potential hazard which is minimized by human awareness and possession of skills in movement and in handling equipment and tools. Thus accident prevention can be approached in a positive way, rather than by frightening people out of undertaking any worthwhile activity. [3,4,5]

Minimal Medical Knowledge

The example of the chance occurrence of appendicitis in a camp cited above shows that part of personal responsibility is to be able to recognize the significance of symptoms and to ask for medical help for their diagnosis and treatment if necessary. It is not realized that the primary diagnosis of illness is made by the patient himself, or by those in charge of him. The distinguishing of symptoms which are purely functional in origin -- for example the aches and pains that come from bad posture, the breathlessness that comes from lack of exercise, or the headache that arises from muscular tension, due to the ineffective handling of anxiety — from symptoms due to organic illness depends upon a fundamental understanding of normal physiology supplemented by experience. To take effective action, there must also be a knowledge of the way in which health services operate. This constitutes a problem when camping abroad where it may not be so easy to summon an ambulance with a '999 call'.

First Aid

There are also emergency situations in which people in the patient's company will have to take action themselves. This is conventionally termed 'first aid'. Although full-scale first aid training needs regular application and will not appeal to all members of the community, everybody should be able to arrest serious bleeding, to restore the airway, and to apply mouth-to-mouth artificial respiration, to apply external cardiac massage, and to organize the scene of an accident in such a way that the patient is protected from cold and further injury and unnecessary pain while skilled assistance is being obtained. In addition to cultivating these elementary skills, a judgment will have to be formed when they are appropriate. [6]

Coping with Stress

There is a considerable contrast between the ordered disciplined life of a camp in which children voluntarily obey the instructions and accept the authority of the teacher, and the adult world with its intense competitiveness, where stresses arise from personal conflicts between loyalties, obligations, and the desire for satisfaction and the innumerable opportunities and encouragements for self-indulgence which are increasingly regarded as normal expectations.

In the biologically vulnerable phases of life, such as adolescence and middle age, the pressures exerted by modern society form the background of behavioural problems which individuals attempt to solve or to compensate for by the excessive use of alcohol, by the abuse of drugs and by sexual behaviour in which sexuality is divorced from affection and responsibility. Whereas the community takes care of the environmental problems such as those encountered in camping, the personal problems arising from the need to achieve satisfaction are much more difficult to solve, and they must be solved by the individual himself. While all responsible people would agree that there is much that needs changing in our present society, it can never become perfect; there will always be anomalies, and aggression will make its appearance in different forms. The most effective way to change society on a long-term basis is to promote the maximum degree of emotional security in the community. An analogy with infectious diseases is appropriate. The serious killing and maiming infectious diseases have retreated before a policy of immunization in which the majority of vulnerable individuals are immunized specifically against these infections. In the same way, if we secured at least an eighty per cent rate of optimum emotional security in the community, the hazards to mental and social health involved in aggression, violence, the use of toxic substances, and perhaps the spread of sexually transmitted diseases would diminish. This is a positive way of tackling social problems which are traditionally approached in a negative way by condemnation or moral exhortation. Health behaviour in these terms thus adds up to a general life-style.

Authority or Reason

The relevance to health education is that, whereas in former times the healthy life-style was cultivated largely as a result of example reinforced by adult authority, young people are no longer willing to accept dogmatism and direction of their lives. We can appeal to reason however by presenting objective studies of the factors known to promote positive health. Thus the behavioural pattern of the authoritarian model can be followed but by reasoned acceptance rather than by simple obedience.

Moses was able to impose a code of hygiene and personal conduct on the early Israelites as a part of their religion, and the camp leader also can insist upon conformity to the life-style appropriate to camping in virtue of the authority conferred on him by consent. Health education in preparation for adult life with responsibility should preferably aim at stimulating the deductive powers of pupils and the formation of judgments based upon an understanding of human needs. We now have precise information regarding needs for physical health and well-being and protection against disease, and also for our emotional lives. Because of our current behavioural problems in society there is an intellectual confusion about the nature of human needs and the ways in which satisfactions can be achieved. Man's nature includes the fact that his performance improves with effort, whether this is in the physical, intellectual, or emotional field. If he is deprived of the opportunity of effort by taking short cuts, such as for example the abuse of drugs in order to alter mood, he is prevented from taking the road to true health. The identification of a healthy life-style with any particular social class is misleading and largely irrelevant. An awareness of a healthy life-style is not dependent upon any level of income or economic development, or of education. It is not incompatible with any type of culture and it offers no threat, which is so often imagined, to the pop culture which is so prized at the present day. The fact that one of the most successful pop music stars is identified with an official campaign to persuade motorists to use seat-belts should be a reassuring point in this connection.

QUESTIONS

1. What are the likely hazards during the course of a pop music festival? What steps should organizers take to prevent them and to cope with those that arise?

2. The patient is the first person to make a diagnosis. Discuss this statement.

3. In what ways may personal conduct endanger the health of others? The general principle of public health has been to make the environment fit the man. The nature of contemporary health problems suggests that we may need to make man fit the environment. Discuss this in relation to mental health.

4. What opportunities exist in the school to equip children to accept personal responsibility for their health?

5. 'The only way that a teacher can opt out of teaching health education is by resigning from his post'. Do you believe this? Give your reasons.

6. 'It is the civic duty of all adults to be able to carry out "life saving" first aid.' How would you deal with:—
   a. A pupil who has just been rescued from the swimming-pool but is not breathing?
   b. A pupil who is bleeding profusely from a severe cut on his leg?
   c. A pupil who has been knocked unconscious?
   d. A pupil who had just scalded her forearm badly?

7. 'For good or otherwise, the teacher is the most effective visual and aural aid.' Discuss this statement.

8. Are you prepared to draw up a list of examples of personal irresponsibility for a teacher. How can you reconcile these yourself when teaching about personal responsibility?

REFERENCES

1. Norton, E. (1972). *Hygiene in the Home*. London: Mills and Boon.
2. Christie, A. B. and Christie, Mary G. (1971. *Food Hygiene and Food Hazards*. London: Faber and Faber.
3. Medical Commission on Accident Prevention. (1970). *Education for Hazards*. London.
4. Backett, E. Maurice. (1965). *Domestic Accidents*. World Health Organization, Public Health Papers No. 26. London: HMSO.
5. Ward-Gardner, A. and Roylance, P. J. (1970). *New Safety and First Aid*. London: Pan Books (with Esso).
6. Nelson, A. (ed.) (1971). *Medical Aspects of Home Accidents*. London: Medical Commission on Accident Prevention.

FURTHER READING

Bergel, F. and Davies, D. R. A. (1970). *All about Drugs.* London: Nelson.

Claridge, G., (1970). *Drugs and Human Behaviour.* London: Allen Lane.

Draper, E. (1972). *Birth Control in the Modern World.* Harmondsworth: Penguin.

Fletcher, C. M. (1965). *Commonsense about Smoking.* Harmondsworth: Penguin.

Grewer, Eira (1965). *Everyday Health.* London: Pergamon Press.

Grewer, Eira (1968). *Caring for your Health.* London: Pergamon Press.

Loraine, John A. (1971). *Sex and the Population Crisis: An Endocrinologist's View of the Twentieth Century.* London: Heinemann.

Office of Health Economics. (1970). *Alcohol Abuse.* London.

Stapledon, Sir George. (1971). *Human Ecology.* London: Charles Knight.

Statham, R. (1973). *Venereal Diseases and Modern Society.* London: Priory Press.

Which. (1970). *Contraceptives.* London: Consumer's Association.

Williams, Lincoln. (1967). *Alcoholism Explained.* London: Evans.

FILMS

Title	Colours B/W	Running time	Distributor	Date
Birthright	B/W	24 mins.	Concord	1959
Every Baby a Wanted Baby	Colour	35 mins.	K. R. Industries Ltd., Hall Lane, Chingford, London E4	1968
Breathing for Others (Part 1 of Emergency Resuscitation)	Colour	12 mins.	Guild Sound & Vision Ltd., Kingston Road, Merton Park, London SW19	
Give them Air	Colour	20 mins.	Guild Sound & Vision Ltd., and Ministry of Defence (Navy), P.O.S.T. H.M. Naval Base, Portsmouth Hants.	
Emergency Resuscitation	Colour	50 mins.	St. John Ambulance Ass., 10 Grosvenor Crescent, London SW1 and Guild Sound & Vision Ltd.	
It's Your Choice		20 mins.	N.A.V.A.L.	1972
A Time for Decision	Colour	16 mins.	Concord	1967
Smoking and You	Colour	11 mins.	Central Film Library	1963
Profile of a Problem Drinker	B/W	29 mins.	Canada House Film Library; and Concord	1957
Understanding Stresses and Strains	Colour	10 mins.	Walt Disney Productions	

FILMS (*Continued*)

Title	Colours B/W	Running time	Distributor	Date
The Eye of the Beholder	Colour	25 mins.	Guild Sound & Vision Ltd.	
Narcotics — the Decision	Colour	35 mins.	British Temperance Society	1968
The Addict Alone	B/W	26 mins.	Concord	1967

FIRST AID

Title	Colours B/W	Running time	Distributor	Date
Your Health (this is a series of films each dealing with a special aspect of children's health. It is a guide for 8—11 year-olds to healthy routine — diets, personal hygiene, care of teeth, accident prevention etc. The scene is a family summer camp. USA).	Colour	10 mins. each	N.A.V.A.L.	1966
Don't Let Him Die (for secondary schools. British)	Colour	19½ mins.	Guild Sound & Vision Ltd. and Ministry of Defence (Navy), Principal Supply and Transport Office, Section 7B3/0572, HM Dockyard, Portsmouth	
Emergency Resuscitation (demonstrates mouth-to-mouth respiration)	Colour	14 mins.	Stewart Films Ltd., 82/84 Clifton Hill, London NW8	1963
Most Precious Gift (this deals with simple precautions that must be taken at home)	B/W	20 mins.	Gas Council	1963
Sleepy Heads (for 5—11 year-olds. This stresses the importance of sleep. USA)	Colour	10 mins	N.A.V.A.L. and Boulton Hawker Ltd., Hadleigh, Ipswich, Suffolk.	1966
Busy Bodies (USA)	Colour	10 mins.	N.A.V.A.L. and Boulton Hawker Ltd.	1970

FILMSTRIPS

Title	Distributor
Becoming More Independent	Concordia Publishing House Ltd.
Dating is not a Private Affair	Concordia Publishing House Ltd.
I'm in Love	Concordia Publishing House Ltd.
Its Good to be Part of a Family	Concordia Publishing House Ltd.
Learning to Communicate	Concordia Publishing House Ltd.
Learning to live with Brothers and Sisters	Concordia Publishing House Ltd.
Parents can be a Problem	Concordia Publishing House Ltd.
When you start to Date	Concordia Publishing House Ltd.
When the Real Thing Comes Along	Concordia Publishing House Ltd.
Where Do I Fit In?	Concordia Publishing House Ltd.
Who Sets the Standard?	Concordia Publishing House Ltd.
Family Planning	Camera Talks Ltd.
Sex and Society	Common Ground Ltd.
Dangerous Droplets	Camera Talks Ltd.
Problems of Lung Cancer	Camera Talks Ltd.
To Smoke or Not to Smoke	Camera Talks Ltd.
Vaccination and You	Diana Wyllie Ltd.
Vaccination and Immunisation	Diana Wyllie Ltd.
Immunisation	Encyclopedia Britannica Ltd.

CHAPTER 8

Evaluation

Health education has, as one of its principal aims, the influencing of attitudes to health and the modification of behaviour. It is therefore imperative that its effectiveness should be measured, and the technical term, *evaluation*, applies not only to the measurement of effectiveness in changing behaviour or attitude, but also upon the effectiveness of methods and the overall planning of campaigns or experiments. It must be added that health education should also enjoy a status as a subject of cultural value, as a liberal study. To impose a rigid scheme of evaluation based on an expectation of immediate results would be undesirable. Nevertheless, with the present-day preoccupation with health problems which are the result of deviant social behaviour or group behavioural patterns, for example, smoking, drug abuse, alcoholism and sexual disorders, it is reasonable to accept that, if money and time is to be spent on these activities, then some practical result must be demonstrated.

Association between Events

To understand the process of evaluation, it is necessary to grasp the principles underlying the association of events which are influenced by a number of variables. In the previous chapter, the example was given of ways in which personal responsibility could be accepted for the preservation of health. The ticking off of a check-list was a crude attempt at evaluation but no general conclusions could be drawn. If we take the occurrence or non-occurrence of diarrhoea and vomiting as one criterion of evaluation, it would be necessary to know what were the probabilities of this infection occurring. If the camp was located in an organized camp site with piped chlorinated water, showers, and water-closets, then the probability of the occurrence of gastro-enteritis would be low. If on the other hand the camp site was dependent upon streams for water supply, requiring attention to sterilization of water and the sanitary disposal of excreta, then the probability of gastro-enteritis occurring would be much higher. We would have therefore to be certain we were comparing like with like in drawing any conclusions from the fact that in this particular summer camp, no child suffered from gastro-enteritis.

What are the Criteria of Success?

In the evaluation of a summer camp, it would also be necessary to decide what were the criteria of success. In the case we have cited, the criteria of success were relevant to the skill and knowledge and experience of the teacher in charge. It cannot be said, however, that attending this summer camp necessarily confers a higher status of health on the children. It is likely that none of their brothers and sisters or friends who did *not* attend the camp suffered from diarrhoea and vomiting. On the other hand, some of those who stayed at home might have contracted para-typhoid fever from eating contaminated ice-cream. A non-availability of ice-cream or the assurance by the teacher that the supply was hygienically sound would have conferred an additional protection on the children who attended the summer camp, but this again could have occurred by chance. All that can be concluded from the evaluation of this particular summer camp is that as regards this group of children under the charge of this particular teacher and camping in a particular site, there were no accidents or a preventable illness. Assessment of well-being on return from camp will be an entirely subjective one.

Operation of Chance

The problem of evaluation in health education, therefore, is that we are confronted with many variables and inter-related or even disparate factors. This means that evaluation has to be planned carefully as an experiment using statistical methods for analysis of data and comparison where possible with controlled situations where health education was not practised. To cite the example once again of our summer camp, if there had been a hundred summer camps taking place at the same time and no diarrhoea and vomiting had occurred in any of them, then the results obtained by any one teacher would not be significant. Similarly, diarrhoea and vomiting may have occurred in a number of camps purely by chance; on the other hand, if it had occurred in ninety-nine camps and not in our particular camp, then our teacher's result would be highly significant.

It will be remembered that in the first chapter we quoted the experience of James Cook who had succeeded in voyaging around the world with only a minimal loss of crew. Anson's voyage which had been disastrous from the point of view of mortality and disability can be regarded as a controlled situation. It would not be ethical of course to set up a controlled situation for summer camps; on the other hand, there are many situations in health education where it is ethical to observe a controlled group in which nothing out of the routine is done and comparing them with the group who have been subjected to a planned health education campaign.

All health education experiments and campaigns must star with feasibility studies. This means that the disease or hazard which is to be prevented by health education must be one that is directly associated with patterns of human behaviour. A useful model is indicated by the diagram below.

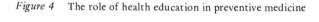

Figure 4   The role of health education in preventive medicine

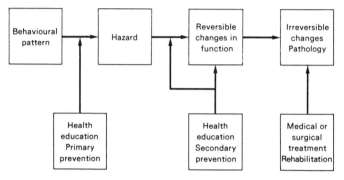

Collection of Data

The ideal at which we aim is to intervene by health education before the behavioural pattern has collided with a particular hazard. It is also useful to be able to identify groups particularly at risk. For example, in the case of education to prevent drug abuse, research such as that conducted by Wigfield showed that most at risk were the sixth-form group. Many students were found to be unaware of the dangers of drugs. In this case the preliminary information was obtained by the use of a questionnaire, an example of which is given below.

Questionnaires are the most frequently used methods of data collection in the preliminary stages of evaluation of health education. Wigfield used the information on the questionnaire as a basis of his research into attitudes of drug abuse amongst young people attending a secondary school, a college of further education, a technical college and the sixth-form society of two independent, and two grammar schools. [1] Apart from his conclusion, already

Table 8. Questionnaire on drug dependence.

1. What drugs taken by addicts have you heard of? ....

2. What dangers do you know of each of these drugs?

3. Do *you* personally know anyone taking drugs? (Please tick √)

        Yes ....

        No ....

If yes, what drugs did they take? Where did they get them? (Please tick √)

        Coffee bar ....

        Party   ....

        Pub   ....

        School   ....

        Street   ....

        Other   ....

4. Have you ever been offered drugs? (Please tick √)

        Yes ....

        No ....

If yes, where? (Please tick √)

        Coffee bar ....

        Party   ....

        Pub   ....

        School   ....

        Street   ....

        Other   ....

What drugs were you offered?

5. If you were offered drugs would you try them?

        Yes ....

        No ....

If yes, why would you?

6. Why do you think young people take these drugs?

7. Where did you first hear about drugs? (Please tick √)

        Television   ....

        Radio   ....

        Newspapers   ....

        Talk in School   ....

        Books   ....

        Friends   ....

        Parents   ....

        Other, please state ....

Source: Wigfield, W. J. (1972). 'Survey of Young People's Attitudes to Drug Abuse'. *Community Medicine*. **129**:139–41.

mentioned, as to the vulnerable group, he found that hallucinogenic drugs were the most popular; many students were unaware of the dangers of drugs; and it appeared that young people who first heard about drugs from lectures in schools are less likely to experiment with them than are those who are informed about drugs by the mass media.

This stage of evaluation then gives us guidelines as to the feasibility and the value of health education in this field, and justifies a policy which includes this subject in the general health education curriculum. These conclusions are based on data and their analysis, and are not dependent upon prejudice or subjective judgment.

Health education to prevent children taking up smoking, or to persuade those who have started to drop the habit, invariably commences with an investigation of the level of knowledge, attitudes, and experience by the use of questionnaires completed anonymously and then analysed. The design of the questionnaire is very important and requires the application of statistical experience, particularly as the process of data analysis will depend upon the right data being collected in the right form.

Baseline Observations

The preliminary collection of data also enables us to form a baseline from which to measure any change of behaviour or attitude as a result of the health education process. It is important, for example, to know how many children smoke, at what age did they start, do their parents also smoke, how much do they smoke, whether they are content to continue smoking, or whether they would like to give it up, and a number of other variables, examples of which are shown in Bynner's study of the young smoker. [2] This method of data collection is applicable to those subjects of health education which are relevant to behavioural patterns and are influenced by value-judgments. It is essential to be able to define the terms of reference of the experiment in such a way that numerical values can be assigned for the final statistical analysis and the drawing of conclusions.

Choice of Method

Having decided that a health education campaign or experiment is feasible, and is likely to produce some positive results, it is then necessary to decide upon the choice of method and materials to be used. Watson's experiment in Edinburgh using five different methods of approach on the subject of smoking is a classic example of the evaluation of the effectiveness of methods. [3] It is necessary to approach this part of the study objectively and to be prepared for some surprises. For example, in Watson's investigation, the didactic lecture appeared to be more effective in converting smokers into non-smokers, and group discussion was more effective in changing attitudes to smoking. So-called psychological methods were found to be ineffective, or even have a paradoxical result. The variables to be considered are the intelligence level and social background of the children concerned. If a topic to be covered in the experiment was likely to produce considerable conflict between the home background and school, this must be allowed for. Some methods of health education depend upon a high degree of verbal ability and capacity to participate. Thus the impact of a television programme on the subject of venereal diseases will vary according to the type of school and the age-group who are exposed. [4] These are matters which should come into the preliminary evaluation when making a decision as to method.

Table 9. Ranking of methods

Method	Ranking of Methods in 3 Aspects			Final Average Ranking
	Behaviour	Knowledge	Attitude	
Didactic	1	3	3	2
Group Discussion	2	2	2	1
Psychological	3	4	1	3
Total Project	4	1	4	4
Control	5	5	5	5

This illustrates the principle that in ranking methods in order of effectiveness the objective of the exercise must be defined.
Source: Watson, L. M. (1966). 'Studies of Health Education Methods'. *Scot. Hlth. Bull.* **24**(1).

Pre-testing of Materials

Evaluation also includes the pre-testing of materials, and this is particularly important where films and other visual aids are to be used. These may have meanings completely different from those the makers of a film intended. It has been found, for example, that films on smoking, which appeal to a non-smoker, so irritate smokers as to cause them to completely reject the health message. In health education as presumably in all branches of education, one has to distinguish between the job satisfaction of the teacher and the effective communication with the pupil. Appraisal panels are useful, but they do entail the drawback that appraisal may not be completely objective and it is certainly no substitute for detailed communications research which reveals so often that a visual aid is less meaningful to the pupils than to those who designed and produced it.

Experienced teachers have found, however, that, despite their tendency to subjectiveness, appraisal panels can be useful pointers, especially when the panel rejects the film or other visual aid. In a notoriously difficult area — drug abuse — a typical appraisal of a well-meaning film by six separate groups of sixth-form pupils produced the consensus that the film was 'ultra sentimental', 'corny', acceptable perhaps to parents, or alternatively to pupils under fourteen years of age. It would seem to be idle to attempt to present such a film to the age-group who might be most in need of it.

Communications Research

An example is a research project which was designed to test the reaction of a group of teenagers to a film on venereal diseases. [5] This research concentrated on communication of essential information and the comprehension of certain aspects of venereal diseases, and the reactions of the audience to this treatment of the subject matter. The test required the co-operation of 233 boys and girls aged thirteen to fifteen; the film was screened under strictly controlled conditions and immediately after the showing a series of specially designed questions was administered. The parents of the children accompanied them to the showing and afterwards, separately from the children, they answered questions designed to assess the reaction of the film from their point of view. After the screening of the film in the ordinary way, the groups were shown a number of 'stills' in which questions were asked as to the exact meaning of the diagram or picture.

Eighty per cent of the parents considered the film to be suitable, and a small majority, fifty-five per cent, considered that more should have been included in the content of the film and they indicated that their opinions ranged from the need for emphasis on moral principles to the giving of a list of local VD clinics in the area. Certain sequences in the film were misleading, according to the pupils' reaction, and it was clear the film did not give a clear indication of how venereal diseases can be contracted. It was also necessary to find out whether any of the aspects of the film, for example, the showing of clinical features, was upsetting.

The procedure of pre-testing materials is now well founded in health education practice. Thus alternative designs of poster or alternative treatment by film or slides can be shown to a sample of the population at whom the message is aimed. The sample must be carefully stratified in order that it is comparable in all respects with the general population who will receive the message. Criteria for stratification include social class, level of education, verbal ability, and taste reflected by usual reading matter (for example, do the group read *The Times* or the *Daily Mirror*), age, and sex. The test situation must be carefully controlled and similar observations made in controlled groups.

When a comprehensive school health education programme has been prepared, it is necessary to determine priorities. One method is to conduct a survey of children's interests and several examples of these exist in the literature. From the teacher's point of view this is an objective measurement which provides a guideline for where to start in a health education programme. The children's interest may not coincide with the teacher's own ideas of what is a priority, but it would be a mistake to take no notice of them It is essential to secure active interest from the beginning, and this is most likely when topics are chosen which reflect a child's own health needs. Such inquiries can be made again by questionnaires completed anonymously. Noseworthy (personal communication) secured the co-operation of about 600 pupils aged 11—16 who submitted ten questions which had a bearing on health. The predominant interests are set out in the following table.

Table 10. Health interests of children aged 11—16 (1966)

Age Group	Interest as stated by pupils
11—13	Diseases — especially cancer, smoking, sexual intercourse, child birth, menstruation.
13—14	Masturbation, 'cohabiting', infidelity, homosexuality, alcoholism, incest.
14—15	Human relationships in general, personal in particular. Dental caries, acne, communication problems with parents, Venereal Diseases.
15—16	Personal relationships, heavy petting, contraception, drugs, adolescent moods, advertising, menopause, personal problems including slow development of penis, or breasts.

In attempting to interpret the meaning of these findings it must be understood that the questionnaires were completed anonymously, but the responses reveal a degree of sophistication (the enquiry was conducted 7—8 years ago) for which the mass media must be to a certain extent responsible. The range of interests is wide and would present a problem of classification in the process of curriculum development. Similar experiments have been carried out in colleges of education.

Having established the baseline of behavioural pattern, attitude, and level of knowledge, and having selected the method considered to be most appropriate after pre-testing, it is then necessary to repeat the observations originally made before the experiment in

Table 11. Comparison of characteristics of all quitters and non-quitters

		Age		Sex		Married	Social class		Diagnosis			Number smoked each day	
	No.	Mean	SD	M	F		Manual worker	Non-manual worker	Relevant	Irrelevant	Uncertain	Mean	SD
Quitter	9	41.3	11.8	6	3	9	9	0	3	6	0	17.2	9.7
Non-quitter	182	40.3	14.6	115	67	144	131	51	54	124	4	15.8	7.7
Total	191	40.3	14.4	121	70	153	140	51	57	130	4	15.9	7.7
		$t = 0.20$ $p = 0.50$		$x^2 = 0.05$ $p = 0.82$		$x^2 = 2.33$ $p = 0.14$	$x^2 = 3.46$ $p = 0.08$		$x^2 = 0.04$ $p = 0.85$			$t = 0.54$ $p = 0.50$	

SD = standard deviation.
Source: Porter, A. M. W. and McCullogh, D. M. (1972). 'Counselling against Cigarette Smoking: A Controlled Study from General Practice.' Practitioner. 209:686.

order to detect whether there has been any change. There are now two sets of data and the problem is to assemble them in such a way that they show trends or patterns, and then to analyse them for significance.

Presentation and Analysis of Data

Statistical tools are the valued ally of modern health education. It is necessary therefore to be familiar with statistical procedures, even if one assigns their application to more skilled hands. Here is not the place to give any details regarding statistical techniques, and the reader is referred to standard works on the subject, particularly those which deal with the use of statistics in biology and sociology. It is necessary however for the health educator who wishes to evaluate his work to have a sound grasp of the principles of frequency distribution, and the calculation of standard deviations, and the application of tests of significance, i.e. tests which can distinguish between an event that would occur by chance and one that is in association with the health education procedure. The principle underlying any test of significance is the difference between what is expected, and what is observed. In some cases the health educator may start with a null hypothesis, i.e. it may be assumed that health education has nothing to do with the change of behaviour at all. An example is given below (see Table 11) in which a general practitioner started with a null hypothesis that counselling patients against smoking would have no effect at all. [6] Perhaps to his chagrin, he found that his null hypothesis was only too true and that the figures in the table and the calculation of tests of significance proved this. Of the nine patients who did stop smoking during the period of the experiment, four had received no counselling at all, and the results were therefore not significant.

It is necessary to present data in such a way that they can be studied and analysed. The first step will be tabulation of results, and here we are producing in tabular form what is virtually a frequency distribution, which can be examined more easily when it is converted into a graph. It is necessary to understand the nature of the so-called normal curve, standard error and deviation, and the significance of skew distribution. The standard baseline study for understanding a normal curve is the tabulation of heights of a number of individuals. Because the human race is characterized by infinite variability, all measurements, whether they are crude, such as the measurement of height or weight, or whether they are of microscopic proportions shows the same degree of variation spread over a normal curve. It must be remembered also in health education that we are frequently measuring parameters, i.e. variables which of themselves present some variability.

Table 12. Distribution of stature in 117 males

Absolute height (in.)	Measurements from working origin at 67 in (x)	Number of men observed (f)	Contributions to the sum (fx)	Contributions to the sum of squares (fx²)
61	−6	1	−6	36
62	−5	3	−15	75
63	−4	6	−24	96
64	−3	8	−24	72
65	−2	13	−26	52
66	−1	18	−18	18
67	0	19	0	0
68	1	14	14	14
69	2	14	28	56
70	3	9	27	81
71	4	5	20	80
72	5	4	20	100
73	6	2	12	72
74	7	1	7	49
Totals		117	+15	801

Source: Bailey, N. T. J. (1969). *Statistical Methods in Biology.* (5th impression). London: Unibooks, English Universities Press.

Figure 5 The diagram shows the observed distribution of the heights of 117 males, exhibited in the form of a histogram (rectangles), together with a fitted 'normal' curve (smooth curve)

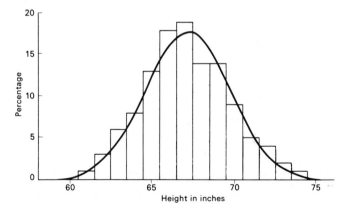

Source: Bailey, N. T. J. (1969). *Statistical Methods in Biology.* (5th impression). London: Unibooks, English Universities Press.

Table 13. Drug-taking among Helsinki School Children

	No. of pupils	Per cent
Non-takers	1,857	75.0
Occasional takers		
One time = 1x	173	7.0
2—10 times = 2—10x	253	10.2
Regular takers = over 10x	125	5.1
(Not stated)	67	2.7
	2,475	100.0

Source: Hemminki, E., Rissanen, A. and Mattila A. (1972). 'The Opinions of Helsinki School Children on the Dangers of Drugs'. *Hlth. Educ. J.* **41**(1):115.

A typical presentation of 'raw' data.

Table 14. Advantages and disadvantages of drug-taking according to the schoolchildren (percentages)

	Disadvantages percentage					Advantages percentage			
	1	*2*	*3*	*4*	*5*	*6*	*7*	*8*	*9†*
Non-takers	53	38	7	8	4	5	5	1	1
*1x	38	24	8	4	1	4	9	1	—
*2—10x	32	24	11	4	1	7	10	3	1
*Over 10x	30	18	8	8	2	8	20	4	—
Total	49	35	8	7	3	6	6	1	1

Code†

1 = endangering health (mental, physical).
2 = becoming dependent.
3 = self-deception, alienation.
4 = wasting money.
5 = demoralization.
6 = escaping problems.
7 = good feeling.
8 = improving personality.
9 = medical therapy.

Refer to Table 2 (column 1).

Source: Hemminki, E., Rissanen, A. and Mattila, A. (1972). 'The Opinions of Helsinki School Children on the Dangers of Drugs'. *Hlth. Educ. J.* **41**(1):115.

These authors solved the problems of how to present figures showing a large number of variables by assigning numerical values to characteristics.

Sampling

Where large numbers of individuals are involved, the usual method is to draw a sample — say, one in eight, or one in ten — which is then stratified according to the age and sex structure or other characteristics of the whole population. Small samples, which are genuinely random and stratified, facilitate the data analysis and at the same time produce estimates of probability of the occurrence of events and significance of associations which can be regarded as applicable to the whole population from which the sample was drawn.

In the design of experiments for the evaluation of health education, mathematical ability is less important than an understanding of the general principles which govern the association of events, their frequency, and their variability. It is the reasoning that goes into the planning of the experiment which determines whether the conclusions will be valid. Where large numbers are involved, the use of calculating machines or computers is essential, and here it is necessary for the designer of the experiment to consult with the computer programmer in order that data can be presented in a suitable form. This aspect of health education provides many opportunities for teachers of mathematics to collaborate with their colleagues on the general science or liberal studies side.

Simple Experiments

All will not have the facilities or even the aptitude for conducting such elaborately controlled experiments. Examples of scientific investigations by teachers are rare. This may be partly due to the omission of research techniques from the curriculum in colleges of education, but also because there is pressure to complete schemes of work in traditional subjects in a limited time. There are signs of change, but it will probably always be advisable to secure the co-operation of professional colleagues outside the school who have had the training in research methods. However, less sophisticated evaluation procedures can be carried out which are still useful as guidelines to effectiveness of communication. An example is the setting of a recall of information test, usually by asking children to write an essay on a health topic that has been demonstrated to them by exhibitions, films, or other educational means. Thus in a comprehensive school one month after an exhibit on the dangers of smoking had been installed in the school for a week, the headmaster announced without warning over the public address-system that pupils would be required to answer certain questions which he then read out. The results were mainly an indication of a recall of information but this was some measure of the impact which the exhibit made on the pupils' minds. Not only was there an accurate recall of the information but pupils revealed which aspects had made most impression. For example, bottled specimens of cancerous lungs appeared to have influenced the pupils in their decision not to take up smoking.

Eriksson used a similar method to evaluate the effectiveness of a visit to a school by a specially equipped mobile unit as part of an anti-smoking campaign. [7] In this experiment control studies were conducted on a school over 200 miles away. Pupils were asked to complete a questionnaire and the following is a selecton of the various responses:-

72% agreed that smoking was the cause of lung cancer, with 7% disagreeing and 22% answering 'don't know'. Of the external influences that would persuade children not to smoke, parents took first rank – 46%. This was followed by television viewed at home – 35% (a surprising finding and it is not clear exactly what it means); posters – 31%; newspapers – 22% (at this time newspapers were publishing articles on smoking and health but the advertising campaign had not started). Teachers came last with 16% of pupils stating that the teacher's influence would persuade them not to smoke.

A total of 1,224 pupils aged 11–12 years took part in the experiment: 598 boys and 626 girls. 82% of the total declared that they would not take up smoking.

QUESTIONS

1. Design an experiment to show the effects of a dental health education with seven-year-old children.

2. Of a class of forty children aged 5–6, 50% are only children. Discuss the way in which a planned statistical enquiry could show the significance of this observation – if any.

3. How would you organize the pre-testing of a film on nutrition aimed at eleven-year-old children?

4. What criteria are necessary when planning an exhibit on population for a secondary school?

5. Granted that changes in attitude, and consequently in behaviour, are difficult to measure, how would you attempt to evaluate the results of teaching a topic of your own choice?

6. In evaluating a film what would you look for? Why is it absolutely necessary to preview a visual aid before using it with your pupils?

7. Have you been involved in any attempts to evaluate a teaching technique? If so, please give a brief account of the procedure adopted and the results and conclusions drawn.

REFERENCES

1. Wigfield, W. J. (1972). 'Survey of Young People's Attitudes to Drug Abuse'. *Community Medicine.* 129:139—41.
2. Bynner, J. M. (1969). *The Young Smoker.* London: HMSO.
3. Watson, L. M. (1966). 'Study of Health Education Methods'. *Hlth. Bull.* (Scotland).
4. Brown, R. L. (1967). 'Some Reactions to a Schools' Television Programme on Venereal Disease'. *Hlth. Educ. J.*26 :108—16.
5. Dalzell-Ward, A. J. (1970). 'Forward Planning in the UK for Anti-VD Programmes'. *Brit. J. Ven. Dis.* 46:159—61.
6. Porter, A. M. W. and McCullogh, D. M. (1972). 'Counselling against Cigarette Smoking: A Controlled Study from General Practice'. *Practitioner.* 209:686.
7. Eriksson, A. W. E. (1966). 'A Questionnaire Evaluation of the CCHE Smoking and Health Campaign'. *Hlth. Educ. J.* 25:177.

FURTHER READING

Roberts, J. (1970). 'Evaluation Methods and Techniques of Health Education'. *Hlth. Educ. J.* 29(4):125—8.

Biology and Statistics

Bailey, N. T. J. (1969). *Statistical Methods in Biology.* (5th impression). London: Unibooks, English Universities Press.

Bradford Hill, A. (1967). *Principles of Medical Statistics.* London: Lancet.

CHAPTER 9

Health education in schools-planning and organization

Continuing Education

People of all ages and at every level of education need some form of health education throughout the whole of their lives. Health education is a supreme example of the need for 'continuing education', a concept which has recently been developed by UNESCO. We all have crises involving personal health or the health of others at periods during our lives, and it is possible to identify certain biologically vulnerable periods, such as pregnancy, early infancy, adolescence, middle age and old age. Some of the crises can be averted by changing health behaviour in advance of the anticipated event — this, for example, is the basis of the so called 'pre-retirement education'.

In the life continuum the school represents a very small sector in terms of years, but it is the sector in which health education is most likely to be fruitful if it is planned with the intention of offering a 'carry-over' value into adult life, even as far as old age. Health education in the pre-school years should ideally be imparted by mothers. This is the case in literate homes where the mother devotes herself to her children, and is not distracted by the needs of outside employment. However, about 50% of mothers of small children now work outside the home, and this is a trend which is likely to increase. This will now place the onus on the nursery school for starting the process of health education which can then be continued throughout the remaining stages of school life to be reinforced in adult life in an incidental way.

There has always been a tendency for girls to be better informed about health matters than boys. This is partly due to the fact that home economics teaching has included the basic principles of nutrition and good hygiene, and for at least half a century it has been considered important that girls should be instructed in the hygiene of menstruation. This is sometimes confused with 'sex education'. Girls are also interested in parentcraft lessons and it is only recently that these have been extended to boys in an experimental form. During pregnancy and while they are caring for young infants, women have the advantage of instruction and guidance from health visitors who are the primary and most important health educators in the community at large.

Guiding the Child through his Experience

One task therefore in the future planning of health education in schools is to redress this balance and to ensure that boys also have an opportunity of interpreting their personal experiences in terms of health concepts. Health education is virtually the guidance of the child through experience and for the most part it will be carried on incidentally by every teacher in the school. In the field of human biology teaching in a junior school, there is of course a place for formal didactic instruction supplemented by the pupil's own efforts and for which he can be equipped with a variety of interesting material.

All teachers are involved with health education from the infant school as far as colleges of further education. The way in which they tackle this task will depend very largely upon the social conditions of a particular school and the degree to which the standards of the school differ from those of the community which it serves.

School and Community

It is an axiom of health education practice that a study is made first of the community, in which the community's own goals, level of knowledge, and attitudes are assessed, and then health education is planned accordingly. This is illustrated by accounts of health education campaigns in developing countries where social organization is so simple, and goals and aspirations are so closely identified with the levels of social and educational development that the lessons seem too obvious. The classical example is that of a community to whom a road, enabling them to export their produce and so gain cash to improve their living standards, is relatively more important than the reduction of infant mortality by attention to better child care.

Health Education must be Meaningful

In the communities of Western Europe too, the same problems are presented. Health education differs from other subjects taught in schools in that it can offer no career advantages, and with the exception of the G.C.E. 'O' and 'A' level in human biology, it offers no examination prospects, although schools may also submit their own syllabus for Mode 3 C.S.E. It is therefore not meaningful to the pupil or to his family in conventional terms, such as providing an additional qualification for the obtaining of employment.

Although many subjects in the traditional curriculum may not be meaningful to the majority of pupils, for example, English literature, there is nevertheless, an appreciation by those of average intelligence that they are unlikely to obtain well-paid employment, unless they can read and write and express themselves clearly. Mathematics too, which to many in the past may have seemed an abstract subject of little meaning, now takes on a glamour because of its relationship to computer programming, an occupation which is enthusiastically pursued by an increasing number of young people, not only at the programmer level, but at a lower level, such as punch card operating. The manipulation of numbers therefore can now be made much more meaningful in real terms.

To children in normal health, free of defect, reasonably well fed and adjusted at their own social level, the end-product of health education may not be meaningful, and the pursuit of this study may be of interest only to those who are academically inclined. The content of health education is intellectually stimulating and satisfying and can produce a high level of job satisfaction for the teacher. There is another disadvantage, which does not apply to subjects in the school curriculum generally, in that health education may implicitly criticise the standard of living and behaviour of the child's family. As we have seen in the chapter on health consequences of behaviour, cultural patterns have a profound effect.

A Threat to a Familiar Life-Style

Cultural patterns on the other hand are so deeply rooted that they are rarely radically disturbed by succeeding generations, and even the high standard of living now enjoyed by the majority of people in Western Europe does not seem to have affected certain cultural patterns which have an impact on health. If health education is seen by the child to be a threat to his familiar life-style which confers on him emotional security, then he will reject it. On the other hand, increasing numbers of adolescents in particular are gaining emotional security from lessons, discussions, conferences etc., dealing with the topics of personal relationships, drugs, and handling stress. Not only does the methodology have to be worked out which can avoid this confrontation between cultures, but it is most important that the family be taken into consultation and should be made aware of what the child is being taught.

Consultation with Parents

Where parent-teacher associations exist, the opportunity should be taken to hold meetings which can be addressed both by teachers and by outside experts, such as doctors and nurses, who will work with the teachers, so that the parents can have an idea of the importance of health education, and how it will be taught in the school. The familiar objection that parent-teacher associations involve only a minority of exceptionally dedicated parents must not be allowed to act as a deterrent to this practice. People learn from their peer groups and if there is a small well-informed group of parents as a result of membership of the parent-teacher association, then ideas will spread from this group in their contacts with their neighbours and friends. In families where free communication between children and parents is encouraged and enjoyed, the children also will enlarge their parents' horizons, but the problem will remain of homes where such communication is not encouraged. This has distinct relevance to parent education.

Channels of Communication

As we have already seen, there are many channels of communication on health matters at the present day. The daily press, magazines, television, and radio are all carriers of information, some of it nowadays increasingly in the field of criticism of the health services and about personal health behaviour. The advertising industry also advertises health in some cases, for example, urging people to consume more first-class protein, and ill health in other cases, for example, advertising for tobacco, alcohol and carbohydrates. The adult who has had a thorough experience of health education at school will be able to benefit from the one and reject the other.

A Universal Need

Health education should apply to all schools, and there is no reason to believe that the stream which is occupied with more academic subjects with the intention of proceeding to higher education has any less need of health education than the others. In schools, and in streams of comprehensive schools, where the academic programmes are of primary importance, there is an understandable reluctance on the part of teachers to spend any time on subjects which have no examination value. In some respects, pupils undertaking an academic course are less vulnerable as judged by research into health behaviour in the field of sexual behaviour and smoking. It is the less educationally able and ambitious child who tends to be sexually promiscuous or to smoke. It is possible that this could apply also to

use and with the excessive consumption of alcohol at too
age.

er, the picture of health breakdown later in life amongst
professional classes shows that they too would have benefited from
an understanding of the general principles of health protection and
promotion. Sexual disorders in marriage, for example, affect the
well-educated and professional classes, as well as the others; in some
cases more so because there are more reasons for conflict and
impotence. The effective handling of anxiety in stress situations
applies to everybody, and in general we should aim at health
education being available to all pupils in all kinds of schools in a
form appropriate to age and stage of development and to the social
situation from which the child comes.

Not a 'Timetable' Subject

Health education very seldom appears on the timetable as a subject.
At a secondary level of education, however, there is an increasing
tendency for responsibility for health education to be taken by
teachers concerned with liberal studies or social studies as well as by
science teachers, and teachers of home economics and religious
education.

In the infant school it has been traditionally assumed that health
education is largely a matter of inculcating good personal habits, of
cleanliness of skin, clothing, and the environment. Where the school
environment is superior to that of the home, then a considerable
contribution can be made by the introduction of the child to the
new and more comfortable ways of life which it is hoped he will be
able to adopt for himself later on. In the present day, however, with
the great improvement in housing, it is very likely that the school
environment is inferior to that of the home. This is one instance
where the environment of most older pre-war schools tends to
defeat the efforts of health education, for example, matters such as
washing the hands after going to the toilet. Deficiencies in a school
environment can often be used in a teaching situation to illustrate a
point or act as a focus for discussion.

The Infants' School

The teacher can reinforce personal habits which should have been
learned at home, or if they have not been learned, she can make a
start with the child at the age of five. The whole of the organization
of the infants' school can be used as a model for learning. It is
important that the school caretaker and the cleaning staff, as well as
the school meals staff, should be taken into consultation and
invited to co-operate in the health education process. The child can
then learn the experience of well-being as a result of clean skin, of

clothing that has been tidily stored during the day and is free from dust, and of the importance of ventilation of the classroom maintenance of an equable temperature, and the prevention of the stirring up of dust which is a vehicle of respiratory infection. Teaching children to blow their noses correctly, one side at a time to avoid back pressure to the ears via the Eustachian tube, is a very important aspect of personal hygiene.

The routines and rituals which are a necessary part of the school's day can be interpreted to the children in health terms. School meals provide an opportunity for a practical experience on balanced nutrition, and the teacher will have been trained to exercise patience and restraint in the case of individual children to whom the school menu is unfamiliar and therefore threatening. It is important that the school meals staff and lay helpers should also understand the psychological aspects of nutrition. Children must be protected from bullying to eat their food, or to eat foods for which they have an instinctive dislike. The provision of water for drinking during meals is also important as this has an impact on oral hygiene by its cleansing action on the teeth. Young children also tend to be very thirsty, and old-fashioned ideas that water drunk with meals is harmful must be dispelled.

Some children may need virtually retraining in toilet habits, but all of them need to understand the importance of personal cleanliness and the danger of the conveyance of infection by hands which have not been washed after defecation. As dysentery tends to be an endemic problem in many schools, scrupulous cleanliness of water-closets is essential as is the provision of washbasins, and the children can co-operate by using them in a cleanly way, but they can also have explained to them the reasons why they are disinfected and why the caretaker and his staff take such care of these premises.

Health education in the infants' school need not stop at this level. The infants' teacher, by her own demeanour, care of her person and skilful handling of situations, can convey a good deal of information informally. She is frequently faced with situations such as a child suddenly being sick, or wetting its pants or becoming ill in some other way. The manner in which she handles the situation will convey to the other pupils the need for sympathy and compassion and the preservation of personal dignity.

The presence of a handicapped pupil in the class is an advantage to normal pupils, as well as to the handicapped. The need for compassion and tactful assistance to the handicapped without depriving him of the opportunity of developing personal skills will prove excellent models for behaviour towards less fortunate people later in life. The normal child will also realize how valuable is his own health.

The infants' teacher is also likely to be confronted with a sudden discovery of sex-play between two children or in groups of children. The way in which she handles this situation is of itself an important lesson in sex education. The teacher needs her own security to be maintained, however, and the handling of situations such as those described should be a topic of discussion at staff meetings and with the head teacher to make it clear that the classroom teacher will be supported in the action she takes. These are topics also which would be usefully discussed in parent-teacher associations.

As regards sex education, there is a continuum of development which starts with auto-eroticism in the infant, an awareness of the pleasure associated with the genital region, giving place to a stage of curiosity, to a desire to experiment with another person accompanied by strong fantasies, and finally, if maturity is achieved, to a stage when sexual behaviour is meaningful only in terms of a personal relationship.

Just as no one expects the child to make a leap from the learning of arithmetical tables to a study of trigonometry, so no one can expect the child to make a sudden leap into adult maturity. All these stages must be passed through if development is to proceed to the final optimal stage of 'sex' as part of a personal relationship with acceptance of personal responsibility for partners. We are therefore faced with a problem of how to guide children through the inevitable experiences through which they pass, and to interpret them according to the level which we assume they have reached. We have already done a good deal in the child welfare centres to encourage mothers to accept infants' play with their genitals, somewhat pompously described as infantile masturbation. The modern young mother can now accept this without feelings of guilt or embarrassment or feelings that the child has already made a start on the road to promiscuity.

To satisfy the stage of curiosity, however, requires a good deal of courage on the part of parents and of teachers. Intellectually orientated homes manage this by the acceptance of displays of nudity at bath times or other appropriate times, and books such as *Peter and Caroline* provide for the educated mother an excellent opportunity of explaining the anatomical functional differences between the sexes in terms of affection and relationships. We know however that the majority of children do not come from such homes and that their own attempts to satisfy their curiosity are frequently met with by dismay followed by punishment and repression which remains as a built-in chronic trauma which may affect their lives for ever. There is also the distinct danger that sexuality may become attached to the aggressive qualities which lie in every human being alongside the qualities which are the opposite of aggression. The mother's task should be to deliberately attach sexuality to affection, compassion, gentleness, sense of responsibility etc.

The infants' teacher can reinforce this teaching, or if it has not been attempted, can make a start on it herself, and the nursery school and infants' school seem to be ideal situations in which curiosity about sex can be satisfied legitimately and under conditions of security.

So far we have been concerned with habits and behaviour, but it has been shown recently by Boustead, that it is possible to introduce simple intellectual concepts of human biology at the infants' school level. [1] This author conducted an experimental course of health education in an infants' school, and was able to introduce the idea of the cellular structure of the body. This is most important as attempts at health education at the secondary stage are frequently frustrated by the pupils having no idea at all of the way in which the body is constructed of cells differentiated and grouped to form organs and connective tissues. This gives rise to quite ludicrous misunderstandings with regard to the biology of conception.

One advantage which the teacher in the infants' school enjoys is that the child is relatively home-centred and that the elementary lessons in health education will be more meaningful to him than at the secondary stage when the life-style of his accepted peer group takes precedence over that of the home. On the other hand the child in the primary school is dependent upon his mother for his standard of personal hygiene, nutrition, and general care. To maintain the standard which he has learned at school may involve a considerable extra burden on the mother, which she had not anticipated.

Once again boys tend to be at a disadvantage because of a tradition that they should not be involved in household chores, whereas girls are encouraged to do their own laundry and to assume personal responsibility for their own care at an earlier age. This is another instance where the teacher will need to study the community served by the school as the first guide for planning the health education curriculum. In the early stages of secondary education the child is more receptive to intellectual ideas as at the moment they do not conflict with his chosen behavioural pattern. It has been observed, for example, that children of between eleven and twelve readily assimilate information about smoking. In general it seems desirable for factual human biology teaching to be completed at the elementary stage before the onset of puberty.

The Junior School — Human Biology

In the more formal organization of the junior school, human biology teaching can be carried on both systematically as a subject in its own right, supplemented by representation through other subjects. The volume of the content of human biology is considerable and if dealt with in detail would occupy the whole of the school time. However, we can set ourselves a target by saying that at the age of eleven or transition to secondary education, boys and girls should have a grasp of the elementary principles of the following aspects of human biology:-

The human body as a going-concern: i.e. its innate tendency to healthiness; its reaction to challenge, stress, and activity; the principles of homeostasis; the function of the oxygen-transport system; and the dominance of the body by the central nervous system and hormonal influences.

Nutrition: energy needs, balanced diets, food groups, vitamins; digestion, absorption, and metabolism, *the body's defences* against bacteria and powers of repair; *the cycle of conception*, reproduction, development in utero, and birth; *growth and development.*

The physical environment: i.e. the effects of climate, geography, heat, cold, humidity, light, noise and radioactivity. This would include toxic substances, poisons of all kinds, including poisons used by man, such as tobacco and alcohol.

The biological environment: the interdependence of man on other life-forms, including bacteria; the life-cycle of parasites — intestinal and skin parasites: louse, itch mite; house flies and fleas; mode of transmission between animals and man and hygienic precautions to prevent this; the distinction between harmful bacteria and those which bear a useful part in life; the importance of conservation.

The social environment: the family, the neighbourhood, the working environment, the crowd; examples of the way in which the greatest danger to man today is man himself.

Emotions: this is best explained as 'feelings', for example, anger, worry, quarrelling, pleasure, excitement, violence; this will introduce the general principles of human relations.

Accident prevention: including introduction to first aid; this should also include road safety, cycling proficiency tests, and maintenance of bicycles.

Simple ideas on population: these can introduce elementary statistics showing the way in which populations are numbered and events taking place in populations can be assessed numerically.

Relation to Children's Interests

The teacher's task will be to select aspects of these subjects which are meaningful in terms of human behaviour and which can be imparted as far as possible in a practical way. There is obviously an overlap with several other subjects, and here co-operation between specialists and class teachers is essential. A preliminary study of the children's own interests will provide guidelines for an approach that will be meaningful. In some cases, it will be children's own experience; in other cases, it will be interest in adult activities, those involving technology of all kinds, recreation and sport. Examples are: the physiological adaptation needed for space travel, which requires the direct application of applied biology through technical means, i.e. the preservation of oxygen-tension and the normal atmospheric pressure to which the body is adapted, protection of astronauts from the stresses imposed by rapid acceleration, and the way in which they can be trained to combat the feeling of weightlessness; in the case of sport, the need for training and adaptation for altitudes which was a problem involved in the World Olympics held in Mexico City. Recreation, such as camping and water sports, riding, and the keeping of domestic animals all provide approaches to human biology that will enable the pupils to deduce the general principles from the practical experiences they are discussing.

Control of the Environment

An opportunity can be taken also to explain the technical ways in which the environment is controlled, so that adverse effects on health are avoided. This introduces the environmental health services concerned with the protection of food and water supplies and the disposal of waste, noise abatement, and the protection from radio-activity. The study of the environment of London Airport and the way in which it is controlled by its staff of technical experts can provide examples of all of these subjects.

The Emotions

The introduction of the emotions at this stage of education has the advantage that the general principles of human relations and the role of the individual personality in the conduct of relationships with others can be understood before the stresses and conflicts associated with adolescence appear. It may well be that if the children were well grounded in these general principles of handling their own emotions before puberty then many of the conflicts traditionally associated with this biologically vulnerable period of life might not make their appearance.

This is a topic which can only be conducted by discussion and participation methods. Didactic talks to children on their feelings will undoubtedly be loaded by value-judgments and may appear to be moral exhortation. However, discussion in groups of why people are angry, why they are worried, how they will behave when faced with a challenge, what causes a feeling of happiness and well-being, can help a child to understand motivation. The first step on the road to mental health is to understand one's own motivations and to be prepared to confront reality, rather than to avoid a threatening challenge.

It is for the teacher to organize ways of imparting this information, but in general it may well involve group discussion, role-playing, and preferably the stimulation of ideas by the use of short thematic films. Discussions on violence can also be conducted with the older age-groups in the junior school. All children today are aware of violence in the community. It is communicated to them every day, both in fact and in fiction on the television screen, in the newspapers and in their own reading material. Whereas society has always tried to protect children against confrontation with sex, no censorship of violence has been imposed. This is one of the great paradoxes of modern society which arises from a lack of general understanding of the nature of sexuality and of the nature of aggression. It cannot therefore be objected that children in the junior school are too young to discuss violence and cruelty. These discussions will of course be taken up later at the secondary school stage.

Biology and Aesthetics

On a more positive plain, it may also be an advantage to consider the question of beauty in the context of human biology and health education. All living forms have their own beauty, and the human form has a beauty which is bound up with strong emotions. Each of the components of the human form has a beauty of its own, as will be appreciated by the study of the cellular architecture of organs. Perhaps one of the most serious deprivations of society of the present day is the growing deprivation of a sense of awe and respect for living forms. There is a dangerous tendency to 'reductionism' i.e. reducing life to merely chemical events or mechanical events. These are important factors in forming value-judgments which all responsible people should bring to bear upon contemporary problems, such as abortion, artificial insemination, extra-corporeal cultivation of the human foetus and organ transplants.

Health education should introduce the child to the three primary values of goodness, truth, and beauty in a meaningful practical form. Health and perfection of form and function are beautiful, disease distorts and is ugly. Behaviour which ignores truth and wounds the feelings of others is also ugly. The child can be encouraged to apply the primary test of whether goodness, truth, and beauty are represented in a behavioural pattern, and whether this is associated with healthiness or whether departure from ignoring these values is associated with disease. This introduces the question of ethics into health education, but it is an ethic which has no religious or class bias. It can therefore be regarded as immaculate in the present day, where there is an ever present anxiety not to impose one cultural pattern upon another. The capacity to perceive and appreciate beauty is a human characteristic. It is highly significant and a test for this capacity is incorporated in the Térman-Merrill intelligence rating. The child is expected in the pre-school phase of development to be able to distinguish between beauty and ugliness and the results of the tests when evaluated show that this capacity for distinction is significant. The claim therefore that every teacher is a teacher of health education is fully substantiated even in the case of the teaching of art.

Materials and Methods

The teacher in the primary school today is fortunate in that a wealth of material is now provided for the age-group seven to eleven. Books are available, providing a basic content for the study of the subjects we have outlined above, and there are also films, film strips, and slides. It is therefore possible for the teacher to build up a learning environment which the child can use to supplement the talks and discussions in the classroom. The project method of learning also lends itself very easily to human biology teaching. There are many agencies with which children can communicate themselves in order to obtain additional information to supplement organized visits, for example, to food factories, waterworks or museums which contain exhibits which are related to personal or environmental health. Children's natural desire to sketch, draw, paint, and model can also be exploited for human biology teaching. In the case of certain aspects of the subject, for example, the cycle of reproduction, it has been found that it is an advantage for the children to take home their sketches and notebooks so that the parents can be aware of what they are learning. In the case of one junior school, this enabled the relatively advanced teaching of the cycle of sexual reproduction without causing offence to parents which would have obstructed the project.

The Secondary School

A new dimension appears at the secondary stage of education. Whereas the pupil in the junior school can study human biology coolly and objectively because he is not consciously involved, once puberty is reached, boys and girls become self-conscious about their health and development. There is no indication that one generation solves the personal problems of adolescence for the succeeding generation. It is remarkable that the magazine *Boys' Own Paper* which continued in publication for about eighty years was answering the same questions concerning spotty skins and seminal emissions to the end of its life, as it did during the 1880s. It is at puberty and in the years that follow that boys and girls become aware acutely of the differences between people which are the result of the biological variation which is most strongly represented in the human species. Self-consciousness about health includes a concern for prestige and status and the desire to appear as mature and sophisticated as possible. Health education after puberty, therefore, will necessarily include reassurance about personal growth and development which may well call for a personal counselling service as many subjects may be too painful for individuals to raise in a group.

Personal Problems of Adolescents

The need to deal with these personal problems was recognized early in the development of health education, and today there is ample material to help the adolescent and his teacher. The code of personal hygiene learned in the infants' school is now no longer sufficient. Girls have the additional problem of menstrual hygiene and require detailed advice on matters such as the use of internal vaginal tampons and the so-called vaginal deodorants. There is a need too for attention to 'masculine hygiene' not only for well-being but important from the point of view of prevention of cancer of the cervix of the uterus. It has been known for over fifteen years that there is a significant association between a poor standard of cleanliness of the penis and the occurrence of cervical cancer in wives or female consorts. [2] Both boys and girls are troubled by acne, and some boys are troubled by a delay in physical development compared to that of their peers. They are no longer dependent on their mothers for general care and maintenance, and indeed they would resent being so. At the same time, many require stimulation and constant surveillance in order to maintain good standards of personal hygiene.

Guilt and conflict about sexual emotions and sexual experiences bother the adolescent today, as formerly, and indeed there may be a greater stress because of the degree of permissiveness about sexual behaviour which offers no guidelines and few limitations on conduct.

Apart from sex, there are preoccupations also with athletic performance, social skills, and in an increasing number of cases, weight control. Studies have shown that when left to themselves and provided with money, adolescents, eschewing the school dinner, buy starchy and carbohydrate foods which satisfy immediate hunger, but which do not provide a balanced diet with protein for the replacement of wear and tear. The sleep rhythm is also disturbed, particularly by parties and other social engagements at week-ends and the desirable biological rhythm of the day and night which is certainly cherished by those who are forced to break it, like long-distance travellers, undergoes considerable disturbance.

In addition to the natural preoccupation with himself, the adolescent also has a well-developed social conscience which is revealed at the present day to an extent unheard of before. Tiglao summed up the changing contemporary scene simply when she referred to the twentieth century as an age of transition in which the developed society is shifting from an industrial to a postindustrial or 'technotronic' society. [3] This applies to the countries of the E.E.C. and other European regions, as well as to the United States, while the *Third World* on the other hand is beginning to move from an agricultural to an industrial economy. Already in certain countries of the *Third World*, in North Africa for example, behavioural problems amongst young people are beginning to appear and are taking on a character similar to that which we find in our own society.

Tiglao draws attention to the communication network which, although it has 'shrunk' the world, has widened the gap between the developed and the developing world. She goes on to say that through modern means of communication, the social elites of the less developed world have come into contact with the advanced world and have assimilated and emulated the life-styles of the latter. In the meantime the masses of the people are more literate, more politically conscious — encouragement having been given by transistor radio and other means of mass communication — and they are experiencing a revolution of rising aspirations. Youth suffers from changes in social values and when newly-awakened desires are frustrated, they tend to feel rejected, and they develop a hostility towards society. This Tiglao believes is the basis of the present day youth unrest and activism. This calls for education and counselling and time should be allowed in the curriculum for free discussion with the teacher and with visiting adults from outside the school of these contemporary problems.

Equipping the School-Leaver

The felt social concern of modern youth is an effective bridge between the satisfaction felt as a result of gaining knowledge in the primary school and its application on leaving school to adult life.

Here again we can make a list of the topics on which the school-leaver should be well informed:

> preparation for parenthood
> the problem of world population
> the problem of minority groups in society
> the reasons for sexual promiscuity and the accidents that follow, i.e. sexually transmitted disease, unmarried motherhood, abortion
> contraception
> self-medication and the abuse of drugs
> smoking, the abuse of alcohol, violence and aggression as symptoms of social sickness
> human relations and how to handle anxiety effectively
> social and health services and how to make effective use of them
> personal responsibility for the maintenance of health.

Most of the content of health education at this stage lies in the area of personal responsibility. It is a far cry from the simple life of the camper outlined in a previous chapter to the complicated life of a breadwinner and parent in the E.E.C. countries. It is urgent that all children leave school with the attitude that health is a valuable asset to the community as well as to themselves. They should be able to resolve the conflict between the needs for productivity and economic growth and the needs for a full life in which leisure and personal relationships are considered precious. They should also be able to distinguish between efficiency in purely mechanistic terms and in terms of cost-benefit and efficiency that permits latitude and flexibility, and is achieved without paying the price of unhappiness and discontentment. They should learn how to handle those whose aggressiveness takes the form of deliberately destroying the security and serenity of others, often in the name of progress.

We have already pointed out that health education is needed throughout the whole continuum of life, and it is unrealistic to imagine that much ground will be covered during the four or five years of secondary education. This places a premium upon the concentration on behavioural and attitude aspects of the subjects that go to make up the content of health education.

Responsibility for Health Education

The planning of health education in schools includes also the problem of who is to do the teaching. There is a general reaction nowadays against the introduction of outside speakers, however distinguished they may be in their own professions. Nevertheless the partnership with the doctors and nurses of the school health service should be regarded as a very valuable asset to a teacher of health education. Similarly, in project work, it will be necessary to cultivate personal relationships with administrators of health services and other organizations which are concerned with environmental control or the promotion of health. Individual experts can frequently join with the teacher in giving an account of their professional duties which then makes the theoretical concepts of health care more meaningful.

In the infants' school there is no problem, because the teaching would invariably be done by the class teacher. The versatility of the infants' schoolteacher should be highly appreciated by the community and it is perhaps too little realized how important she is in giving children the first grounding in health education. In the junior school, general science teaching will usually cover subjects of human biology and ecology, but as will be explained later, there is an incidental component to all subjects on the curriculum which can contribute to health education. At the secondary school level, there is a trend towards health education's coming under the aegis of the teacher with special responsibility for liberal or civic studies.

An account by Larter of the remarkable experiment of a health week in a comprehensive school shows what can be done by a team of four teachers of social studies and English in co-operation with a large number of outside experts in organizing a comprehensive health seminar. [4] This experiment is interesting in several ways, not least the fact that the final sessions were conducted by the pupils themselves, each group having an obligation to put up a speaker with a prepared paper on one of the subjects studied during the week. It was possible also to bring the pupils into contact with administrators of hospitals, medical officers of health, public health inspectors, marriage guidance counsellors, general practitioners, and consultant health educators who played a part in the team-teaching project. The learning environment was also set up for the pupils to use themselves, and the afternoons during the week were allotted to private study using charts, slides, books, and exhibits. On the final day the groups and their spokesmen were putting the final polish to their reports. Visiting experts sat at tables around the hall and were available for individual consultation, and this opportunity was eagerly taken by many children.

The concept of team teaching therefore as regards health education in the secondary school will probably always need to include experts who are not on the staff of the school, but who contribute their personal experience in co-operation with the regular teachers. In less ambitious projects than the one described, it is also useful to organize a dialogue between the teacher and the doctor, nurse, or public health inspector.

The main justification for inviting an expert to assist in teaching is that the content of health education changes continually. Familiarity with the up-to-date situation comes most readily from actual practice in the health professions. It is too little realized that the biological sciences are not exact and that medicine is the least exact of all. Medical shibboleths are being disturbed all the time by the findings of large-scale research employing statistical methods of control. Teachers can best become acquainted with current interpretations of medicine in health education terms by regular professional contact with their medical colleagues of whom the school medical officer and nurse are closest.

QUESTIONS

1. When planning a health education programme would you consider inviting 'outside' specialists to take part in the teaching sessions? If so, in what way would you use them?

2. When planning an integrated programme how would you avoid giving the impression that the other subjects are being made the handmaidens of health education?

3. Team teaching is proving to be a very efficient technique. What combination of subject teachers would you like to have in your team and why?

4. Do you consider that conferences (day or half-day) for pupils on one or more health topics have a place in a programme? What are the advantages and disadvantages? Give an account of how you would organize one to deal with the problems of 'obesity' and the problem of drug abuse.

5. What is your attitude to having health education as a discipline in its own right in a school curriculum?

6. What different types of teaching techniques would you employ in your health education programme spanning the first five years in secondary school?

7. What areas of study would you include in a health education programme and why?

REFERENCES

1. Boustead, M. C. (1973). 'Health Week in an Infants' School'. *Hlth. Educ.J.* 32(1):12.
2. Wynder, E. L. (1955). 'Environmental Factors in Cervical Cancer'. *Brit. Med. J.* 1:743.
3. Tiglao, T. V. (July-September 1972). 'Planning for Health Education in Schools'. Supplement to *Int. J. Hlth. Educ.* 15(3).
4. Larter, J. (1971). 'A Health Seminar for Fifth-year Students at a Comprehensive School'. *Hlth. Educ. J.* 30(1):25.

FURTHER READING

Elliott, Daphne and May, E. T. (1967). *Health Education:Patterns for Teaching*. London: MacMillan.

Tanner, J. M. (1971). *Education and Physical Growth*. London: University of London Press.

Turner, C. E. (1966). *Planning for Health Education in Schools*. London: Longmans.

Ungoed-Thomas, J. R. (1972). *Our School* (Life-Line Series). London: Longmans.

FILMS

Title	Colour B/W	Running time	Distributor	Date
Blocks to Communication (USA Television)	B/W	30 mins.	Concord	
Fair Teachers	B/W	60 mins.	Concord	1961
It's a Battleground	B/W	40 mins.	Concord	1969
A New School of Thought	B/W	25 mins.	Concord	1969
The School in Contact	B/W	25 mins.	Concord	
Summerhill Swimming Pool	B/W	10 mins.	Concord	1968
Who Cares?	Colour	20 mins.	David, Sevenoaks School, Sevenoaks, Kent. Publicity Officer, National Children's Home, 85 Highbury Park, London N5.	

CHAPTER 10

Health education through other subjects

Biology

Biology, understandably, has a major contribution to make to the background of health education. This is not in respect of the systematic study of zoology and botany, but rather in the opportunity that is offered for deduction and the drawing of conclusions which can be applied to personal and community life. For example, the cycle of reproduction which will have been accepted as a fact in the infants' school with talks of animal and human babies and their parents is now shown to have a material basis. Similarly, the child in the infants' school will have appreciated that people vary in size and colour, both of eyes and skin, and that they resemble their parents and their brothers and sisters. The material basis for heredity and the infinite variation that characterizes the human race can now be shown in a study of genetics in which the chromosomes bearing an infinite number of genes are seen to make a contribution from each parent to the future child.

BIOLOGICAL COMMONSENSE

In general, it is possible to inculcate a kind of 'biological common sense'. This is an attribute needed in our modern communities where people make judgments on human affairs employing analogies from the physical sciences with which they are more familiar. Expectations are either unrealistic and over optimistic, or on the other hand they are pitched too low in the absence of a confidence in the human organism to adapt to handicap or to adverse conditions. An appreciation of the variation observed in the human race and of its importance to the stability of all societies should be acquired before leaving school. As we have already pointed out in the first chapter, scientific progress in the biological field in the twenty-first century will call for an informed democratic participation in policy-making.

We have seen that it is possible to teach infants about the cellular structure of the body. Biological studies in older age-groups can examine the life of the individual cell and the way in which groups of cells are integrated into organs which subserve functions of the various systems of the body. This will be the basis for the understanding of normal replacement of cells from wear and tear, of the phenomenon of growth and development, and of the defence which cells put up against invading bacteria or other foreign materials. The action of poisons is also explicable by an understanding of the internal life of the cell.

THE NEW LOOK IN EVOLUTION

The study of evolution which usually forms part of a school biology course should abandon its preoccupation with Darwin and Mendel and consider the process of evolution in the human being. This is important in view of the recent introduction of fundamental changes in the way of life for which there has not been time for adaptation. We have already referred to the consumption of refined carbohydrates; it may well be that the consumption of tobacco which is very recent in evolutionary terms has revealed a failure of human adaptability. The sedentary nature of modern life has also produced its problems. Mass communication is the most recent innovation of all, and its effect upon mental health and human thought, action, and attitude is worthy of study in evolutionary terms.

With an understanding of the biology of human reproduction, it is a short step to an understanding of modern techniques for the control of reproduction and population, and also the disorders which arise from the maternal environment while the foetus is developing. The thalidomide tragedy is only one example. A search is now going on to identify adverse effects of any drugs that may be taken during pregnancy, and self-medication during pregnancy is certainly unwise. There is also the effect of virus infections of the mother, and with an understanding of human embryology, the importance of the first three months during which, as it were, 'major decisions' are taken for the formation of limbs, organs, and the nervous-system must be understood. The ways in which conception can be avoided either from abstinence from sexual intercourse to the taking of a contraceptive pill and including within the range all other mechanical and chemical devices present no difficulty when the child knows how fertilization occurs and the route taken by the male sperm towards the advancing ovum.

The phenomena of growth and development provide excellent material for biological studies that can be related to common experience. Examples are the differences in growth rates between the sexes and the variations within the normal expectation of growth shown by individuals. The initiation of growth by the growth hormone has already been outlined (chapter 3). Rates of growth differ in various organs and it is significant that the brain grows fastest of all.

Children can study their own growth by making records of heights and weights and the phenomena of human growth with its spurts, its filling out, and springing up phases can be compared with the linear growth of animals such as mice.

PLANT LIFE

Biology does not consist entirely of zoology, and the study of plant life also has a direct application to health. Plants used as food, those which are harmful to man, or those which threaten growth and development, plants which he can use in many ways including as a source of drugs, and plants which give him pleasure, can all be considered. The application of biology to agriculture is an attractive way of considering human nutrition. The concept of 'calories per acre' offers opportunities for discussion as to the choice of crops and the right use of land. The favourite topic is the comparison between the calories obtained from cereal crops and those obtained from livestock. This will introduce the question of first-class protein in the diet, i.e. a protein containing the requisite number and variety of amino acids, as well as mineral salts and vitamins. A topical subject in view of the threat to health from the consumption of tobacco is the use of land for this crop. Already a joint committee of FAO and WHO has discussed the possibility of government subsidies to farmers who convert their tobacco crops into edible crops. The economics of agriculture and food production and distribution are highly relevant to human nutrition, and modern food technology which can provide a balanced diet throughout the whole of the year without seasonal variations is an indispensable need for industrialized societies.

BIOLOGY AND DISEASE

Biology is the science of life, and as the German pathologist Virchow pointed out over a hundred years ago, disease itself is life, i.e. the disease process is a 'vital' one owing to action between parasite and host cell, as in the case of infections and infestation, or between the cell and a chemical hazard, or the degeneration that follows from disuse or misuse of organs and structures. [1] This introduces the total field of human ecology which includes other living forms whose survival depends upon man as a host. The study of bacteria comes naturally into the study of biology, but all bacteria are not harmful, some in fact are useful and necessary, like those in the intestine which play a part in the synthesis of vitamins. The study of enzymes provides some clues to the action of certain drugs, particularly the drugs of addiction, like heroin, which appear to enter into the enzymic activity of the brain as substitutes.

THE CANCERS

It is suggested by some authorities on health education that the school is a suitable place for an understanding of the nature of cancer. There are in fact many types of cancer — it is better to refer to 'the cancers' and to avoid the unnecessary emotive effect of discussion of these diseases which account for far fewer deaths during a year than does heart disease. There is an increasing knowledge of the causation of various cancers in different sites of the body. Some of this knowledge is directly applicable to personal life. One can cite, for example, the relationship between poor personal hygiene and the occurrence of cancer of the cervix of the uterus. This association was discovered by epidemiological techniques as long ago as 1955, was reconfirmed in several countries since then, and in 1969 was found to have an infectious basis when it was discovered that herpes virus could be transmitted by sexual contact.

In industry, cancers caused by prolonged contact with carcinogenic substances have been prevented by enclosing the process or by providing the workers with protective clothing and masks. The question of smoking and lung cancer is now widely known and a study of the chemistry of tobacco and the products of combustion give some clues for speculation at least on the possible carcinogenic substance.

The changes occurring in individual cells which lead to malignant growths are interesting and are likely to be studied and understood by boys and girls in the secondary school entirely divorced from the emotion which this matter raises in the adult mind. The emotive effect these diseases have is due to a lack of biological commonsense in the present adult generation. New growth affects every living organism in the universe, even fungi, and it has been observed in every era, even in fossilized remains.

Physical Education

Physical education provides opportunities for a study of exercise physiology, the function of the nervous-system, and the skilful use of muscle groups so that unnecessary strain is not placed on any part of the skeleton, fatigue is minimized, and later in life degenerative diseases such as arthritis will be prevented. The development of sports medicine provides the teacher of physical education with many exciting and fascinating topics to discuss with the pupils.

There is for example the problem of adaptation to high altitudes which had to be faced by the medical officers and trainers of the Olympic teams at the Mexican Olympics in 1968. The use of electronic radio telemetering in-training swimmers is an attractive introduction to the understanding of the physiology of the heart and circulation. The fact that we all of us possess 'venous pumps', which have already been referred to, should be learned in the school gymnasium.

PRESERVING HEALTH BY PHYSICAL SKILLS

The prevention of accidents in the home and at work will be advanced by a better understanding of the importance of physical skills. Common faults in lifting heavy weights, for example, are to lift them with the knees straight, which imposes a severe strain on the relatively weak muscles of the spine. The thigh muscles are the strongest in the body, and can therefore bear most weight so that weights should be lifted with the knees bent. Attempting to lift very heavy weights above the level of the shoulders is often a cause of accidents, and muscle fatigue, which sets in very quickly when muscles are cramped and cannot obtain an adequate oxygen supply, causes a falling off of skilful performance as well as increasing the risk of accidents.

Ergonomics, which is applied in modern industry, also has a domestic application, and should be understood thoroughly by girls and boys before they enter adult life. Here is another example of the inequality between the sexes as regards educational opportunity. Because most boys are being trained for an industrial occupation, they have a greater opportunity of learning the skilful and safe use of muscle groups. Girls on the other hand will not have this advantage, and may not even take craft lessons at school, and when they are running their own homes, they are extremely vulnerable to accidents due to lack of wisdom in lifting or climbing.

MOVEMENT AND PERSONALITY

The teacher of physical education can also make a contribution to the understanding of personality as expressed by bodily movement. There is a need for a new perception of our body image. The study of the skeleton as a dead and static thing is of little help, and a great advance could be made if it were possible to study cinema X-ray films. It is not sufficiently appreciated how beautifully adapted the human body is for a social role and for the various skills it is required to undertake. These vary from the hewing of stone and coal to the manufacture of watches and micro-electronics and the creative tasks involved in the arts and music. None of these could be performed on all fours, and in addition, the quality of human life is enhanced by face-to-face confrontation.

The human body can be considered in a series of segments which are mobile and flexible but which can be locked together in groups or as a whole for the purpose of stability. The segments are the head and neck, the torso, the lower limbs from hips to knees, then from knees to ankles, and finally the feet, which are themselves segmented.

THE SEGMENTED BASIS OF POSTURE

A series of curves produce the characteristic silhouette of the human body. This is distorted by faulty posture and slack muscles. The key to posture lies in the head and neck and in the buttocks. Holding the head high results in the other segments falling into line, while a good tone of the buttock muscles ('tucking in the tail') will tilt the pelvis back and will produce that slight external rotation of the knees which is necessary for the proper shape of the feet.

The problem of flat feet therefore starts in the hips which control external rotation. The feet are segmented in such a way that they can either be completely mobile, or alternatively, each is converted into a half-dome by the raising of the inner arch. Two half-domes placed together form a rigid firm platform which can bear the whole weight of the body and also take the weights which are carried. The teaching of foot health starts by the teaching of posture, and a foot which cannot be freely flexible and at the same time maintain its inner arch and the arch beneath the heads of the metatarsal bones will suffer from the pressure of foot-gear and the general wear and tear of walking and standing. At the same time, shoes which do not allow mobility of the feet, and particularly the exercise of the small intrinsic muscles which maintain the arches, or which cause unnecessary strain, like the casual shoe which can only be kept on the foot by contraction of the great toes and the 'high platform' shoe, will lead to a variety of foot defects.

FOOT HEALTH AND HYGIENE

Foot health is an aspect of personal hygiene which comes within the purview of the teacher of physical education. The need for cleanliness, the prevention of ringworm infection, and verrucae, the importance of cleanliness before entering a swimming-bath, of the taking of showers after exercise, and the regular washing of clothing which is used in P.E. can all be emphasized. The general hygiene in the gymnasium and the swimming-pool, or indeed of the playing-field, provide practical examples of health education. The teaching of first aid could also come within the P.E. curriculum.

The teacher of P.E. can also co-operate with his colleague, the teacher of biology, in discussing examples on nutrition and athletic performance. An opportunity can be taken of topical events, such as the major international or national games and the news items which are eagerly read on the general life-styles and habits of individual stars. One might say in summary that physical education in its modern form can make a substantial contribution to health education. The snide remark about 'talks on anatomy on wet afternoons' when play outside is impossible should be forgotten.

English Literature

THE SOCIAL ROLE OF AUTHORS

It has often been suggested that English literature provides an opportunity for incidental health education. This has been very superficial, however, referring merely to the reading of fiction or drama in which some of the characters suffer from tuberculosis, an almost inevitable event in the nineteenth century, or are handicapped in one way or another. The idea that the teacher should then break off the lesson and discuss the particular disease is jejune. Such an approach ignores the social role of the writer and playwright which is to interpret life as he has experienced it, and to help the reader to an understanding of human relations, motivation, and behaviour. English literature therefore has its major contribution to health education in the field of mental health. It is not insignificant that Wordsworth himself referred to 'mental physiology' as a basis for some of his major works.

LITERATURE AND MENTAL HEALTH EDUCATION

The contribution of English literature to mental health education depends upon a premium being placed upon those authors and playwrights who are most skilful at depicting human relationships, particularly relationships between the sexes and the tensions and conflict which arise from competition. The modern book, *Games People Play*, which is a brilliant exposition on devious human behaviour, has collected together and has classified the various manoeuvres that people undertake in order to give one impression while intending something quite different. [2]

Prejudice against authors on grounds of class bias or permissiveness must not be allowed to conceal the value they have from the point of view of an understanding of human behaviour. Somerset Maugham, for example, is excellent in this respect. Shakespeare is frequently cited as providing such opportunities, and they certainly seem to be concentrated in one play, *Hamlet*, which anticipates the Rorschach personality test in the soliloquy regarding the cloud, as well as role-playing with a view to stimulating insight into motivation. We should not ignore the English translations of foreign literature, in particular the plays of Ibsen and Strindberg and the short stories and novels of Chekov. Cohen points out that Balzac antedated Freud by fifty years by drawing attention to man's internal organization. [3] In some ways, nineteenth century society in Continental Europe appears to have been in advance of English society and the women depicted are much freer of speech and behaviour than their contemporaries in English literature. Poetry too has a great value, and we have already mentioned Wordsworth who had an idea of his own work as an explanation of emotional processes and human behaviour, and in our own day, T. S. Elliot, ranks very high in this respect.

One of the purposes of mental health education is to secure identification with various models. This does not mean that the models are necessarily good or bad, but they do represent the vagaries of human behaviour. An adolescent boy or girl could easily identify with characters in fiction and drama, and a discussion of this identification would assist to achieving an insight into motivation. Drama has a particular value in this respect, but a word of caution is necessary here. In selecting pupils to play various parts, the teacher should have regard to the emotional stability and adjustment of the pupil concerned, and should consider whether the identification which will occur as a result of playing a role may be disturbing. However, this does introduce the technique of role-playing which, as will be explained later, is a very valuable one in mental health education.

Mathematics

We have seen how mathematical techniques are applied to epidemiological studies and to interpretation of the results. This is probably the clearest possible demonstration that mathematics is concerned with events, associations and tests of significance. All the usual mathematical procedures and calculations can be used in exercises designed also to show how indices of health and disease in a community can be recorded, measured, and analysed.

STUDYING FREQUENCY DISTRIBUTIONS

For example, frequency distributions can be studied both by tabulation and then translation of the tables into histograms or curves. The normal curve which is drawn as a result of the plotting of the frequency of the distribution of characteristics like height, weight, blood-pressure etc. reinforces the teaching of the variation of the human race in the biology syllabus. There are also many examples of where observations can be analysed by contrasting what was expected, and what was observed. This will offer the pupil a direct confrontation with the need for caution in drawing conclusions from a series of observations. The fact that biology and its applied aspects are not exact sciences has not yet been grasped by the population at large and yet this is a basic lesson to be learned before an informed judgment can be made on contemporary events.

DEMOGRAPHIC STUDIES
Mathematics can also be used for the study of population problems, population distribution and general demography. The technique of clustering can be used, either by spot diagrams, or by the use of spot maps. For example, it can be shown in which areas of a town places of infectious disease occur. This is a practical technique which has been used frequently by medical officers of health in order to identify particularly vulnerable areas of their boroughs. In the days when tuberculosis was a common problem, for example, it was possible to isolate certain wards of a borough by showing how the incidence of tuberculin-positive skin tests clustered in these districts, leaving others relatively free.

EVALUATION OF MEDICAL TREATMENT
In order that pupils may be able to form mature judgments on new medical discoveries, simple exercises showing the effect of treatment on various conditions can also be used, applying mathematical tests of significance. This is the modern way of testing new drugs, so that it can be assured that it is the drug itself having an effect, and not other factors. Pupils taking advance courses in mathematics can also study multivariate analysis which is directly applicable to the evaluation of health education procedures where so many factors may have an effect upon the result.

There is ample material for the teacher of mathematics to use for such exercises. The annual reports of the Chief Medical Officer, Department of Health and Social Security, as well as the frequent reports from the Office of Population Censuses and Surveys, provide tabulated material which can be made more sophisticated in various ways turning it into graphs, histograms, 'pie' charts etc. It is possible also to use this material for individual calculations of significance and for the identification of priorities in public health problems. The use of this material would also enlarge the pupil's horizons in that he would be aware later on as adult that there is a continual medical and social and demographic audit of his country and that the results are available to the public and can be consulted at any time.

General Science

INTELLECTUAL CONTRIBUTIONS BY PIONEERS
The history of science has a contribution to the health education curriculum, provided that it is not confined to biographical detail

which is traditionally the case. The lives of individual pioneers and discoverers should be shown as meaningful in terms of steps taken towards the present highly technological systems of health care. The obvious examples are the discovery of the microscope and the observation of living forms by van Leeuwenhoek; the discovery of the cell by Schwann; the development of organic chemistry by Liebig; the discovery of the relationship of bacteria to infection by Pasteur, who also laid the basis for immunization, and the application of this knowledge to surgery by Lister who invented antiseptics, later of course to give place to aseptic surgery.

There are two other pioneers of fundamental medical science whose lives and work are little known, outside the medical profession. These are Claude Bernard who discovered the principle of homeostasis, and Rudolph Virchow who founded the science of pathology by study of the microscopical events taking place in the individual cell. It was Virchow who was first to identify the point of no return when a physiological change in a cell became a structural and organic change, resulting in death of the cell, and perhaps death of the entire organism.

Another figure little known outside the field of medicine was Frascator of Verona who concluded from his clinical observations that disease was caused by small particles passing from the sick to the healthy. As this observation and conclusion were made long before the discovery of bacteria, it was a feat of genius. Frascator also wrote a poem entitled *Syphilis*, a romantic story of a Sicilian shepherd who thereby bequeathed his own name to a notorious disease! Syphilis in Frascator's time was known as the 'Morbus Gallicus'. A teacher could stimulate a very lively discussion on this contribution by Frascator alone, including the claim that syphilis was a 'French disease'.

PHYSICS AND HEALTH

Environmental control is a matter of technology which is based mainly on physics and chemistry. The teaching of physics offers an opportunity of the understanding of the way in which the cooling power of the air is controlled and measured. The wet and dry bulb thermometer for example, used traditionally to measure the relative humidity of the air, is used practically in the form of the whirling hygrometer that is used in factories and mines and other places where it is necessary to control the humidity. The relevance to health lies in the fact that when humidity is too low there is a sense of discomfort and the nasal mucus membranes are irritated and colds and respiratory disease are more frequent. When the humidity is too high, the air is saturated with water vapour and cannot absorb the sweat which should be evaporated from the skin. Another factor in the cooling power of the air is air movement and a number

of experiments can be conducted in the classroom at the cost of
minor discomfort to the pupils to reinforce these points regarding
ventilation.

VISION AND THE ENVIRONMENT
The study of light also has always included an elementary knowledge of the physics of the eye. Unfortunately this is presented in so
static a form that the eye is regarded merely as a refracting device.
The correction of this view has been supplied by H. C. Weston's
beautifully turned phrase, 'the eyes are a pair of fenestrated orbs,
housing a crowd of receptors, turning this way and that, seeking the
stuff of vision'. [4] We do in fact have to work hard to see, and we
have to deliberately look for something to see. The voluntary
muscles controlling the movements of the eyes which move in
parallel and are reciprocally innervated can undergo fatigue as a
result of adverse conditions for seeing. This includes illumination
which can be measured precisely in lumens per square foot, and
different levels are prescribed for different visual tasks.

THE VISUAL TASK
Visual tasks can be analysed according to whether they require near
or distant vision, the observation of moving objects, or doing work
on materials with poor coloured contrast, for example, sewing black
cotton on to dark cloth. The physiology of vision involves the
posture, and the posture of the head and neck and the angle
subtended between the eye and the object to be seen are matters of
personal hygiene. The avoidance of glare from shiny surfaces and
the difference between critical and casual vision are all matters that
can be studied in the physics class. The use of lighting to maintain
optimum conditions for seeing with the minimum of eye strain, at
the same time producing a pleasing effect, and the use of colour, are
matters largely neglected in the domestic scene, although they are
taken note of in industry.
    (The study of heat will be linked with the study of ventilation
referred to above.)

SOUND AND HEARING
The study of sound involves the physiology of the ear but also that
of the part of the brain receiving nerve impulses from the inner ear
so that they are built into a pattern and analysed. The communication between the throat and the ear by the Eustachian tube is
equally important from the point of view of prevention of infection – this has already been mentioned in the case of the infants'
school child. There are pressure effects which result from a train
entering a tunnel, or an aircraft taking off or landing. The act of
swallowing to equalize the pressure is now familiar to most people,

now that air travel is so common, and in the early days, boiled sweets were handed out in order to stimulate swallowing.

Noise abatement is a contemporary problem of environmental control, and pupils can learn how to measure noise levels using the decibel scale. Audiometry, whereby hearing can be tested accurately in different frequency bands, is carried out by the school health service, and the school medical officer can be asked to co-operate in making apparatus available so that this can be studied in the physics class.

CHEMISTRY AND POLLUTION

In the measurement of pollution and its control, the methods and the instruments involved are those derived from physics and chemistry, and there are innumerable opportunities for studying these problems practically by visits to waterworks, sewage works, factories, and other places where measurements of this kind are required as a routine.

The science of chemistry is basic to an understanding of bio-chemistry, or the chemical events occurring in the body, as well as to the development of modern drugs. It is also important from the point of view of food analysis for monitoring of basic food values in foodstuffs, and the prevention of pollution in the atmosphere. In using these topics for study, the basic lessons of chemistry can be applied. The chemistry of tobacco tar is a topical study.

Art

We have already referred to the importance of aesthetics in considering human biology. The teaching of arts, including both the practice of artistic techniques as well as the appreciation of works of art, should provide many opportunities for the study of the external form of the human body and its functions, of posture and of appreciation of aesthetics. All the classical models of painting and sculpture provide perfect examples of surface anatomy and it may also be impressive for pupils to realize that the human body observed for example by Leonardo da Vinci is identical to the one that they can observe today, even though the modern artist of course has deserted the conventional representation of contours.

THE CATHARTIC VALUE OF ART

In the stage of sexual development where curiosity is giving place to sexual fantasy, there may be a case for deliberately allowing this fantasy to be expressed in practical art. All children make drawings with a sexual content. It has been conventional to confiscate these and to administer punishment. Children then produce their drawings on walls and public lavatories and other secret places causing defacement of public property which is so often deplored. It is possible however that they are expressing a felt need, and that under mature guidance, the art class may be a suitable medium for this natural expression of fantasy which is cathartic in character.

The clandestine nature of such expression is probably the most harmful aspect as it causes tension and unnecessary excitement. If such expression is accepted however as a normal process, and if it is given adequate guidance and criticism, then it may well contribute to mental healthiness as regards sexual instincts. It is already a common practice to use the drawings and paintings of small children as diagnostic material. Perhaps only timidity and fear of being thought too *avant garde*, or of releasing forces which could not be controlled, have prevented people from applying the same interpretations to the pictorial fantasies of older children and young adolescents. On a practical plane children can also design posters.

Home Economics

The contribution of domestic science to health education is traditional but in the present form of teaching of home economics a much wider scope presents itself in the field of the teaching of nutrition, including budgeting, in accident prevention in the home, and in the control of the home environment to produce the maximum of comfort and safety.

NUTRITION EDUCATION

The teacher of home economics can present the facts of a balanced diet containing food groups, protective substances and mineral salts in terms of dishes which are familiar to the pupils. In view of the rising costs of food, it is important that the cheapest ways of obtaining the necessary nutrients should be demonstrated and also how further economy can be effected by careful storage, preparation, and cooking.

The tendency to use foods of convenience, which has been encouraged by the increasing numbers of married women who work outside the home, brings with it an additional responsibility for the care of such foods and for their proper handling in accordance with the instructions on the wrapper before being presented for consumption. The dangers of food spoilage now include the possibility of the ingestion of toxic substances, for example, potatoes affected by blight are now suspected as being responsible for developmental abnormalities when they are consumed by pregnant women. The spoiling of foods by fungus also may be responsible for the production of allergies including asthma.

FOOD HYGIENE

Food hygiene is a proper topic to be included under the heading of home economics and here there is an overlap with the biology syllabus which should have prepared pupils for an understanding of the nature of bacteria, the way in which they multiply and the conditions they need for survival. The general principles of the prevention of food poisoning are the prevention of contamination of food at source, during distribution and storage, followed by thorough cooking so that any bacteria that may be present are destroyed by heat. The subtle relationship between time and temperature must be understood in order to deny the bacteria the opportunities for multiplication.

Thus, ideally, food that has been cooked at a high temperature should be eaten at once. If some of it is to be stored for consumption later on, then it must be cooled as rapidly as possible and preferably stored at a low temperature in a refrigerator. Sources of contamination of food from human beings include intestinal infection conveyed by the hands where people have been careless after defecation, and have not washed their hands, and from the skin, in particular, the skin lining the nostrils. Seventy-five percent of the population are carriers of the staphylococcus in the nose, which if it gains entrance to food can produce a toxin which is heat resistant and which will cause one form of food poisoning.

CARE OF CLOTHES AND FABRICS

There are many lessons in domestic hygiene which can be included under the heading of home economics. Care of clothes and of fabrics and their correct laundering requires some knowledge, judgment, and skill,, and with the widespread use of detergents, some care is necessary in the use of the latter as they tend to cause dermatitis or other allergies in susceptible people. The reasons why fabrics undergo discoloration when in contact with the skin must be explained frankly, as contamination of undergarments from urine, faeces or discharges can not only be unpleasant for the wearer, but also can be a source of infection for other people in the household. Experiments have been conducted on volunteers, half of whom have had a bath and have worn clean underclothing, and the other half have worn clothing for a considerable time and have omitted to take a bath. Ordinary movements in the two groups have been observed, and it has been found that in the second group there is a widespread distribution of bacteria from the clothing to the surrounding atmosphere. Because there is a continuous movement of a current of warm air over the front surface of the body, there is a tendency for bacteria to be distributed from the nose to the region around the anus. All attempts at personal hygiene are obviously futile unless clean underclothing is worn regularly.

Teachers of home economics will prepare their own syllabuses which can include these and many other points that are relevant to health education. They will be assisting in inculcating healthy attitudes which will have a carry over value into adult life, and in this respect, it will be important for boys to enjoy this part of the school curriculum, as well as girls. Experienced teachers of home economics have remarked on the congenial atmosphere which develops among small groups — not more than twenty pupils — who are pursuing home economics. Such a situation is conducive to dicussions in a homely atmosphere. For some years now in the upper social groups, men have been accustomed to do their own personal laundry which has been made possible by the introduction of drip-dry fabrics. This practice is not so common in the lower social groups where the whole burden for personal laundry falls upon a mother who is already very hard pressed and usually working outside the home as well. The ideal would be for all people from puberty onwards to be able to cope with their own personal washing, so that they can achieve a high standard of personal hygiene, without imposing a burden upon their mothers or wives. It should be a personal code of practice that dirty underlinen is never worn a second time, although it appears from surveys in industry that faecal contamination of underlinen is a frequently observed event.

History

It is true that history contains many interesting references to plagues and large-scale epidemics, as well as to individual maladies suffered by monarchs and statesmen. This however is history from an antiquarian point of view. It is less important that Napoleon is said to have lost battles through having cancer of the stomach than that he shrewdly observed that nutrition is the source of energy and stamina for an army — the famous 'army marching on its stomach' aphorism.

THE NINETEENTH CENTURY

From the point of view of the understanding of modern health and social services, the social history of the nineteenth century is easily the most important source of study. There is a substantial body of literature providing information on this subject. The history of the factory acts and the amelioration of severe working conditions is fairly well known, but the history of sanitary reform is probably less well known. Even this branch of history sometimes mentions princes. For example, the Prince of Wales, later Edward VII, was a member of a Royal Commission on Housing in 1884 and signed its report. Housing commissions, the organization of local government to take responsibility for sewage-disposal and the control of epidemics, and the growth of voluntary societies to relieve poverty and sickness and to provide medical care for the needy, are all part of the nineteenth century scene. Study of these events shows that clearly they are linked with measures such as the reform bills and the factory acts.

Geography

The study of geography can include observations of the way in which infectious diseases pass from continent to continent along the various routes of travel. Smallpox, for example, can travel very rapidly from countries of endemic origin, such as India, to Europe as a result of air travel, and since the Second World War, it has been imported into the United Kingdom numerous times in this way. Cholera too has made its reappearance in Europe as a result of air travel.

DEMOGRAPHIC GEOGRAPHY
The study of geography in its physical, economic, political, and social aspects offers an opportunity of understanding the ways in which civilization has organized its affairs to protect health. The traditional medical officer of health was often a geographer in his own right as evidenced by the kind of annual report which used to be written. It was a statutory requirement to give a review of the sanitary circumstances of the borough, and in this review many medical officers of health would describe centres of population, lines of communication, industry, water supply, and climatic conditions, in addition to the demographic details involved in an audit of the community's health.

There are many opportunities in the study of world geography to apply the same principles. For example, there are parts of the world where the background natural radio-activity is extremely high; this includes even Aberdeen in the United Kingdom, as well as a desert in India. Climatic conditions prevented many regions of the world from being populated until techniques could be invented to overcome the effects of climate.

An interesting comparison can be made between Lancashire and India. The cotton spinning industry was established in Lancashire in the nineteenth century and depended on the natural humidity of the air to prevent the breaking of the woven threads. The high humidity, coupled with the severe industrial conditions of the day, contributed very largely to a high level of respiratory illness, including tuberculosis. When India started to spin its own cotton, the health hazards of the workers there were concerned mainly with heat exhaustion, aggravated by the high humidity which prevented the evaporation of sweat and diminished the cooling power of the air. The pursuit of geography will find many examples where altitude or climate or natural barriers such as mountain ranges have created living conditions which have an effect upon health. A classical example is the endemic goitre found in Switzerland and formerly in parts of Derbyshire due to a lack of iodine in the drinking water.

WATER SUPPLIES

The provision of an abundant clean water supply is a problem in which geographical features dominate. Study of the world's water resources reveals that there are many parts of the world where the supply of water is less than adequate for basic needs. The question of whether water could be obtained from desert areas by the use of atomic energy for deep bores is one which should excite the imagination. Water supply is also bound up with the question of afforestation and soil erosion. The colonization of virgin lands will often depend upon a successful solution of this problem.

ECONOMIC GEOGRAPHY

The problem of protein lack in many developing countries, particularly in the African countries, raises the question of economic agricultural geography. Even the question of smoking and health can be tackled from the point of view of whether it is economic and socially desirable to devote so many acres for the cultivation of tobacco and whether these lands could be diversified. These can be studied as part of a geography syllabus. The use of organic fertilizers, of pesticides, particularly D.D.T., and the possible toxicity resulting to man and animals, are also problems of developing countries where the use of such chemicals has been an attractive proposition in view of the high rate of depredation of crops by pests of all kinds. Desalination of sea water or other brackish water supplies is now a technical possibility and there are several areas of the world where this is being carried out.

As regards the geography of the United Kingdom, social geography plotting the migration of populations from the former industrial areas to the south-east and the original reasons for the siting of industry are all questions having a bearing upon the community health. Reports of medical officers of health of up to a century ago are usually filed in most public libraries and pupils will find particular interest in studying these reports of their own areas.

Religious Instruction

All the great world religions have advice to offer on health, both from the point of view of environmental control, and also personal hygiene. In addition, they all have some guidance on the question of human relations. In the case of the Christian religion, a good deal of what is studied under the heading of religious instruction is of course the history of Israel and of the Middle East and much of it reflects the Graeco-Roman-Judaic culture which Europe has inherited. There is a tendency for the Christian religion also to be confused or identified with social issues, but in modern times these will usually be considered under the heading of liberal studies or social studies.

RELIGION AND MENTAL HEALTH
The Christian faith has most guidance to offer in the field of mental health, because the philosophy of Jesus respecting the laws which govern inter-personal relationships have been confirmed by psychiatrists and social psychologists and even, it may be said, by sociologists in recent times. The Christian faith therefore offers direct guidance on respect for personality and the way in which people should behave to each other, based on principles of what is now recognized as psycho-dynamics. The teacher of religious instruction therefore need not think that it is necessary to concentrate on those books of the Old Testament which set out the Mosaic law as applied to the prevention of the spread of illness. That this is of interest is undisputed, but a more practical value in modern times is a study of the nature of man himself as envisaged in the Christian faith.

There are three main aspects. Christians believe that man was created in the image of God which therefore places a degree of expectation on his behaviour. Secondly, they believe that he is inherently sinful. For many this is unacceptable but all recognize that we are capable of evil, as of good. In all personalities, the two capacities co-exist. Thirdly, man is endowed with free will. Perhaps the most succinct guide to emotional maturity can be found in the Sermon on the Mount and an interesting discussion could be conducted on the meaning in modern terms of 'meek and poor in spirit'.

Buddhism and Islam, as well as Hinduism, all have a separate contribution to health education. In all of them, the basic hygienic principles are conveyed in the context of religious law and in their precepts of personal hygiene, all demand daily baths, clean clothes, and brushing of the teeth. Buddhism even proscribes dry sweeping, and we know today that this prevents the dispersion of dust containing organisms, yeasts, and moulds which cause respiratory illness. Carcinoma of the cervix of the uterus is unknown in Jewish women who practice rituals designed to preserve cleanliness before and after sexual intercourse. Circumcision practised amongst Jews and Moslems offers an additional protection to the women against the contraction of carcinoma of the cervix. [5]

Hinduism attaches the greatest importance to family life, and in orthodox Hindu families small girls aged seven to twelve learn parental duties like growing seeds, watching them germinate, and undergoing some small personal sacrifice during the process. Yoga is also a branch of the Hindu faith, and when the practice of yoga is analysed according to anatomical and physiological principles, it would appear that it has a great value in inducing muscular relaxation and at the same time speeding up the venous return from the limbs.

In many schools in the United Kingdom today, teachers will be confronted by a class containing children who belong to all of these faiths. They will therefore be well experienced in teaching their subject without causing misunderstanding or giving offence. The health education element need not be isolated because if the subject is taught according to its basic principles the implication for a code of human behaviour should be obvious.

Social Studies

LIBERAL AND SOCIAL STUDIES

It has been remarked earlier that teachers of social or liberal studies have often been responsible for the planning of health education programmes in a school. This subject has a special contribution to make, particularly now that the behavioural sciences have developed as a part of general sociology. The studies of the social services at the present day, often reinforced by the older pupils undertaking voluntary social work, such as helping care for old people, offer an important contribution to health education.

PROBLEMS OF LEISURE

There are however more sophisticated studies that could be pursued. Population and demography, migration and the level of technical and social services required in a modern community are all related to the general idea of the community's responsibility for health. The use of resources for leisure and recreation, the balance between urban and rural communities, and the impact on communities of discoveries such as oil in the North Sea or North Sea gas are all important. With the increasing availability of leisure, there is the equal difficulty of making a purposeful use of that leisure, particularly in areas which are deprived of natural resources.

MEETING POINT OF RELIGION AND SOCIOLOGY

Social studies can be a meeting point also of geography and religious instruction, when we consider the problem of population. Catholic and Marxist thinkers share the opinion that Malthus was wrong in his prognostication that the growth of population would outgrow the supplies of food and other resources. It has been suggested that such a doctrine would merely serve to prevent the development of world resources for human benefit, and exponents of family planning are frequently described as neo-Malthusians.

It is nevertheless apparent that in the time-interval between resources being thoroughly developed, for example, the development of protein supplies mentioned above, a good deal of suffering will occur. In modern industrialized communities, such as those of the E.E.C., the expectations for amenities and resources for each individual are very high and over-population puts a considerable strain upon them. It may be seen even in the question of medical services at the present time, certainly in the United States of America, where large sections of the population who have not the means to contribute to voluntary insurance schemes are frequently deprived of medical care altogether.

A debate on what is the right approach to population control and resource development necessarily involves value-judgments and a teacher of religious instruction would be expected to make a contribution on what is the nature of man, a subject which also concerns a teacher of social studies. In other words is it a good thing in itself to produce as many human beings as possible and then find resources to meet them, or is it better to have fewer human beings who can enjoy a higher standard of living? How far does selfishness or greed come into this, and are there other motivations for producing children, other than raising a future generation to shoulder the burdens of the present one? Such a question would require the background of geography, religious instruction, and social studies for an adequate discussion.

Craft

The expression of creative instincts and the development of personal skills involved in a craft are undeniably beneficial to emotional well-being and mental health. From this point of view instruction in a craft gives every boy and girl something which will be useful to them in adult life, in home-making for example, but it will also give them a physical skill which will contribute to their personality and sense of prestige.

The teaching of craft also involves the teaching of safety precautions, the kind of accident prevention which does not inhibit action, but which places a high premium upon personal skill. Thus the care of tools, the prevention of fire in a workshop, the prevention of accidents when handling machine tools — this applies particularly to the care of the eyes — all give the child an extension of domestic experience which is necessary for accident prevention.

Engineering has now made a substantial contribution to medical care and teachers of craft could ensure that their pupils have information regarding the design of equipment to help the handicapped, and the engineering principles which are put into use here. Apart from the technical interest in such matters, there should be a carry-over into the human interest in the handicapped themselves, and a sense of the community spirit which is required to help them.

It is in these main subjects outlined above that the contribution to the health education curriculum comes. This used to be called incidental, but it has been seen that all these subjects make a contribution in their own right, and it is not necessary to create a diversion from the main topic in order to point the way to the application of this knowledge to the promotion of health and the prevention of disease. It should be possible for the child when confronted with every subject he meets in school to realize that the factors relating to health and disease are indivisible, and how medical-care systems play only a relatively small part compared with industrial, economic, and social development, when this is carried out with biological commonsense.

QUESTIONS

1. If it were not possible to have health education lessons, how would you propose that health education be done in a school?
2. In what ways may useful information in the report of the Chief Medical Officer of the Department of Education and Science, or any other reports, be used in the teaching of health education?
3. In the majority of mixed secondary schools girls have greater opportunities than boys to learn about the practice of healthy living. How do you account for this and how would you overcome the problem in planning a scheme?
4. How would you seek the co-operation of a variety of subjects to teach each of the following topics:-
   a) Nutriton b) Pollution c) Personal Relationships d) Personal Responsibility e) Dental Health?
5. What precautions are necessary in the use of drama? Make a list of authors, playwrights, and poets, who, in your opinion, offer most guidance on human personality and relationships.
6. Plan an experiment designed to demonstrate the importance of warmth, ventilation, and humidity in the classroom.

REFERENCES

1. Virchow, R. (1858). *Cellular Pathology*. Berlin.
2. Berne, E. (1968). *Games People Play*. Harmondsworth: Penguin.
3. Cohen, J. (1970). 'Comments on Literature and Mental Health'. Chapter 4 in *Homo Psychologicus*. London: Allen and Unwin.
4. Weston, H. C. (1949). *Sight, Light, and Efficiency*. London: H. K. Lewis.
5. Wynder, E. L. (1955). 'Environmental Factors in Cervical Cancer'. *Brit. Med. J.* 1: 734.

FURTHER READING

Human Biology
Brierley, J. (1967). *Biology and the Social Crisis*. London: Heinemann.
Brierley, J. (1970). *Natural History of Man*. London: Heinemann.

Brierley, J. (1973). *The Thinking Machine*. London: Heinemann.
Brimble, L. J. F. (Part 1, 1958; Part 2, 1966). *Physiology, Anatomy and Health*. London: MacMillan.
Oria, M. and Raffin, J. (1968). *Studies in Human Biology*. London: Blandford.
Oria, M. and Raffin, J. (1968). *Social Biology and Hygiene*. London: Blandford.
Family Doctor Series. (1962). *How Not to Kill Your Husband*. London: Allen and Unwin.
Family Doctor Series. (1965). *How Not to Kill Your Wife*. London: Allen and Unwin.
Family Doctor Series. (1968). *How Not to Kill Your Children*. London: Allen and Unwin.

Books for pupils

Probert, A. J. (1973). *Parasites*. (Biology Topics). Harmondsworth: Penguin Educational.
Rutherford, Margaret (1969). *Man with Two Environments*. London: Longmans.
Stoneman, C. F. (1973). *Space Biology*. (Biology Topics). Harmondsworth: Penguin Educational.

For Age-groups 6–12
Health and Growth: Six volumes, graduated for ages 6 to 12. A comprehensive account of biological and social factors concerned with human health. Includes material on mental health. Originally USA, obtainable from the publisher: Scott Foresman Company, 32 West St, Brighton BN1 2RT.

Nutrition

Basic Nutrition (Four teaching programmes). (1970). Oxford: Pergamon Press.
Gawthorpe, Lilian M. (1966). *Food and Nutrition*. Amersham, Buckinghamshire: Hulton Educational.
Reinsh, Ernest (1971). *Diet You can Live with*. London: Angus and Robertson.
Wells, Dilys (1970). *Eating to Live*. London: Times Newspapers.

Ecology

Arvill, Robert (1969). *Man and Environment*. Harmondsworth: Penguin.
Bugler, J. (1972). *Polluting Britain: A Survey*. London: Pelican Books.
Ehrlich, Paul R. and Ehrlich, Anne H. (1970). *Population, Resources, Environment: Issues in Ecology*. Reading: W. H. Freeman.
Lawreys, Alec (1969). *Man and his Environment*. London: Aldus Books.
Perry, G. A. (1970). *Approaches to Environmental Studies*. London: Blandford.
Report of the Royal Commission on Environmental Pollution. (1971). London: HMSO.

Sex Education

Bevan, James (1970). *Sex — The Plain Facts*. London: Faber and Faber.
Corner, George W. (1953). *Attaining Manhood*. London: Allen and Unwin.
Gosblow, J. (1970). *Science and Your Body*. London: Blond Educational.

Hummel, Ruth S. (1967). *Wonderfully Made*. St Louis: Concordia Publishing House.

Kind, A., Kind, R. W. and Leedham J. (1969). *Sex and Your Responsibility*. (Five programmes). London: Longmans.

Schofield, Michael (1970). *The Sexual Behaviour of Young People*. Harmondsworth: Penguin.

Sharman, A. (1960). *From Girlhood to Womanhood*. Edinburgh: E. and S. Livingstone.

FILMS

Title	Colour B/W	Running time	Distributor	Date
HUMAN BIOLOGY				
(See also Personal Responsibility)				
Your Body during Adolescence	B/W	10 mins.	McGraw Hill	
Then One Year	Colour	20 mins.	N.A.V.A.L. and Concord	1971
Human Reproduction	B/W	20 mins.	Concord	1966
Homosexuals	B/W	25 mins.	Concord	1966
The Important Thing is Love	B/W	50 mins.	Concord	1971
The Nervous System	Colour	18 mins.	Gateway	1968
Blood and Circulation	Colour	10 mins.	Guild Sound & Vision Ltd.	
Breathing and Respiration	Colour	10 mins.	Guild Sound & Vision Ltd.	
Digestion and the Food We Eat	Colour	10 mins.	Guild Sound & Vision Ltd.	
External Respiration	Colour	14 mins.	Rank Film Library	
Elimination	B/W	14 mins.	Rank Film Library	
Organization of the Body	B/W	15 mins.	Rank Film Library	
About the Human Body	Colour	15 mins.	Gateway Film Library	
Senses of Man	Colour	18 mins.	Gateway Film Library	1968
Your Digestion	Colour	12 mins.	Unilever Film Library	
No Toothache for Eskimos	Colour	5 mins.	Unilever Film Library	1952
Tooth in Time	Colour	18 mins.	Unilever Film Library	
Where There's a Will	Colour	28 mins.	Unilever Film Library	1961
Your Mouth	Colour	16 mins.	Unilever Film Library	1969
Out of the Mouths	Colour	25 mins.	Unilever Film Library	1970
Thirty Two of Her Own	Colour	22 mins.	Guild Sound & Vision Ltd.	
Your Food and Teeth	Colour	10 mins.	N.A.V.A.L.	
Your Skin	Colour	16 mins.	Unilever Film Library	
Your Hair and Scalp	Colour	14 mins.	Unilever Film Library	
Your Digestion	Colour	12 mins.	Unilever Film Library	
Your Feet	Colour	15 mins.	Unilever Film Library	1965
Lets Keep Our Teeth	Colour	20 mins.	Unilever Film Library	1952
Nothing to Eat but Food	Colour	18 mins.	Unilever Film Library	1962
Room for Hygiene	Colour	16 mins.	Unilever Film Library	1961

F I L M S (*continued*)

Title	Colour B/W	Running time	Distributor	Date
Insects as Carriers of Disease			Walt Disney Productions Ltd.	
Fly About the House	Colour	9 mins.	Central Film Library	1949
Physics and Chemistry of Water	Colour	20 mins.	Unilever Film Library	1966
Your Teeth			Unilever Education Section	
Dental Care			General Dental Council	
About Your Teeth			Health Education Audio-Visual	
Keep Smiling			General Dental Council	
Blood			M. Ray, 36 Villiers Ave., Surbiton, Surrey	
Circulation			M. Ray	
Digestion			Rank Film Library	
The Human Body			Hulton Educational Publications Ltd.	
Elimination			Rank Film Library	
Nervous System			Rank Film Library	
Sense Organs			Educational Productions Ltd.	
Respiratory Organs			Rank Film Library	
Posture			Common Ground Ltd.	
Teenagers Feet			Camera Talks Ltd.	
Acne & Dandruff			Diana Wyllie Ltd.	
Menstruation			Camera Talks Ltd.	
Premenstrual Syndromes			Camera Talks Ltd.	
Artificial Respiration — Expired Air Method			Royal Life Saving Society	
Respiratory Resuscitation			St. John's Ambulance Association	
Immunity			Camera Talks Ltd.	
Life Saving First Aid:				
1. Not Breathing			Camera Talks Ltd.	
2. Bleeding			Camera Talks Ltd.	
3. Unconscious			Camera Talks Ltd.	
First Aid at Home			Camera Talks Ltd.	
Posture				
How do you sit and stand?	B/W	12 mins.	Rank Film Library or Ed. Foundation for Visual Aids	1968
Foot Health				
The Fives (British) (for girls 8—12)	Colour	7 mins.	Dept. of Audio-Visual Communication, British Medical Association, B.M.A. House, Tavistock Square, London WC1	1970

F I L M S *(continued)*

Title	Colour B/W	Running time	Distributor	Date
Small Bones (for children 8—12; this illustrates the physiology of feet relevant to footwear)	Colour	20 mins.	British Medical Association Film Library at above address	1963
X-Ray Motion Picture of the Foot	Colour		Ealing Scientific Ltd.	
Dental Health				
Oral Hygiene — Your Teeth			Eothen Films International Ltd.	
The Teeth (on the development, structure and care of teeth)	Colour	11 mins.	Rank Film Library	1945
Look After Your Teeth	Colour	13½ mins.	Eothen Films	1967
Tons of Teeth	Colour	15 mins.	Oral Hygiene Service, Hesketh House, Portman Square, London W1	
Growth and Development — Puberty				
Exploring Your Growth (USA; secondary schools only)	Colour	11 mins.	Boulton Hawker Ltd., Hadleigh, Ipswich, Suffolk	1966
Boy to Man (USA)	Colour	16 mins.	Boulton Hawker Ltd.	1962
Girl to Woman (USA)	Colour	18 mins.	Boulton Hawker Ltd.	1962
Ecology				
Environment (Parts 1 and 2)			Diana Wyllie Ltd.	
Water Pollution			Diana Wyllie Ltd.	
To Survive			National Audio Visual Aids Library	
Conservation and Balance in Nature	Colour	18 mins.	Concord	
Population and Pollution	Colour	17 mins.	N.A.V.A.L.	
A Matter of Attitudes	B/W	30 mins.	Concord	1968
Rubbish People	B/W	18 mins.	Concord	1969
NUTRITION				
Fats and Proteins			Common Ground Ltd.	
Food and Health			Common Ground Ltd.	
Good Food for Good Health			Camera Talks Ltd.	
Milk — From Farm to Consumer			Camera Talks Ltd.	

F I L M S (*continued*)

Title	Colour B/W	Running time	Distributor	Date
Nutritional Values			Camera Talks Ltd.	
Food Free from Germs			Camera Talks Ltd.	
Food Infections			Camera Talks Ltd.	
How to Slim and keep Slim			Camera Talks Ltd.	
Elementary Dietetics			Camera Talks Ltd.	
Good Health to You			Camera Talks Ltd.	
Carbohydrates and the Calorie			Common Ground Ltd.	
Our Daily Bread (Brady)	Colour	30 mins.	Concord	1971
Talking about Kitchens	Colour	17 mins.	Unilever Film Library	
Obesity (Psychosomatic Conditions)	B/W	28 mins.	Concord	1961
Foods and Nutrition	B/W	11 mins.	N.A.V.A.L.	1949
Proteins and Health	Colour	27 mins.	Flour Advisory Bureau, 21 Arlington Street, London SW1	1966
Another Case of Food Poisoning	B/W	15 mins.	Central Film Library	1949
Introduction to Nutrition	Colour	10 mins.	Guild Sound & Vision Ltd.	1962

SMOKING

(See also Personal Responsibility)

Title	Colour B/W	Running time	Distributor	Date
Smoking and Health — Report to Youth	Colour	13 mins.	N.A.V.A.L.	1969
Dying for a Smoke	Colour	11 mins.	Central Film Library	1967
The Drag	Colour	9 mins.	Concord	1967
Let's Discuss Smoking	B/W	16 mins.	Concord	1964
Beyond Reasonable Doubt	Colour	25 mins.	British Temperance Society	1964
This is Your Lung	Colour	16 mins.	Tenovus Cancer Information Centre	1963
Time and Two Women	Colour	18 mins.	Cancer Information Centre, Cardiff	1956

SEX EDUCATION

Title	Colour B/W	Running time	Distributor	Date
Phoebe	Colour	40 mins.	Concord	1964
Preparation for Parenthood	B/W	17 mins.	Rank Film Library	
Steps towards Maturity and Health	Colour	10 mins.	Walt Disney Productions	
To Janet — A Son	Colour	50 mins.	Farleys Infant Foods Ltd. 8 Galleymead Road, Colnbrook, Slough, Bucks.	1962

F I L M S *(continued)*

Title	Colour B/W	Running time	Distributor	Date
In Step	Colour	11 mins.	Random Film Library Ltd.	1970
The Confident Ones			Random Film Library Ltd.	
Story of Menstruation	Colour	10 mins.	Walt Disney Productions	1959
Family Planning			Camera Talks Ltd.	
Focus on the Family			N.A.V.A.L.	
Human Reproduction			Common Ground Ltd.	
Sex Education (Parts 1 and 2)			Camera Talks Ltd.	
Birth			Camera Talks Ltd.	
Male Reproductive System			Camera Talks Ltd.	
Female Reproductive System			Camera Talks Ltd.	
Genital Diseases			Camera Talks Ltd.	
Influence of Menstruation			Camera Talks Ltd.	
Sex Education Series			Camera Talks Ltd.	
Anatomy and Physiology Series (2; 4; 10; 15; 16; 17)			Camera Talks Ltd.	
The Endocrine Glands			Camera Talks Ltd.	

VENEREAL DISEASES

Title	Colour B/W	Running time	Distributor	Date
Genital Diseases			Camera Talks Ltd.	
Venereal Diseases			Camera Talks Ltd.	
About VD			Health Education Audio-Visual	
Venereal Diseases			Concordia	
Opportunity Knocks			Kay Film Strips	
How was I to Know			Kay Film Strips	

DRUGS AND ALCOHOL

Title	Colour B/W	Running time	Distributor	Date
The Chemical Tomb	Colour	20 mins.	British Temperance Society	1969
L.S.D. — Insight and Insanity	Colour	20 mins.	British Temperance Society	1968
Narcotics — Pit of Despair	Colour	25 mins.	British Temperance Society	
Drugs and the Nervous System	Colour	18 mins.	N.A.V.A.L.	1967
False Friends	Colour	9 mins.	Guild Sound & Vision Ltd.	
Hooked	B/W	20 mins.	N.A.V.A.L.	1965
Monkey on the Back	B/W	30 mins.	Concord/National Film Board of Canada	1956
New Drugs — Same Needle	B/W	30 mins.	Concord	1969
Some Grains of Truth	B/W	25 mins.	British Film Institute	1967
Alcohol and the Human Body	B/W	11 mins.	Rank Film Library	

F I L M S (*continued*)

Title	Colour B/W	Running time	Distributor	Date
Bottle and Throttle	Colour	12 mins.	British Temperance Society	
From 5—7.30	Colour	28 mins.	British Temperance Society	1962
To Your Health	Colour	10 mins.	Central Film Library	1956
Just for Today	Colour	30 mins.	Alcoholics Anon.	
Drugs and Health			Encyclopedia Britannica	
The Birth of a Drug			Diana Wyllie	
Drug Dependence			Camera Talks Ltd.	
Drug Abuse (3 strips)			Encyclopedia Britannica	
Drugs in our Society (6 parts)	Colour		Concordia	
1. Tobacco — The Habit and the Hazards				
2. Alcohol — Decision about Drinking				
3. R.X. — Not for Kicks				
4. Narcotics — Uses and Abuses				
5. Marijuana — A Foolish Fad				
6. L.S.D. — Worth the Risk?				
Smoke or Not to Smoke			Manchester Regional Committee on Cancer, Kinnard Road, Manchester	
Pot or Not?			Health Education Audio-Visual	

FIRST AID
(see also Personal Responsibility)

Title	Colour B/W	Running time	Distributor	Date
Emergency Resuscitation	Colour	50 mins.	Guild Sound & Vision Ltd. and St. John Ambulance Assoc., 10 Grosvenor Crescent, London SW1	

ROAD SAFETY

Title	Colour B/W	Running time	Distributor	Date
Ballad of the Battered Bicycle			Petroleum Films Bureau, 4 Brook Street, Hanover Square, London W1	
Defensive Driving			Petroleum Films Bureau	
Over the Road			Petroleum Films Bureau	
Pedestrians (6 filmlets)			Petroleum Films Bureau	
Look Alert — Stay Unhurt	Colour	14 mins.	Guild Sound & Vision Ltd.	
Mind How you Go	Colour	12 mins.	Gateway Film Library (C.F.L.)	1973

F I L M S (*continued*)

Title	Colour B/W	Running time	Distributor	Date
Accidents don't Happen	B/W	10 mins.	Rank Film Library	1954
Ten Little Schoolboys			Camera Talks Ltd.	
HUMAN RELATIONS				
Head of the House	B/W	37 mins.	Concord	1956
(made in the U.S.A.)				
Making a Decision	B/W	6 mins.	Concord	1957
Courtship	B/W	59 mins.	Concord	1961
Learning to Live	Colour	20 mins.	Guild Sound & Vision Ltd.	1964
The Challenge to Leisure	B/W	30 mins.	Concord	1967
Understanding — Stresses	Colour	10 mins.	Walt Disney Productions	
and Strains				
FAMILY HEALTH				
Healthy Families (for	Colour	11 mins.	Boulton Hawker Ltd.	1958
primary schools, USA)				
FOOD HYGIENE				
Clean Food	B/W	16 mins.	Central Film Library	1957
By Whose Hand?	Colour	16 mins.	Central Film Library	1962
WATER				
Let's Look at Water	B/W	20 mins.		
(U.S.A.)				

TAPES

The X Factor (VD)	Infotape Productions,
	50 Frith Street, London W1
A Matter of Life (Contraception)	Medical Recording Service,
Stop before you Start (Smoking)	Writtle, Essex
Drugs in School (for adults)	

CHAPTER 11

Mental health

The term mental health is a useful label to identify those activities in health education which are concerned with the development of an adequate personality, the promotion of good relationships in groups and in the community, and assistance to the individual to achieve the maximum possible social satisfaction. In this context, mental health is not concerned with severe mental disorder requiring psychiatric treatment, and although we must acknowldge the debt to the child guidance service for much of the content of mental health education, we are not concerned here with any conditions requiring remedial treatment. One of the difficulties in this area of health education is language, but it is possible to describe people's emotions and the way in which they behave without resort to overtechnical language. We must commence then with definitions.

Definitions

We are concerned with:

1. The way in which a person behaves.
2. The way in which the group makes him behave.
3. The effect on feelings (a) personal, (b) group.
4. The resulting reaction by the individual or by the group.

In describing behaviour, it is better to substitute 'expected' for 'normal'. Human beings show as wide a range of variation in personality and behavioural characteristics as they do in other biological features. More than this, the effect of culture on behaviour has always to be taken into account and presents us with another variable. It therefore becomes impossible to talk about normal behaviour without reference to variation of the individual from the mathematical norm and variation in cultural patterns.

Compensation for Inner Emotional Tension

Analogies are useful. For example, it could be said to be 'expected' when blood flows after cutting the skin. It is also 'expected' for someone who has severe guilt feeling to attempt to project his guilt to another person by aggression. It is also 'expected' for a person to behave in such a way that he imagines that he is distracting public attention from the reason for his guilt, although in fact this may not have been perceived by anyone around him. To cite another analogy, if a child has a short tendon behind the heel and cannot easily bring the heel to the ground, he rolls his foot inwards in an attempt to reach the ground. He can walk after adopting this manoeuvre, but the cost is distortion of the segments of the feet, strain on ligaments and muscles and eventually severe foot defects. In the same way, people adopt behavioural patterns, speech, and actions which compensate for some inner emotional tension. This also is to be 'expected', and for a long time, such people may pass as 'normal', but when they are put to the test and the test may be a crisis in personal relationships, or in occupation, then the emotional deformities they have created by their behaviour begin to appear.

An understanding of what is the 'expected' behaviour in a person faced with the need to discharge guilt or to compensate for some inadequacy is an important factor in considering the way in which groups make people behave. The emotional environment will be much improved if everybody had the capacity to perceive behaviour that appeared to be anti-social or irritating, or even bizarre, as a reaction for some inner emotional strain. This is very important when faced with sudden aggression in the community. An aggressive traveller may provoke a latently aggressive railway official who responds with counter-aggression and when the next traveller approaches him, the latter then gets the full force of the official's anger. There is a chain reaction often starting in the home before setting out for work, which passes rapidly around a group, often to come full circle on the return from home. An example in the school setting would be when a pupil, through some trivial misdemeanour, may trigger off an emotional reaction in a teacher because the latter may have some unresolved personal problem — e.g. marital, financial, sexual, or professional — which has caused inner emotional tension.

Conceptual Models

Watts has described the causes of emotional breakdown as being the result of three main factors: [1]

1. Unrelieved anxiety.
2. Unresolved depression.
3. Inadequate personality.

Health education is concerned with the problem of inadequate personality, but fortunately personality can be improved at any time of life, although there is an advantage if the child has certain emotional needs supplied to him during early infancy. The school provides an excellent opportunity for the strengthening of inadequate personalities, provided that its organization and relationships are structured according to the general principles underlying emotional security.

Emotional security is characterised by a series of capacities, as follows: [2]

1. There is no handicap of inner emotional tension.
2. It is possible to live and work with other people without making them break down.
3. Human relationships are enjoyable.
4. Events are seen as they really are, and are not distorted in perception by feelings of insecurity.
5. It is possible to tolerate criticism without breaking down.
6. It is possible to co-operate with a group of people, subject to this being morally acceptable.

None of us scores highly on all these qualities all the time, and it is reassuring to know that everybody suffers from defects of these capacities when faced with crisis situations, as a result of passing through biologically vulnerable phases of life, or as a result of fatigue and illness. Although it is not advised that people should attempt to score their own personalities, according to these characteristics, it is nevertheless helpful to examine one's behaviour and motivation in this light. This is the first step to understanding the way in which we behave, the way in which groups make us behave, and the effect upon our feelings and the feelings of those around us.

Variation

We have already referred to the infinite variation to be found in human beings. Whenever any biological characteristic can be measured and the measurements are plotted in a frequency distribution, it falls into a normal curve. This is true of personality characteristics and of behavioural patterns related to them. Some of these may be genetically determined, and some psychiatrists assert that there are people who are born with a built-in anxiety neurosis. The characteristics which are known to vary by genetic determination, include intelligence, and probably the capacity for imagery. Research into the assessment of people's capacity for visual imagery suggests that this capacity is distributed at random throughout the community in a normal curve. Both intelligence and imagery are important factors when considering the way in which people behave in a relationship with others and as a result of stress and crisis. Otherwise people differ infinitely in personal experience. Every home has a uniqueness, and although behavioural patterns have cultural resemblances, even they vary in individuals.

Environmental Factors

Variations in the environment must also be taken into account. These include socio-economic level of the family, whether there is only one parent, sex of individuals, the number of siblings, and their rank order. Experienced teachers are aware that these factors are vital in taking decisions about a child's educational future. The six capacities listed as forming together a structured personality can be regarded as potential qualities which grow when stimulated. Their growth in the child is therefore dependent first upon the child receiving consistent affection and parental care with an opportunity of returning the affection.

Affection should not be 'one-way' and the child who is said traditionally to be 'smothered' by excessive maternal care is one who is being deprived of the opportunity of exercising his own capacities for affection. Further growth of the capacities for emotional security depends upon regular stimulus and opportunities for exercising these capacities in the face of a series of stresses and anxieties which are inseparable from the human condition and are far better looked upon as natural challenges. To use another analogy, a child must jump over a number of hurdles, but the height of the hurdles must be adjusted to the child's age and ability.

Vulnerable Age-Groups

There are certain phases of life in which there is particular vulnerability to stress. This is in infancy; on entering school; at adolescence when the latent sexuality then becomes revealed to the boy and girl; in pregnancy, particularly when the couple are very young; and at various crisis points in life which now occur to whole groups of people, rather than to individuals. We referred in the first chapter to the problem created by redundancy in industry. Old age also is a biologically vulnerable phase of life, because there is a weakening of the physical organism with a diminishing capacity and loss of powers of adaptation and compensation, coupled with poverty either real or relative, the feeling of rejection, and the disappearance of the sense of purpose in life.

Parental Roles

We may therefore consider the factors concerned in the growth of personality both in the positive and in the negative way. As regards children, the growth of personality is as much a task of parenthood as the supply of adequate nutrition, clothing, and protection from common danger.

To be adequate as parents and as teachers, and to help to promote personality, parents and teachers have to understand the usual reactions that children display when faced with frustration, fear, or anxiety. It is usual for example for a small child to test out the security of the tie of affection with his parents by deliberately wilful acts of aggression or disobedience. It is interesting to observe that in residential childrens' institutions, one child usually takes on this function for the group. Such a situation is not uncommon, either, in a class of children in an ordinary school when insecurity exists by reason of conditions, attitudes of some of the pupils, or, it must be said, by inefficient teaching. During infancy and early childhood, parents have to be exceptionally careful to avoid creating fear and anxiety in the child whose organism is not yet sufficiently robust to tolerate it. Fears related to too early toilet-training lie buried in the personalities of hundreds of thousands of adults at the present day, giving rise to various disabilities of a psycho-sexual nature and carrying with them that feeling of guilt which is the genesis of inner emotional tension. Doctors and health visitors working in child welfare centres have succeeded in recent years in teaching the modern views, thus encouraging young mothers not to associate toilet-training with goodness or badness.

Models of Behaviour

However the most important factor in the child's personality development is the model of behaviour which his parents and sibling show. If the reaction to a family crisis is calm and constructive and anxiety is channelled into positive action, then the child will have learned that you do face crises without avoiding the issue and that you apply your experience and energy to solving them. If on the other hand, a crisis, whether it is domestic, financial or marital, causes widespread alarm and dismay and there is no constructive action, the child will have learned that this is the way you behave when faced with a threat. It is commonplace to observe that many children and adults are too easily threatened, and in this case the compensatory reaction is one of withdrawal, rather than aggression.

This has been learned early in childhood by observing the model of behaviour presented by the parents and other adults. We have already seen that health education involves non-verbal communication, and in the infants' school, the classroom teacher has an opportunity to show a healthy model of reaction to situations that arise. It should be possible by observing children's play and physical activities to detect a child who turns away from difficulty, the child that meets contact with another rougher child by stretching the arms out with the hands held in protest, rather than engaging combat, or just running away. Later in school life, the teacher of physical education also has a contribution to make to personality development when faced with individual cases of timidity, absenteeism from P.E., or avoidance of contact situations.

Understanding Anxiety

It is necessary to understand the nature of anxiety and the way in which people are equipped to handle it. Anxiety and stress are not in themselves undesirable, they are a driving force in society, as well as in the physical environment which provides the challenge for human activity. It is when they become overwhelming, causing physical symptoms and loss of satisfactory performance, verbal, intellectual or physical, that anxiety becomes a problem.

The hypothalamus at the base of the brain contains the terminals of nervous circuits originating in the frontal lobes, the higher centres of thought and emotion. The pituitary gland, also, is linked with the brain by circuits passing through its thin stalk. It is the hypothalamus that sounds the alarm when anxiety becomes uncontrollable fear. The medulla (core) of the adrenal gland responds to the direct stimulation by the sympathetic nervous system by pouring out adrenalin causing a rapid heartbeat, rise of blood pressure, pallor of the skin, and a feeling of tension in the abdominal organs. The adrenal cortex too protects the body against stress and this part of the adrenal is indirectly influenced by the nervous system via the pituitary. In a wild animal, this is a useful alarm system, which is then followed immediately by flight, i.e. violent physical activity in which these hormonal and circulatory changes are put to good use. In the human being, flight or fight becomes impossible after childhood, and the tension therefore remains. When the acute stage of anxiety has passed, there is chronic anxiety which is converted into muscular tension causing severe headaches or pains in other parts of the body (the back is particularly vulnerable in women) leading to loss of skill, which may make a person accident prone for example, as well as to loss of skill in general social and work performance. Close contact with a person suffering from acute or chronic anxiety shows that this tends to be 'infectious', it causes tension in others who are involved either personally or in the work situation. On the other hand, emotional security is also 'infectious' and the insecure gain from regular contact with those who have handled their anxiety effectively, and who have a reasonable 'score' of the capacities of the kind outlined above.

Normal Swings of Mood

We all experience swings of mood from elation to depression and back again, and for the most part, moods which maintain a balance between elation and depression. At times the swing of mood is natural, e.g. success produces justified elation, and bereavement or disaster produces justified depression. It is only when the swing of mood occurs without justification that it can be considered an aspect of mental ill health. This is highly relevant to the current problem of drug abuse.

Health education in this field aims at imparting personal skills which children can then use in schools, and later in the adult world, in order to minimize harmful stress, and to handle anxiety effectively. These skills can be learned throughout the whole of school life, but they become much more important in the secondary school where there is little time left to prepare the boy and girl for the aggression and stress which they will meet in the adult world. Moreover, the use of language is essential for understanding concepts such as motivation, so that it is necessary to await the development of intellectual capacities and educational experience before this type of health education can be tackled seriously.

Participatory Methods of Learning

Experience shows that it is seldom possible or desirable to impart this information didactically. This is *par excellence* a case for the use of group discussion and for participatory techniques, such as role-playing. The most fruitful discussions will ensue when the pupils have been provided at an earlier stage of their school life with relevant factual information on the principles and practice of healthy living. There are a number of short cartoon films available explaining the nature of stress and anxiety both in the individual and in communities, and these are useful if they are merely a means for promoting discussion.

It has to be accepted that it is impossible to discuss problems of personality and mental health without involving value-judgments. The teenager's natural propensity to criticize society will be given full reign here, and this must be expected and encouraged. There is also however an opportunity of encouraging informed criticism by discussion of the way people behave in order to achieve a satisfaction. Satisfactions themselves can be discussed on a value basis as to those which are legitimate, and those which are not admissible if the needs of the community are to be protected. Once again, the value of the infinite variation of human nature is relevant. For the balance of societies, there must be groups of people who have different characteristics and who are distributed at random.

For example, the value of the nonconformist is frequently mentioned, and many regret the dwindling numbers of eccentrics in our society. How many nonconformists and eccentrics can we afford without disturbing the balance of society as a whole? The presence of such people in smaller groups, such as youth clubs, can also have an effect. The capacity to absorb members who diverge from the norm is probably one indication of a healthy social group. We are also faced in Western Europe with a problem of substantial minorities with specific cultural characteristics, aims, and aspirations, as well as insecurities and fears. How can these be protected and helped without damaging the interests of others? There are always dangers inherent in social systems where relatively small but powerful groups can join forces to dominate the rest. Historically, this was a basic principle of the doctrine of the balance of power in Europe, and it appears to have relevance today.

Violence

The problem of violence, whether related to sexual misbehaviour or not, is one which we know to our cost cannot be settled by repression. Taking a long-term view, violence should diminish when there are fewer severely insecure people in the community. Discussions on violence and cruelty could be handled very effectively by senior pupils in secondary schools, and should form part of a curriculum for education for mental health. Where environmental factors are important, those of course will be discussed and remedies suggested, but this must not allow the avoidance of the central problem that mental health, like the Kingdom of God, is within us, is concerned with our innate behavioural patterns which are mainly learned and conditioned as a result of experience.

Film clips from box-office type of films which show aggressive and anxiety reactions well could be useful teaching material in the right hands. Role-playing, using a tape recorder where possible, the playing back of a recording and discussing it in the light of the theory of personality and human relations has the added value that it contrives an emotional experience under controlled conditions in which it can be analysed by those undergoing it themselves.

It is clear that education for mental health is relevant to many other aspects of health education, particularly parentcraft and sex education. Sex is of itself a stress, and the handling of the instinctive sex drive is frequently attended by conflict, guilt, and anxiety. Hormonal disturbances and imbalances in the body at adolescence increase the biological vulnerability to stress, but this will not be helped merely by telling adolescents about the way in which their organs of reproduction suddenly come to life, and develop, become capable of conception, as well as the giving of physical pleasure. They will need also to understand the association between feelings of love and affection or anger and aggression with their physical sexual feelings.

QUESTIONS

1. Outline a mental health educational programme for the secondary school.
2. What preparations should the teacher have for mental health education?
3. What are the potentially dangerous situations in school life from the point of view of the development of emotional insecurity?

FURTHER READING

Brierley, J. (1973). *The Thinking Machine*. London: Heinemann.

Cohen, J. (1970). *Homo Psychologicus*. London: Allen and Unwin.

Dalzell-Ward, A. J. (1967). 'Health Education for Mental Health'. *Hlth. Educ. J.* 26: 192-203.

Davies, N. and Heimler, E. (1967). 'An Experiment in Assessment of Social Function'. *Med. Officer.* 117:31.

English, O. S. and Pearson, Gerald H. J. (1965). *Emotional Problems of Living*. London: Allen and Unwin.

English, O. S. and Pearson Gerald H. J. (1951) *Emotional Disorders in Children*. London: Allen and Unwin.

May, A. R., Kahn, J. H. and Crossholm, B. (1971). *Mental Health of Adolescents and Young Persons*. Report of a technical conference. World Health Organization, Public Health Papers No. 41. London: HMSO.

National Association for Mental Health. *Questions on our Mind*.

Oakshott, E (1973). *The Child under Stress*. London: Priory Press.

Ratcliffe, T. A. (1967). *The Development of Personality*. London: Allen and Unwin.

Watts, C. A. H. (1958). 'Management of Chronic Psychoneurosis in General Practice.' *Lancet*. 2:362.

FILMS

Title	Colour B/W	Running time	Distributor	Date
Mental Illness (Panorama Programme)	B/W	50 mins.	Concord	1966
My Brother David	B/W	30 mins.	Concord	1971
Once Upon a Time	B/W	17 mins.	Concord	1969
One in Every Hundred	B/W	50 mins.	Concord	1966
Out of the Shadows	Colour	20 mins.	Concord	
Stress	B/W	30 mins.	Concord	1966
The Stress Theory	B/W	10 mins.	Concord	1956

FILMS (*Continued*)

Title	Colour B/W	Running time	Distributor	Date
A Way of Caring	B/W	40 mins.	Concord	1969
Three in Every Thousand	Colour	30 mins.	Concord	1972
Angry Boy	B/W	33 mins.	Concord	1951
Being Different	B/W	10 mins.	Concord	1957
The Bridge	B/W	20 mins.	Concord	1958
Feeling of Hostility	B/W	32 mins.	Central Film Library	1950
Feeling of Rejection	B/W	23 mins.	Central Film Library	1950
Out of Tune	B/W	41 mins.	Concord	1951
Relief of Confusion	B/W	28 mins.	Eothen Films	
The Greater Community Animal (cartoon)	Colour	5 mins.	Concord Films, Nacton, Ipswich, Suffolk	1966
Understanding Stresses and Strains (cartoon and live action)	Colour	10 mins.	Walt Disney Educational Materials Co., 83 Pall Mall, London SW1 Y5EX	

CHAPTER 12

Preparation for marriage and family life

Marriage and the rearing of children are of vital importance to the community's health, as well as being a universal way of achieving self-fulfilment. This has attracted the attention of health educators for at least half a century. Attempts at preparation for marriage mostly with adolescents and with engaged couples followed earlier programmes of mothercraft which were concerned with the problems of physical care and maintenance and protection against common danger of the very young child.

Importance of Psychodynamics and Expectations

These efforts were made before we had the advantage of a precise knowledge of psychodynamics and reference back to the chapter on mental health will remind readers that the application of the general principles governing personality action are particularly appropriate when applied to the marriage situation. Marriage is entered into with certain expectations, and a useful exercise with older pupils is to have a discussion on the reasons for marriage and what boys and girls expect from it. Expectations are necessarily idealistic, and they are derived partially from admired models, either in real life or in fiction, or nowadays perhaps more commonly the models communicated to the reading public by the mass media.

It is clear also that conventional premarriage guidance and parentcraft teaching are based on a stereotype which is now under such serious pressure by the modern environment that it should be revised in the light of social change.

Distinction between Gender and Sex

In this field of health education, we are concerned with gender, rather than sex, and there is a subtle distinction which is so often missed. Gender roles in society are qualitatively different from sexual roles, and are more subject to change. The sexual role has not changed, and even though some women may discuss variations of sexual behaviour with their partners the final act of intercourse and conception remain unchanged.

Gender roles are changing all the time. Proportionately, this has affected men rather than women. For example, it is now commonplace for young fathers to share the tasks of the physical care of young children with their wives. It is still the rule rather than the exception for the father to play the role of the principal breadwinner, and in the majority of cases where the wife does make a financial contribution to the home, it is usually in an occupation that is less well paid and less socially prestigious than that of her husband. Although there is talk about the need for women to work at a gainful occupation for self-fulfilment, perhaps in the majority of cases the motive is simply to augment the family income and so obtain the amenities which the couple consider necessary for themselves and their children over and above the subsistence level.

Social Class Influences

There are variations of this situation in the different social classes in the community. In social class 1, there are a few couples enjoying equal professional status and prestige, and in positions of authority in their respective occupations. This applies also in the entrepreneurial classes, such as the owners of family businesses, or in the catering industry. For the remainder of the population, social mobility favours the man and the tendency is for the man to develop socially and to achieve more personal fulfilment as he grows older and more successful in his occupation, and for his wife to remain behind to be either kept out of sight or employed as a social appendage at appropriate occasions. Following the expected pattern of reaction to frustration, the wife either tolerates it and falls back upon activities of her own, or she rebels against it, becomes resentful, and tension arises. It is at this point that sexual problems now appear, and it is interesting that the peak incidence of divorce granted for adultery occurs either in the first five years after marriage, or after a lapse of fifteen to twenty years. [1]

The Influence of Occupation

The pressures on marriage and family life differ qualitatively according to the social class. In the case of skilled and unskilled workers and workers in the middle ranks of management, pressures are mainly economic. While in employment, the rate for the job is paid, and there is usually an opportunity for overtime which produces another strain on marriage and family life, as well as diminishing the quality of life by depriving the breadwinner of the opportunity for recreation. There is also the fear of redundancy and unemployment, and this affects highly skilled workers, as we have seen in the Rolls-Royce and Upper Clyde Shipbuilding disasters.

These are hazards of life which are anticipated and for which adjustment can be made more easily in the modern welfare state with opportunities for retraining or alternative employment, with unemployment benefits, supplementary benefits, and redundancy payments. These blows are softened by a more enlightened society. The effect on marriage and family life in these cases will be due mainly to overwork producing profound fatigue and causing the absence of the father from family gatherings at week-ends and public holidays. It brings in the problem of sexual impotence.

The Organization Man

Much more vulnerable is the boy who achieves a full set of 'O' levels and perhaps one or two 'A' levels and who then decides to make an executive career in industry. The hazard of becoming an *organization man* is a very real one. The modern industrial corporation prefers to employ married men because they cannot easily leave; on the other hand, they can be very easily sacked. Normal aggressions and ambitions are encouraged and advancement is offered but at the cost of an encroachment on personal life and leisure. The ambitious young man usually cannot afford to go home at the normal time. The custom of upper management insisting on being addressed by their Christian names produces a feeling of uncertainty and identity crisis which can be more stressful than the old-fashioned formal relationship.

Not only does the modern corporation like its employees to be married, but in the upper ranks of management, it likes the wives to become organization wives. There is thus encroachment on family leisure, demands for wives to be present at various gatherings at which it is clear they are expected to be as loyal to the organization as their husbands and at the same time they are subjected to the same insecurity which is almost built in to this kind of occupation.

It is not long before such couples find the other couples are their friends because they belong to the organization and hold a certain rank in it. As soon as rumours go round that an executive is due for the sack under whatever euphemism this is described, there is an immediate cancellation of engagements and a falling away of friends.

An Argument for an Alternative Society

This is one of the distressing facts of society and if preparation for marriage is to be undertaken at school, then it is important that the teacher be aware of this, as well as of the other stresses in the outside world. If teachers wish to play a part in the changing of society, then they probably have no better opportunity than in this situation. It is the boy equipped with 'O' and 'A' levels and perhaps later, a University degree, who will fight hard to maintain his position and succeed, and when he does succeed, he will then repeat the process with his subordinates in turn. This perpetuation of insecurity, encroachment on personal liberty, privacy, family life and self-fulfilment probably influences the contemporary arguments for an 'alternative society'.

Our immediate task implies that young people should be helped to understand the emotional nature of the marriage relationship, to come to terms with their similarities and differences on a gender basis, and to approach their own coming parenthood with confidence and anticipation of doing better than their parents did.

Parentcraft Education

Children appear to be interested in marriage and family life from the earliest age, and quite small children play at weddings and at mothers and fathers. However, the appropriate stage at which to commence preparation for marriage and parenthood is in the secondary school, after the child has had the advantage of a general education in human biology which we have described earlier. It is necessary once again to emphasize that no subject that contributes to health education should ever be considered in isolation. When parentcraft was concerned with bathing babies, dressing and undressing them, hours of sleep, preparation of feeds and the like, then this was meaningful to quite young children because they saw these events in their own homes and in those of their friends. In its modern form, however, parentcraft goes far wider in its scope and attempts to equip a future parent with a skill that will take him right up to the point at which his own children are entering adult life.

Behavioural Problems

We have been fairly successful in equipping parents to be adequate in caring for young children up to the age of entering school. The problems occurring later, which are mainly behavioural in character and which require understanding of the nature of child development and emotional needs, have been left to others to tackle, that is schools and Child Guidance Clinics. Unfortunately they have been left to be dealt with at the stage where remedial, rather than preventive, action is required. We have given parents no guidance at all as regards their relationships with adolescent children and their role as parents, but rather we have offered them from time to time abuse and criticism, and have added to their burden of guilt without offering any practical solution. Although it is obvious that one cannot present a whole life-experience to children in the secondary school during a year or two, we can attempt to give boys and girls some insight into their emotions, as expressed in a close relationship like marriage and to direct their attention to the obligations and responsibilities of marriage and parenthood and the pleasure that can be derived from fulfilling them.

The Cycle of Conception

This process should commence after the boys and girls have a sound idea of the cycle of conception, of the way babies are born, and of their material and emotional needs. Family planning obviously comes into the curriculum of preparation for marriage and family life, and this term is used in its widest sense for *contraceptive* techniques are regarded by many in a modern world for the prevention of reproduction, not for its encouragement on a planned and rational basis. Family planning therefore not only includes all methods of contraception, but also problems of fertility and methods of fertility investigation and promotion. This provides an opportunity for discussion of the material resources needed to be adequate parents if every child is to enjoy basic human rights.

Human Rights in Marriage

Human rights extend also to married couples and whether the normal expectations of marriage can be fulfilled will depend very largely upon a wise choice of a marriage partner. Assortative mating is a biological and social reality, and this was demonstrated over twenty years ago by Eliot Slater. [2] Unfortunately, the mating of like with like includes the mating of people with adverse characters and personality disorders, as well as those who are adequate in every respect. The boy and girl may be brought together as a result of pursuit of a common hobby, or on the other hand, as a result of the need to escape from an unhappy home with maladjusted parents, constant strife, and squalor. There are many instances of course where one partner has possessed a more resilient and secure personality, and has been able to help a partner less secure. In the practice of family psychiatry, such partners are often used as domestic 'psychotherapists'; this of course is at the cost of considerable strain to the adequate partner, which is hardly an ideal arrangement. [3]

Background Experience

When two young people meet for the first time and become attracted to each other, they may be quite unaware of each other's background and childhood experience, and yet these factors are those that produce personality structure, which may be adequate or inadequate. As we mentioned earlier, it is only at the time of stress that the personality breakdown becomes apparent. *Some* safeguard against unsuitable people meeting and proposing marriage is provided when people seek partners within their familiar social group, where they have had an opportunity of observing the behaviour and relationships of the person to whom they have been attracted. The place of work would seem to be a very suitable venue for meeting a future spouse. Adolescent boys and girls should be encouraged to enjoy their leisure in mixed groups as far as possible, so that they have an opportunity of observing many individuals until the inevitable mutual attraction begins to show itself.

Support of family and friends and encouragement and approval of marriage is also important, and although there are many couples who have succeeded in breaking away from their families and early social environment, these have probably been people of exceptional qualities of character and personality. Apart from its religious function, a marriage ceremony does in fact signify the blessing of society upon the union.

The Inter-dependent Relationship

The ideal fundamental relationship in marriage is interdependence. Dependence of one partner upon another entirely produces a strain on the one and a feeling of inadequacy in the other, whereas interdependence means that there is an equal sharing of giving and taking of affection and mutual support.

Bearing in mind what we have said above about the problem of social mobility affecting mainly men, any serious educational gulf or difference about life aspiration is likely to cause trouble in the later years of marriage. Authoritarianism and lack of self-control under frustrations are personality characters which will be inimical to a happy marriage and which would have adverse effects upon children.

Decisions on Life Goals

There has also to be a reconciliation between marriage partners on the goals in life which each have set themselves. Ideally, their goals should be identical as there are obviously diverse interests related to gender roles and of gender behaviour which will have to be reconciled. This problem will present itself very early in the relationship even before marriage. Certain recreations and hobbies are divisive. Boys and girls would do best to seek partners who have some interests that they can share, even if these are not all their interests. There is a particular problem with regard to sport. Some sports are entirely male, and girlfriends and young wives are very welcome as spectators, and agreeable social appendages. As wives become older, they are less welcome, and in fact have no role, but also by this time the husbands will have become too old to play this particular sport, and they in turn become spectators, a role they can pursue until old age if they wish to.

Communication between Husbands and Wives

Attention has been drawn in recent years to the problem of lack of communicativeness between married people. Divorces have been granted on a plea that one partner, usually the husband, has failed to start a conversation over a period of many years. In extreme cases, husbands and wives live lives apart, even occupying separate rooms, taking meals separately, and communicating only by written messages.

Verbal communication is basic to all human relationships, and has a particular value in marriage, in that it can be entirely free of inhibition. Sex life is enriched by speech, otherwise it degenerates into a mere automatic habit. By talking to each other, husbands and wives show that they wish to share their experiences and to live each other's lives as far as possible. The increasing social gap between partners already referred to may be one of the causes of breakdown of communication, as there is no common ground left for discussion. In some social classes, there is a stereotype of male behaviour which identifies taciturnity with strength and manliness, and despite the social progress of the last half century, this is still found.

Shared Needs

It is essential that boys and girls understand that they share identical emotional needs, irrespective of gender. For the most part, girls marry with the expectation of a lifelong companionship and women attach more importance in later years to companionship and to the other advantages obtained from marriage. One would have thought that the establishment of co-education which has affected the majority of boys and girls for at least two generations would have gone a long way towards eliminating the unnecessary and artificial differences between the genders. On the other hand, *artificial* differences as opposed to *biological* differences are a result of culture and social pressures, and outside the world of the school, these have remained largely unchanged.

The Need for External Relationships

Despite the closeness of the ideal marital relationship, there is still need of the stimulation of the companionship of people who are outside the relationship. When completely isolated from its neighbourhood, the home is a place at which it may be said that the laws of the land are automatically suspended as soon as the front door is closed. Under such circumstances, people may insult, ignore, and neglect each other, and even commit physical assault without any sanctions being applied. Neglect of children has to be so severe that the children have suffered perhaps permanent trauma before official or voluntary intervention occurs. Similarly, it is unusual for husbands and wives to institute legal proceedings against each other for assault and battery, and many blows are exchanged, even in homes where the educational level is fairly high.

It is therefore necessary for some social sanctions to be applied, however gently, to family life, and these are derived from the friendship with other families. There is a healthy restraint against giving way entirely to frustration, when there is a knowledge that friends may visit at any time and will have to be received in a courteous and genial atmosphere. It is also good for husbands and wives to observe the respect and affection with which their spouses are regarded by others outside the family. It becomes more difficult to abuse anyone who is obviously highly regarded by people whose respect one values.

Influence of the Environment

The pressures of modern society and the way in which it is organized structurally tend to encourage the withdrawal of families into their own homes with little opportunity for further enrichment of their lives by contact with others. The housing estate, the towerblock of flats, the long hours of work, the tendency to spend what leisure is left in decorating, home repairs and other do-it-yourself activities, the escape from home at the week-ends in the motor car which is an extension of home, are all factors causing the family to be indrawn.

If town planners could return to the medieval ideal of the small city, this should provide most of the satisfactions within its boundaries, with the opportunity of an occasional excursion to a more exciting or more scenic place. Families would then enjoy the benefits of daily contact with members of other families, preserving the balance of necessary privacy of the home with the need for regular stimulation and enrichment from outside.

Ideas for Syllabuses

There have been a number of syllabuses designed to prepare the adolescent boy and girl for marriage and family life. An excellent example is that developed by the Gloucestershire Family Life Association and outlined in its second report in 1966. [4] This syllabus is comprehensive and rests upon a basis of human biology but it includes also elementary sociology and ethics. For example, topics include the aggressive pattern, work, authority, politics, and economics. The need for moral standards is included, as also an examination of moral codes. Discussions on standards of behaviour are highly appropriate to the matters we have mentioned above. There is, for example, the problems of bullying, teasing, or exploiting others. The problems of friendship, group loyalty, and patriotism must have a relevance to the tensions encountered by the organization man at the present day. The world of work is examined and the syllabus includes class and racial discrimination. 'Courtship, marriage, and the family' includes discussion of sexual relationships, parenthood, home-making, government of affairs of the home, expenditure, education, and health with particular emphasis on mental health. Religious matters are included and also problems of recreation and leisure. The Association recommends that learning should be through group discussions as far as possible. It is also pointed out that pupils will require definite answers to questions about values and standards.

The National Marriage Guidance Council has a long and distinguished record of helping couples to preserve their marriages but also the Council has included education for marriage for engaged couples in its activities. Both the professional staff and the voluntary, but trained, counsellors are skilled in the practical application of the principles of psycho-dynamics to the marriage situation.

QUESTIONS

1. What are the implications of the phenomenon of assortative mating?

2. Sexual satisfaction in marriage depends on previously established emotional interdependence. Discuss.

3. Draw up a list of possible reasons for marriage and comment.

4. How may education for marriage and family life be included in the school curriculum? When should we start?

5. In dealing with questions of family life how would you avoid giving a pupil the feeling that his parents are inadquate?

6. What are the characteristics you consider to be indicative of a happy marriage?

7. Parents may give their child the impression that the teacher does not know anything about family life. How would you endeavour to overcome this misunderstanding?

8. Young people frequently complain that they cannot communicate with their parents on any emotionally charged topics like drugs, contraceptives,

personal relationships etc. What do you consider to be the reasons for this and how would you try to help these young people?

9. When talking to children about marriage and family life they will ask questions relative to their age. What questions on sexual intercourse, pregnancy, and birth would you expect from

   a. five-year-olds
   b. ten-year-olds
   c. fifteen-year-olds?

10. How would you explain the role of the father to each of these age-groups?

REFERENCES

1. Office of Population Censuses and Surveys. *Statistics on Divorce.* London.
2. Slater, E. and Woodside, M. (1957). *Patterns of Marriage.* London: Cassell.
3. Howells, J. G. (1968). *Theory and Practice of Family Psychiatry.* Edinburgh: Oliver and B.
4. Gloucestershire Family Life Association. (1966). *Education in Personal Relationships and Family Life.* 2nd. ed. Gloucester.

FURTHER READING

Family Doctor Series. (1962). *How Not to Kill Your Husband.* London: Allen and Unwin.

Family Doctor Series. (1965). *How Not to Kill your Wife.* London: Allen and Unwin.

Family Planning Association Publications.

Fletcher, Ronald (1969). *Family and Marriage in Britain.* Harmondsworth: Penguin.

Gavron, H. (1968). *The Captive Wife: Conflicts of Housebound Mothers.* Harmondsworth: Penguin.

Griffith, E. E. (1973). *Modern Marriage.* London: Eyre Methuen.

Hubbard, C. W. (1973). *Family Planning Education, Parenthood and Social Disease Control.* Florida, USA: Henry Kimpton.

Kenyon, F. E. (1973). *Homosexuality.* London: Family Doctor Publications. (Obtainable from chemists' shops.)

Mace, D. (1972). *Sexual Difficulties in Marriage.* London: National Marriage Guidance Council.

Proctor, A. (1953). *Background to Marriage.* London: Longmans.

Report on the Conference on Family Planning for Britain. (1968). *Family Planning.* London: Royal Society of Health.

Sanctuary, Gerald. (1968). *Marriage under Stress.* London: Allen and Unwin.

Sex Education in Perspective by various authors. (1972). National Marriage Guidance Council. (Available from their bookshop: Little Church Street, Rugby, Warwickshire.)

Wallis, John H. (1968). *Thinking about Marriage.* Harmondsworth: Penguin.

Whyte, W. H. (1960). *The Organization Man.* Harmondsworth: Penguin.

Wolff, Charlotte. (1971). *Love between Women.* London: Duckworth.

FILMS

Title	Colour B/W	Running time	Distributor	Date
Marriage under Stress	B/W	30 mins.	B.B.C. T.V. Enterprises	1967
Teenage Marriage	B/W	30 mins.	Film Hire, 25 The Burroughs, Hendon, London	1967

CHAPTER 13

Parentcraft

'Parentcraft' into 'Parent Education'

Parentcraft has been a stable component of health education in schools for over half a century. It has been through an evolutionary stage of development in that time, beginning as mothercraft in an age when such matters were considered to apply only to women and developing later into a wider concept of parentcraft involving fathers and mothers but rather uncertain of assigning a precise gender role to the father. In recent years, interest has centred on what is called parent education, although this is mainly in the field of adult education and has been fostered mainly by the École des Parents movement which started in France in 1929. [1] The International Federation for Parent Education founded in Brussels in 1965 brought together the many 'schools for parents' in European countries and also in French-speaking territories of North Africa, in Latin America, in the U.S.A., and Canada. For the last twenty years, the climate of opinion in training for parenthood has changed and concentration on the basic tasks of physical care and maintenance and protection from common danger has widened to an understanding of emotional needs and of adjusting the home environment to the child's stages of emotional development.

The Cycle of Deprivation

In recent years, attention has been called to the so-called 'battered baby' syndrome which although by no means commonly encountered has been met by doctors and nurses with sufficient frequency to cause alarm. The term applies to situations where babies are brought in to doctors' surgeries or to hospitals with injuries which are said to be accidental, but which on inspection can only have been deliberately inflicted. In 1972, Sir Keith Joseph, the Secretary of State for Social Services, made a speech in which he referred to the 'cycle of deprivation' which has become a challenge to all those in the health-caring professions and in teaching ever since. The cycle of deprivation refers to the perpetuation of emotional deprivation as a result of bad or uninformed parenthood and parental maladjustment. Whereas health visitors half a century ago spent a lot of time among the poorer sections of the community in helping them to compensate for their poverty and basic ignorance about a child's physical needs, it seems as though the same process will now need to be repeated in respect of emotional deprivation.

Fostering Natural Instincts

Parentcraft, as taught in schools, cannot afford *not* to keep pace with this advance of ideas. All the evidence suggests that attitudes towards children and an appreciation of the needs of small children for their proper emotional growth must be understood well before boys and girls actually embark upon parenthood. Some of these needs have already been outlined in the chapter on mental health, and need not be repeated here. When we observe the behaviour of children in the infants' and junior school, we see that there is some natural instinct towards parenthood, and that this is acted out in the games that children play, particularly with the Wendyhouse.

It is at this stage of emotional development that children are more naturally compassionate and are eager to protect weaker creatures, to look after them, and to make them happy. This is one direction in which keeping pets in the classroom can help. At this stage of development, small children can identify the needs of other children with their own needs; they are still in the stage of dependence; they are still home-orientated; they have not so far had sufficient experience to become disillusioned with the world as it really is. An examination of their usual play material and reading matter shows that the mother-centred, child-orientated, home is their ideal, but there is very little guidance on the role of fathers. Only in the case of the books on *Orlando the Cat* does a father figure appear in any other than a shadowy fashion as someone who merely provides the material needs of life. In the Orlando stories on the other hand, the father's role is shown also as a husband role and these stories may well provide basic material for discussion of parental roles with small children.

Involvement of Boys

In the case of younger children, there does not seem to be any difficulty about gender roles and small boys seem to be acceptable to small girls in the roles of fathers. In older boys, there is an understandable rejection of the domestic role, and this constitutes a difficulty for those who have tried to involve boys in parentcraft lessons. This difficulty might be resolved if the appropriate gender role could be identified. The idea that young fathers should simply be 'auxilliary mothers' acquiring the basic skills of nappy-changing, bathing babies, and the like, is not really sufficient. There is a danger that children today are being confused about the gender role of their parents and that the essentially masculine contribution is not appreciated. Ideally, this is support for the mother in every possible way, not only in material terms and in facilities, but also morally and by giving her the same consistent affection which she needs in order to be able to dispense the same commodity to her children.

Deprived Parents

Writers who criticise parents who are not providing consistent affection for their children too often overlook the fact that the parents themselves have been deprived and are now depriving each other, hence the cycle of deprivation already referred to. It is also idle to make an approach to older boys on purely sentimental grounds. They are anxious at this moment to reject their own childhood; they are not in tune with the emotions and needs of younger children, but they will be more likely to understand their role in supplying these when they become parents if they had an idea of how children develop emotionally and socially, and to realize that they themselves have been through these stages, although they were not conscious of it at the time.

The study of child development therefore must rate high in priorities in parentcraft training for both girls and boys. There is an opportunity even in the conventional lessons dealing with physical care. For example, the familiar 'bathing the baby' situation can be exploited to enter into a discussion upon the effect of parental skills and attitudes on children as a result of the kind of care they receive.

Margaret Mead's film *Bathing a Baby in Three Cultures* although made over forty years ago is still valid, because it compares the effects of the Nigerian, United States, and Balinese cultures from the relationships between babies and their mothers and the effect this has upon the future development of the child. It has been found experimentally that this film can be used effectively with C stream girls and that they are able to appreciate the abstract concepts implicit in the film in a way that would have been impossible if an attempt had been made to explain them verbally and didactically.[2]

Society's Evaluation of Childhood

Adolescent boys and, perhaps nowadays, quite a few adolescent girls, do not quite appreciate the high value placed upon childlife by the society in which they live. It would do much to temper the uninformed criticisms of the middle-aged generation if it were pointed out how children's needs have been given priority for nearly a century in our society, which has been made more compassionate and temperate towards these weakest members of our community.

Discussions on child cruelty and the battered baby and news items such as the occasional theft of a baby by a maladjusted young woman would always be useful topics for discussions with older age-groups. Child development can be studied in some excellent films that are available where children's behaviour has been filmed objectively and its interpretation can be achieved by discussion. The law relating to the protection of child health and wellbeing should also form one of the topics of a comprehensive parentcraft curriculum.

Parental Stress

A neglected area of parentcraft is the study of the reactions of parents to their children, it being assumed too readily that the parent is a well-established stable person, able to tolerate any amount of irritation and stress and always smiling and serene in return. This is not true, and perhaps many of the cases of the battered-baby syndrome are due to the parental threshold to irritability being lowered as a result of cumulative stress, emotional deprivation, and feelings of disillusionment about marriage and family life in general. It is known that children do provoke their parents, and although usually the naturally kindly instincts will restrain a parent from reacting in too violent a manner, even kindly parents sometimes strike their children. Nevertheless, skilful parents will create a climate in the home in which the opportunities for provocation are minimized. Perhaps the best example is of avoiding imposing disciplinary patterns which are not practicable and which will never succeed. The loss of face resulting from rebellion against the discipline makes the parent as insecure as the child. On the other hand there is need to emphasize that some boundaries of discipline and limitations of behaviour actually create emotional security in children and even in adolescents.

Emotional Development

The far-reaching effects of parentcraft on the behaviour of adults is another justification for concentrating nowadays on the emotional development of children and guiding them through life experiences in which they need support. It is remarkable how the mothers of youths who are convicted of serious crimes involving physical violence consistently state that their son had always been a *good boy.*

(We might enquire what the term 'good boy' means in this

context.) Sometimes this is a reflection of an attitude in which boys respect no females at all, save their mothers for whom they have an infantile emotional and dependent tie. We have already referred to the fact that in every human personality there are two sets of characteristics and that in a baby they are evenly matched. The aggressive and sadistic characteristics in the baby do not matter much because the child is too small to do much harm; at worst he can be a nuisance. It is by a process of education and socialization in which the main motivation is secure consistent affection that the aggressive characteristics are gradually subdued and channelled into constructive use. This is a process which really only the mother can do, with the father's help, and the example that the parents will offer to the child in their behaviour to each other and to the other siblings in the family and to friends will be an important factor.

Baby-Sitting

The most realistic situation in which to teach these concepts is that of baby-sitting. Perhaps the majority of schoolgirls will baby-sit at some time or another and sometimes they will be joined by their boyfriends and frequently they will receive some kind of reward for this service. They are however acting as child-minders, completely untrained, and the parents who ask them to perform this service for them are usually thinking only in terms of protection from common danger, for example, should the house catch fire, or should the child be accidentally smothered, fall out of bed and the like. These are obviously primary and important factors, but in handing their babies over to adolescent boys and girls for an evening, parents are also risking emotional trauma to their children which may be transient and can be recovered from but which could be cumulative. It is therefore important that teenagers who undertake baby-sitting should know exactly what to do when a child wakes up and cries. The diagnosis of the reason for crying should not be confined entirely to wetness, dryness, hunger, thirst, or any of the conventional causes but should be interpreted also in the light of fear of being found alone without the familiar encircling arms of the mother. The teenage baby-sitter has to be a substitute for these encircling arms, and in the demeanour that he or she shows to the child, a communication will pass between them which will either comfort and reassure the child and cause the crying to cease, or may actually accentuate it. There is always the risk of the teenager's threshold to irritability being suddenly lowered, and this may happen even to the best disposed youngster.

Role of a Substitute Parent

Teenagers who undertake baby-sitting with older children must realize that if the child comes down from bed and asks to have a story read, then it is their duty to do so, and they should read the story with real interest, not in a perfunctory manner showing the child fully that it is boring to them. They must expect to play with the child's toys and even perhaps to improvise stories if asked for. This is essentially the parental role, and this applies equally to either gender. They must be aware of the real terror that a child can experience as a result of thinking it has been abandoned by its parents.

No one should be asked to baby-sit who does not already know the child, and is recognized by the child as a member of the family and trusted by the parents. It is necessary for the baby-sitter to understand the child's private language, the words he uses when he wants to go to the lavatory, or have a drink etc. The baby-sitter must also realize that stern discipline is not appropriate and that less harm will come from nursing and cuddling a child who has got up out of bed, reading stories, playing with him and so on, than will occur if a child is repeatedly put back to bed, simply because the baby-sitter thinks that this is the right thing to do.

The practice of baby-sitting could be encouraged as a valuable experience for boys and girls who will eventually have their own children. No aspect of this experience should incur any risk to the small child who is involved. This applies to all parentcraft training and children should not be used merely as teaching objects or tools of health education for the benefit of older children.

Ideas for Syllabuses

A valuable guide to syllabuses is provided by the National Association for Maternal and Child Welfare. [3] This organization has a parentcraft training scheme extended to many schools in the United Kingdom under the direction of a parentcraft adviser who is responsible to an education committee. The aims of the scheme for the study of child care and human development are stated to be:-

1. To contribute towards the education of young people for family life, parenthood, citizenship, and personal relationships.
2. To teach the basic physical needs of children and all individuals.
3. To show something of the emotional, intellectual, social, and spiritual needs.
4. To implement and clarify knowledge already absorbed.
5. To help the rising generation to be competent to deal with whatever life may bring.

The basic course is intended to provide a foundation for all young people and it includes practical instruction, encouragement of contact with or observation of children, and the teaching of theory.

An understanding of simple anatomy and physiology and the development of the foetus is included, and studies are made of the care of the expectant mother, attitudes to birth, and the birth of the baby itself. Safety and first aid, diet and health, childish illnesses and home nursing and character training form part of the syllabus.

The more advanced syllabuses and examinations are concerned with the study of child care and human development and are progressive. Studies of development include puberty and problems of adolescence, so that the ideal of confronting the teenager with himself or herself can be achieved. In Part Two, the needs of the child include emotional needs, opportunities for play, cultural needs etc. Heredity and environment are studied and physical development is studied at a deeper level. Venereal diseases are included in the topics at this stage. There then follow studies on intellectual development, emotional development, and social development.

Contemporary Problems

Part Three of the general syllabus aims at the study of several contemporary problems, including the battered-baby syndrome. The effects of deprivation, of the child not being wanted, and the child who is specially gifted are included, as well as attitudes to handicapped children and their parents. The management of accidents and first aid is included in the section dealing with childish illnesses.

It is when we come to the section dealing with parenthood that we find an integration of preparation for marriage and for family life. For example, the home, the mother and father, changing roles of relatives with a new baby, the family unit, the one-parent family, and family planning are all included. The problem of caring for other people's children already referred to includes baby-sitting and the problem of children in homes and foster children. Community studies tackle the problems of immigration, social security, budgeting, and communication.

The N.A.M.C.W. scheme is operated in a number of local educational authorities and local resources are used. In order to attain the approval of the studies for entry to the N.A.M.C.W. certificate examinations, approval from the association will be necessary.

Practical Experience

It is required that students will have had experience with children of all ages, including some work in nursery schools, playgroups, or holiday playgrounds, or some work in infants' schools for the over-fives. Local visits to clinics and other institutions and organizations dealing with health are required. The Association recognizes that the study of child care and child development involving discussions of standards of behaviour and culture will be applied by the students to their own lives. Among other things, this will encourage some insight into other people's points of view, parents, relatives, the elderly, teachers, and those in authority. Boy-girl relationships may also be seen in a fresh light.

These syllabuses are followed by classes of girls, boys, and of mixed groups, but mature students may also take the advanced courses. The advantages of the N.A.M.C.W. scheme are that it is possible to cover all levels of intellectual attainment. The award of a certificate for the basic examination, although not a qualification in any way, is an encouragement to girls who may have very little educational success in another direction. The syllabuses can also in a way be regarded as an introduction to general health education, as they open up many avenues for discussion of fundamental issues regarding health, disease, relationships, and behaviour. That they would be of great advantage in conducting the syllabuses for mixed groups would seem to be obvious.

Basic Skills

Of the boys and girls who take these courses and succeed in the certificate, the girls of course will in the majority of cases have the advantage of further instruction from health visitors when they marry and become pregnant. They will however have some basic skill and knowledge on which to build, and their husbands, if they have also been to a similar course, will have an understanding of the support that their wives require and of the attitude that they must adopt towards their future child.

This is of primary importance -- there can be nothing so discouraging as a situation where an expectant mother, or the mother of young children, is given advice by doctors and nurses which she cannot follow at home because her husband obstructs her, or will not help her. In some cases, husbands are supported by their own mothers or mothers-in-law in their opposition and a tense family situation arises which may lay the foundations for bad relationships for the rest of life, which will have an adverse effect on grandchildren.

Where the husband and wife can stand firm in their resolve to carry out advice, however, and can tactfully resist any attempts to interfere with their actions, then the situation can be saved. It may therefore be more important that a boy understands the needs of mothers of young children, and how these may be achieved, than that he should be particularly skilful in changing nappies, manipulating safety-pins, or giving bottle-feeds. It cannot be escaped that gender role is still important in family and social life, and that a clear identification of gender role is an essential factor in the child's emotional development.

QUESTIONS

1. What are your views on (a) breast feeing (b) artificial feeding (c) feeding according to the clock and (d) feeding on demand? Give the pros and cons for each.

2. What part, if any, should habit training play in the first year of life? Have you any views on 'potting' a child?

3. How would you help a child of say two years to distinguish between right and wrong?

4. A time comes when the young child shows signs of wanting to be independent. In what ways would you help it to achieve this aim with confidence?

REFERENCES

1. Dalzell-Ward, A. J. (1961). 'L'École des Parents Paris'. *Cerebral Palsy Bulletin.* 32: 180-82.
2. Porter, D. Lynton. (1957). Personal communication to the author.
3. National Association for Maternal and Child Welfare (1973). Revised syllabus and examinations.

FURTHER READING

BBC. (1964). *Growth and Play.* London: BBC Publications.

Bowlby, John and Fry, Margery (1970). *Child Care and the Growth of Love.* Harmondsworth: Penguin.

British Parent Education Information Circle. *Quarterly Bulletin.* (Obtainable from Mrs. J. Hall M.Phil., B.Sc., 6, Westborough Drive, Halifax.)

Creese, Angela (1968). *Safety for Your Family.* London: Mills and Boon.

Finlay, Frances (1969). *Boy in Blue Jeans: A Woman's Story of her Delinquent Son.* London: Robert Hale.

Frankenburg, C.U. (1970). *Commonsense about Children: A Parents' Guide to Delinquency.* London: Arco.

Kellmer-Pringle, M. L., Davie, R. and Hancock, L. E. (eds.) (1969). *Directory of Voluntary Organizations Concerned with Children* (National Children's Bureau). London: Longmans. (See also other publications of the National Children's Bureau.)

MacKeith, Joseph and Michael (1966). *New Look at Child Health.* London: Pitman.

National Association for Maternal and Child Welfare. (1973). *A Guide to Developmental Studies Syllabus: 1973—75.* (NAMCW publications are obtainable from the Association at Tavistock House North, Tavistock Square, London WC1 9JG.)

Pitcairn, L. (1963). *The Young Student's Book of Child Care.* Cambridge: CUP.

Pitcairn, L. (1968). *Parents of the Future.* Cambridge: CUP.

Pitcairn, L. (1970). *Baby-sitting.* London: National Asociation for Maternal and Child Welfare.

Ratcliffe, T. A. (1967). *The Development of Personality.* London: Allen and Unwin.

Royal Society for the Prevention of Acidents. (1962). *Safety in the Home.* Yorkshire: Educational Productions.

Spock, Benjamin (1969). *Baby and Child Care.* London: Bodley Head.

Stewart, W. F. R. (1970). *Children in Flats: A Family Study.* London: NSPCC.

FILMS

Title	Colour B/W	Running time	Distributor	Date
Motherhood	Colour	20 mins.	Cow and Gate Limited, Motherhood Bureau, Stoke Road, Guildford, Surrey	1968
Their First Year	Colour	30 mins.	Guild Sound & Vision Ltd.	1966
Your Children and You	B/W	28 mins.	Scottish Central Film Library	
Afraid of School	B/W	28 mins.	Concord	1965
Children Growing Up 1. Mother and Child 2. Making Sense 3. Power of Speech 4. All in the Game	B/W	25 mins. each	B.B.C. T.V. Enterprises — Film Hire	1970
Children Thinking 1. Discovering the World 2. The Moon Follows Me 3. 'Cos It's Naughty' 4. Playing the Game	B/W	30 mins. each	B.B.C. T.V. Enterprises — Film Hire	1968
Over Dependency	B/W	31 mins.	Central Film Library	1949
Aggressive Child	B/W	28 mins.	Concord	1965
Angry Boy	B/W	33 mins.	Concord	1965
Girl in Danger	B/W	28 mins.	Concord	1965

CHAPTER 14

The school health service

The question is frequently asked — sometimes even in final examinations — whether, in view of the existence of the National Health Service giving comprehensive care to all age-groups, the school health service is justified in its continuance. It is impossible to answer this question objectively without a grasp of the general principles on which the service operates.

Unique Functions

The superficial resemblance of medical techniques of clinical examination should not mislead an observer into believing that the school medical officer is a substitute for the general practitioner. Neither is the general practitioner an effective substitute for the school medical officer, if the relationship between health and education is to be preserved. The aim of the service has always been to enable children to take full advantage of the education provided for them. The school health service, moreover, is staffed by a team of professionals who exercise surveillance over the health of all school children in order to identify those in particular need and to provide help when necessary.

The team includes doctors with specialist training, dentists, psychologists, social workers, and of course, the teachers themselves. Teachers are directly involved in the working of the school health service from the point of view that the service is designed to help the child to benefit from education and also to help the identification of the child who is at risk of falling behind his peers in the ordinary school curriculum and who is in need of special help, remedial teaching, and follow-on assessment. Although all teachers will feel empathy for the sick or handicapped child, from their professional point of view, they will be interested in the ways in which medical techniques can help such a child to overcome disability and realize his full educational potential.

The First Screening Service

The history of the school health service shows how its method of practice has been adapted according to changing social and medical scenes. It is the first example of a screening service, and in its early years, as we have already mentioned, its main preoccupation was the diagnosis of severe illness and defects and arranging for their treatment. Such a screening function has not come to an end, because with the advance of medical knowledge, disorders have now come to light for which techniques were not available for diagnosis formerly. Nowadays, quite a lot of screening is undertaken before the child enters school.

Screening Before School Entry

All births are notified to the area health authority and health visitors pay at least one visit to the home in which a new birth has been notified. Homes are selected by general practitioners, paediatricians, or community physicians in conjunction with the health visitor in cases where it is believed that constant attention will be required during the pre-school years. Mothers of young children are encouraged to take them for regular check-ups at child health centres where doctors and nurses specially trained in the new clinical science of developmental paediatrics can assess the child's physical and emotional development and intellectual development. They can also diagnose any disorders which would benefit from treatment. During this time mothers receive health education in the management of the normal child and the care of the sick child.

However there is a considerable falling off of attendance after the age of two, so that any disorders which were not detectable or had not developed before that age, may be missed unless the child has symptoms severe enough to require the attention of a family doctor. With the advent of the National Health Service there is no economic barrier to taking a child to the doctor, but there still remains a considerable barrier of misunderstanding in some social groups. General practitioners and their colleagues in hospitals have had a greater opportunity during the last twenty-five years of tackling disorders of childhood. At the time that the child enters school there is a record of information concerning congenital malformations, metabolic disorders, or mental and physical handicap. In some cases it is only the family doctor who would have an opportunity of making a diagnosis.

Assessment of Health in the School Environment

At the time of writing a new concept of medical examination on entry into school is planned. This will be designed to assess a child's developmental progress, learning potential, and liability to develop emotional or behavioural disturbance, or any innate inability to cope with the normal educational curriculum in an ordinary school.

This advance has been stimulated by the findings of clinical research which have demonstrated associations between learning disorders at school and neurological abnormalities or deviations in developmental skills. Behaviour or learning disorders resulting from these abnormalities may not show themselves until the age of nine or even later, by which time the child's performance is very much behind that of his age-group.

The medical examination on entry includes measurements, general physical examination, testing of vision, hearing, speech, and language. Neurological development tests are also carried out and these include motor function, co-ordination, dexterity, perceptual function, and various neurological functions e.g. the range of eye movements, anomalies in the usual tendon reflexes which may suggest defects in neural control of movement, clumsiness etc. When all tests have been carried out, and the information collated together with the parents' own report on the child, the school medical officer then makes a final assessment of the child.

This new method of assessment takes the school environment into account e.g. the first contact with large numbers of children, with teachers and the stress inevitably involved in school life which may have an effect on any disorder that has been detected.

In case of very severe handicap the recommendation for Special Educational Treatment (SET) is one of the most important responsibilities of the school medical officer. The tendency nowadays is to educate handicapped children in normal schools as far as possible and it is mutually beneficial to normal and handicapped alike. There are some however whose handicap is so severe as to require regular medical attendance, nursing, or procedures such as physiotherapy but whose educational potential is the same as that of other children. These must necessarily attend special schools, sometimes boarding schools.

General Picture of the School Child's Health

The general picture of the health of school children in the UK is good, so that major disorders affecting children in this age-group are concentrated in a minority. In terms of mortality, over 50% of the deaths of children in the age-groups 5-9 and 10-14 are due to accidents and, unfortunately, to malignant diseases which, of course, are extremely rare in children. In terms of categories of pupils requiring SET the prevalence in the age-groups 2-19 is remarkably low. For example, delicate children account for 1.3 per thousand pupils, physically handicapped, 1.5, epileptics, 0.1, deaf and partially hearing, 0.9, blind and partially sighted, 0.5, speech defects, 0.03, maladjusted, 1.5, and ESN, 7.8. The report of the Chief Medical Officer of the Department of Education and Science for 1969-70 stated that 50-60% of the defects observed affect the sensory and motor skills and also vision, hearing, speech, skin disorders, and to a small extent nutrition. [1]

New problems have arisen, paradoxically, as a result of developments in medical and surgical treatment. For example, children are now successfully operated on for the closure of spina bifida but they survive with a handicap. The thalidomide deformities and the personal and social problems they raise have received wide publicity but it is less well known that in the early 1950s blindness due to retro-lental fibroplasia occurred in some children who had been premature at birth and who had been exposed to concentrations of oxygen in the incubator that subsequently were found to be too high. Knowledge regarding the effects of the maternal environment on the growing child *in utero* is increasing but there are still many gaps. Congenital disorders of a new character are likely to continue to raise problems in the future.

In the case of defects and disorders already present and which are non-progressive, children will have to learn to live with them for the rest of their lives. With the necessary family support, help from

Table 15. Prevalence of physical disorder in ten- to twelve-year-old children: $N = 3271$

Disorders	Boys	Girls	Total	Rate per 1000
All physical disorders	102	84	186*	56.9
Asthma	43	33	76	23.2
Eczema	15	19	34	10.4
Uncomplicated epilepsy	15	6	21	6.4
Cerebral palsy	9	6	15	4.6
Other brain disorders	6	6	12	3.7
Orthopaedic conditions	6	5	11	3.4
Heart disease	3	5	8	2.4
Deafness	4	2	6	1.8
Diabetes mellitus	1	3	4	1.2
Neuromuscular disorders (with lesions at or below the brain stem)	2	2	4	1.2
Miscellaneous disorders (not specified above)	5	7	12	3.7

*Because of some overlap between conditions the total exceeds the sum of the rates for individual conditions.

Source: Rutter, M., Tizard, J. and Whitmore, K. (1970). *Education, Health and Behaviour* (Report of a survey in the Isle of Wight). London: Longmans. p. 285.

Results of a medical survey conducted on school children aged 10–12 in the Isle of Wight.

doctors, teachers, and friends, they will become skilful in so doing. In some cases there will be emotional difficulties and this applies particularly to diabetes where a child is encouraged to live a normal life and yet has to rely on his regular injections of insulin and his own judgment as to the kind of food he can take, whether he is in danger of hypoglycaemia, and so on.

From what we understand about the principles of mental health, and emotional growth, the school medical officer and his colleagues also have an opportunity of prevention of psychiatric disorders in adult life. Again to quote from the report of the CMO Department of Education and Science, problems associated with puberty and adolescence are largely missed until they reach a crisis point, for example, serious academic failure, behavioural problems, unmarried motherhood, delinquency, or drug addiction. By the exercise of 'medical awareness' problems of puberty can be detected long before the crisis point.

Medical Inspection

The policy regarding routine medical examination has undergone radical changes in the last twenty years. One beneficial result of the traditional routine inspection of all children has been that school medical officers have become the major experts in the assessment of normality — an essential baseline from which to detect departures from the normal. On the other hand, having regard to the limited resources available, and to the intrusion into academic time, the new policies of selective examination which have been adopted by at least a third of local education authorities in England and Wales have much to recommend them. New regulations have been introduced which no longer make entry and leaving examinations statutory and do not lay down a minimum number of routine examinations required. This allows local education authorities far greater flexibility in their policies.

No education authority has actually abandoned the entry examination and this has great value in that the school medical officer can explain to the parents the aims and scope of the school health service, something, perhaps, of which they were not aware and they may not have realized how the service can supplement that given by their family doctors as regards the educational setting. The doctor can also discuss with the teachers any disability which is already existing but which may affect the child's progress. There is a health education situation also in that the doctor can offer personal counselling to parents and in many cases he is available to give talks to groups of parents.

In many education authorities parents are invited to complete a questionnaire before the medical examination. There is one variation of this practice where school nurses visit the home to interview the parents and to complete the questionnaire on their behalf. The information obtained from the parents' own assessment of their child is a valuable contribution to the first medical examination as is of course the teacher's assessment. With the future establishment of linkage-systems for medical records, the school medical officer will also have information regarding conditions that have been observed by the family doctor, by the medical officer at a child health centre, or in hospital.

Children in Special Need

During the remainder of school life, selective medical inspection will concentrate on children in need of investigation and supervision. The advantage of the school health service being manned by full-time specialists is that it is possible to survey the entire school population and to identify the vulnerable groups within it. In that population, perhaps as many as a hundred individual family doctors will have children on their lists, and it would be an extremely difficult task to collect information from all of them in order to piece together the general health picture of the school. Another advantage is that the school medical officer is part of the educational team. He should be a regular visitor to the school, should be well known to all the teachers and can contribute considerably to the content of health education in the syllabus. This is specialist knowledge gained very largely by experience which is not available to the general practitioner, nor could it be expected of him. It will therefore not be sufficient for each individual child to have a school entry examination conducted by his own doctor.

Participation of Parents and Teachers

Selective examination where it is used relies partly upon the completion of further questionnaires by parents, and also the observations made by teachers, school nurses, and the school medical officers themselves. Crisis points in education are frequently associated with departures from health, and the school health service can contribute to the supportive treatment that the child will need at this time. There is therefore a sharing of responsibility and this is to the benefit of the child. It may well be therefore that the majority of children after the entry examination will not need to be seen by any of the school health service team during the remainder of their school life. The examination of leavers however has many advantages from the point of view of health education, and advice on future careers. In some authorities for example, I.L.E.A., it is the custom to issue school-leavers with booklets giving them advice on the protection of their health when they leave school and enter employment.

The records of physicians in charge of student health at universities show that in their case at any rate such advice has not been taken to any extent. There is a need for liaison between school medical officers and physicians in charge of student health services in all institutions of further education. With the setting up of the Employment Medical Advisory Service there will be a further opportunity of liaison with physicians in charge of employment medical services so that the disadvantage of a school-leaver being left high and dry, bereft of personal medical advice on the care of his health will disappear.

Teachers' Anxieties

Teachers can expect to have at least one child in their class during their careers who will be suffering from some disorder such as diabetes, epilepsy, or physical handicap. This will naturally produce anxiety in teachers, particularly those less experienced, and they will find that close contact with the school medical officer and nurse will be a great help in guiding them as to how these pupils should be handled. It is necessary to know just how much of normal school strain a handicapped child can endure and often the school medical officer can be reassuring on this point. He will be able to specify the kind of activities which are beneficial and which will not cause worsening of the handicap. At the same time the school medical officer has the advantage of being familiar with the educational setting and he can therefore anticipate specific hazards with which the child will be faced. It must be remembered that sometimes it is the school itself that is malfunctioning. (Plowden Report).

The school medical officer and nurse are also valuable allies in the case of deviant behaviour at all age-groups. In general, the teacher will be a partner with the school health service in maintaining the health surveillance of the child throughout school life, the detection of disorders which have not appeared before, the modification of the school programme for the child with handicap, and the assessment of the health component involved in educational failure or behavioural disorder. The work of the school health service itself provides a valuable teaching point as an introduction to the child to the National Health Service, and perhaps he may feel more personally involved in this setting than even with the family doctor, and also an explanation to the child of the ways in which medical knowledge and techniques can be applied for the promotion of health.

As it is impossible to generalize on the handling of children handicapped by physical or emotional disorder, the old notion of the health education syllabus for the college of education giving information to help the teacher in the classroom should now be modified. The teacher will find greater benefit from accepting a close professional relationship with the school medical officer and school nurse, who are sympathetic to the teacher's professional aims, and who understand them because of the nature of their own task.

Periodic Screening Process

Although selective medical inspection is now being increasingly used, there are still periodic screening procedures which should be carried out at intervals during school life. These are tests of eyesight, or hearing, measurement of height and weight — this is particularly useful to identify the overweight child — foot inspection, skin inspection, and general surveillance of hygiene, including the detection of verminous infestation which unfortunately is still fairly common. The frequency with which these periodic screening procedures are carried out is a matter for the policy of the local education authority. With regard to the testing of hearing, however, which is carried out by pure tone audiometry, the CMO Department of Education and Science has suggested that it should be done at approximately the ages of seven, ten, and thirteen. The measurement of height and weight has three advantages. Firstly, it provides the material for the anthropometric survey recommended originally by the Interdepartmental Committee on Phyical Deterioration; secondly, it enables an assessment of nutritional needs, and thirdly, it gives early warning of the onset of obesity.

It is perhaps in the case of the obese child that the special value of the school health service can be seen from the health education point of view. The medical officer will be able to make an assessment of the cause of the obesity, and this is not always simple, for example, many obese children do not eat as much as children of normal proportions. The handling of such a case will involve the whole family, it may involve the school meal service, and it may be necessary for the child to attend a special obesity clinic where weight reduction methods include health education.

Special Medical Examination

Provision is always made for special medical examinations on request. Even though a family doctor service is now freely available, many parents will request special medical examination by the school health service; in some cases, family doctors may refer children to the school medical officer because they appreciate that the treatment of a condition may be modified by the school programme and teachers and school nurses often observe changes in an individual child for which they request medical advice, with of course the consent of the parents and the family doctor.

The teacher plays an important part in the teamwork of surveillance, including the request for special medical examination. It is important however that non-medical members of the team should be aware both of the potential and the limitations of medical examination, as carried out in the school clinic or the school itself. For example, although it is now recognized that over-activity may have a neurological basis, this can hardly be detected or assessed in the school clinic, or even the family doctor's surgery.

Assessment Centres

The concept of assessment centres where the school health service works in conjunction with the paediatric department of the hospital is now being developed and this will have the advantage of the pooling of resources, in terms of medical expertise, special equipment, and a multidisciplinary team including educational and social as well as medical workers. The reorganization of the National Health Service and the employment of school medical officers by the area health authority will facilitate the development of assessment centres, particularly now that medical officers are trained in developmental paediatrics, opening up possibilities of new techniques and diagnosis and measures of treatment that have not been available before. This advantage outweighs the disadvantage in that the school medical officer is no longer employed directly by the local education authority. There is no reason to believe however that this administrative change is necessarily a barrier, and school medical officers, as specialists in their own right, will continue to be identified with the educational system.

Contemporary Tasks

The tasks for the modern school health service have been summarized by the CMO Department of Education and Science in the Report already referred to. There are twelve main tasks ranging from watching over the growth and development of the school child, having regard to the effect of the home environment, as well as that of the school, to working closely with family doctors and paediatricians. The range of duties includes the identification of children with specific disorders affecting learning and behaviour, (these are, principally, vision, hearing, speech, and neuro-psychiatric disorders); identification of physical defects at examination of entry; the carrying out of population screening procedures; the establishment of liaison and communication with schools including the interpretation to teachers of the educational significance of what is known medically about a child; and the supervision of school children with various disorders, for example, epilepsy and asthma, or diabetes, to arrange for supplementary treatment. There is also the making available of advice to adolescents who have psychosexual problems or problems of behaviour, for example, those involving the abuse of drugs.

Child Guidance

An important supportive service is the child guidance service staffed by psychiatrists with special experience in problems of children and adolescents, and a team comprising educational psychologists and psychiatric social workers. This is a service to which reference is made principally by school medical officers, although general practitioners may refer children directly. In a well-integrated service, the school medical officer and the psychiatrist who is the director of the child guidance clinic know each other well professionally and take every opportunity to meet and to discuss mutual problems.

The child guidance movement came to Europe from the United States in the early 1920s and although it has undergone considerable evolutionary change since that time, no longer for example relying entirely on Freudian psychology, it has been able to produce a considerable body of knowledge which can be used for health education and, therefore, for the prevention of maladjustment and mental breakdown. Of particular significance is the development of 'child and family psychiatry' and some specialists in this field hold that the designation 'child guidance clinic' is a handicap to the development of the service as it implies that it has the omniscience and omnipotence to guide children, parents, and teachers in the management of disturbances of behaviour. This is not so; it is rather that the professional team – psychiatrist, psychiatric social worker, educational psychologist and psychotherapist – has the capacity to evaluate some of the psychodynamic factors producing the disturbance and they can suggest ways in which these can be modified, provided that the family and school are prepared to accept their own involvement.

This concept has resulted in a greater flexibility of procedure in child guidance work, particularly a flexibility of role of the different members of the team. It is the practice to interview the whole family if possible as it is now recognized that a large proportion of the problems referred to clinics are in fact symptoms of disturbance within the whole family. The child is the presenting problem, but unless the whole family (this may even include aunts and uncles) are included within the treatment-process little change can be effected. Consultation with parents is essential as they are always directly involved and may be primarily involved. It should go without saying that teachers' reports too are most important to the diagnostic procedure. For the most part children will be referred to this service only as a result of personal crisis and to an increasing extent disturbed children can receive help in the school health service with the co-operation of teachers.

The child guidance service itself values the opportunity of consultation with paediatricians as the relationship between emotional and behavioural problems and developmental delays and abnormalities is an area requiring further exploration. This is in accord with the multidisciplinary nature of the professional work carried out at assessment centres.

The concept of 'family psychiatry' is relevant to the health education aims of the 'École des Parents' movement already referred to. The ideal organization comprises a diagnostic and remedial service, an associated research project, and an educational project. The three are interdependent and feed each other with experience and material. In the UK we owe a great deal of progress towards mental health education from the work of child guidance clinics. Some local authorities have already changed the name of their clinics to 'Clinic of Child and Family Psychiatry'.

The School Dental Service

The school dental service makes its own contribution to health education in addition to its primary function which is to inspect all school children at least annually so that pupils and parents may be made aware of any treatment that is needed and advised to obtain such treatment either from the school dental service or from a private dental practitioner.

It is staffed by full and part-time dental surgeons assisted by dental auxiliaries, that is women who have received a two-year training in doing fillings, extraction of primary teeth under local anaesthesia and other minor procedures, all of which have been prescribed by a supervising dentist. Also in the dental team are a small number of dental hygienists who do mainly scaling and cleaning of teeth under the supervision of the dentist. There are also dental surgery assistants who work in the surgery and in cases where the local authority has its own dental laboratory there are dental technicians to make dentures, orthodontic appliances etc. that have been prescribed by the dentist. The co-operation of teachers in every field of dental health education is of course a prerequisite and often it is of a very high order.

All staff of the school dental service are expected to play some part in dental health education and there is emphasis on instruction at the chairside. Because of the co-operation from the school dental service almost all local authorities carry out some form of dental health education. Thus talks are given in the classroom by dentists and dental hygienists and publicity campaigns are frequently undertaken. These usually involve other agencies such as the General Dental Council's health education section, the British Dental Association, and the Oral Hygiene Service. Some local authorities issue free toothbrushes, toothpaste, and beakers to children who have just entered school. The General Dental Council supplies posters, and leaflets, and booklets to schools to encourage oral hygiene, to stimulate interest in the care of the teeth and to persuade children to avoid dangerous sticky carbohydrates and to follow a diet which helps to build sound teeth. The GDC has also produced films, filmstrips, and slides which can be used by teachers.

Local authority dental officers examine pre-school children at child health centres, treatment being given when necessary. Children are also dentally examined on entry into school and subsequently during their school life. This itself has an educational effect as it makes parents aware of the need for regular dental care, and encourages children to accept this as part of normal life. Although as we have seen, treatment is often undertaken by private dentists working in the National Health Service, the school dental officer is the key figure to the maintenance of dental health.

Research

The school health service has a considerable and distinguished record of research during its long life. Health surveys of various kinds have been undertaken by individual school medical officers and by groups of school medical officers sometimes co-operating with doctors from hospitals or university departments of preventive medicine. An example was the study undertaken by the Kent Paediatric Society (now the Kent Child Health Society) between 1949 and 1953. [2] The research group which undertook the work voluntarily comprised a principal school medical officer of an Excepted District i.e. a county district to which the local education authority has delegated administration of the educational services, three school medical officers, two consultant paediatricians, and a director of a child guidance clinic. There was co-operation from the Department of Social Medicine of the University of Oxford and the group set out to make a study of the prevalence of completely healthy children in the 11-12 year-old age-group. One hundred children were identified from about 1,200 in this group and assessment was made not only on the absence of major organic disease, but also on positive factors, concerned with personality, scholastic achievement, and physical development, and stamina. It was interesting that the reports on the children by teachers lead to conclusions which were identical with those obtained by a group personality test.

This is only one example of research projects which have been undertaken by the school health service with the co-operation of teachers leading to improvement in knowledge about the needs of the school child and the ways in which his health can be protected and promoted. Another example of group research was conducted also in Kent in the Medway towns in connection with smoking habits of children aged eleven.

This was a joint project involving the schools, the county health department, the Central Council for Health Education, and the Social Medicine Department of a London teaching hospital. Studies were made of the smoking habits of the children and of the prevalence of symptoms such as morning cough and phlegm. A campaign was conducted in the classroom to inform the children of the dangers of smoking and an attempt was made to measure the effectiveness of this teaching. Amongst other findings it was discovered that children had symptons caused by smoking of an identical nature with those observed in adults. It was concluded that chronic bronchitis had its origin in childhood and that smoking was a cause. The educational efforts had had no effect on the smoking habits of these children and it was suggested that they would have been more effective if it had been demonstrated that smoking was causing ill health and lack of fitness at the time rather than in the future. [3]

With the new opportunities offered by the reorganization of the National Health Service, and establishment of assessment centres and the closer link between hospital departments of paediatrics and school medical officers, the scope of research may be expected to increase. Teachers have an excellent opportunity of co-operating in such research projects, and in fact most of them could not be carried out without their co-operation.

In summary, it will be seen from the foregoing that the school health service has a unique contribution to make to the health of the school child, and is neither competitive with nor an alternative to the family doctor. The adaptation made by the service during the process of social and medical evolution in the last seventy years is significant in the contribution that it has made to the reduction of avoidable illness. This contribution may be expected to increase, and also problems regarding educability of children, such as reading difficulties, behavioural difficulties, and so on, will also be resolved eventually with the help of the school health team. It is perhaps a prime example of the permanent continuing effect of the application of medical techniques outside the conventional therapeutic field.

The relevance to health education lies in the channelled communication between medicine and teaching afforded by the close contact between the school health service team and the school, and also the teaching situation which medical inspection, dental inspection, and periodic screening offer for health education in the classroom. It must not be thought that this contribution is all in one direction. The staff of the school health service also value close contact with teachers and for the most part would not care to be isolated in hospitals or clinics. The fact that medical inspection is carried out on school premises is significant.

Special Education Treatment

Categories of handicapped children defined in the Handicapped Pupils and Special Schools Regulations 1959:

> Blind Pupils
> Partially Sighted Pupils.
> Deaf Pupils.
> Partially Hearing Pupils.
> Educationally Subnormal Pupils.
> Epileptic Pupils.
> Maladjusted Pupils.
> Physically Handicapped Pupils.
> Pupils suffering from Speech Defect.
> Delicate Pupils.

The Regulations specify criteria for ascertainment and finally labelling of a school child as belonging to one of these categories. Readers should consult the Regulations made by the Secretary of State, Department of Education and Science, under the Education Act.

QUESTIONS

1. Should secondary schools each have a matron and/or a counsellor? Discuss the pros and cons.

2. Should routine medical examinations of pupils be increased in frequency or vice versa? In what ways may the teacher co-operate with the doctor on these occasions?

3. What has the health visitor to offer the teacher by way of health practices in school and involvement in teaching programmes?

APPENDIX ONE

Signs of Children at Risk

There are occasions when the caring teacher confronted with a pupil who is at risk may, with the best intentions in the world coupled with his eagerness to help the child, overstep into the realm of the diagnoser and even attempt some form of psychiatric treatment — this must be strenuously guarded against as must the tendency to become emotionally involved. The teacher's role is essentially that of a 'spotter', or scout, for those specially trained to deal with a pupil showing signs of disturbance. A sobering thought which is worth mentioning at this juncture is that the teacher may be at risk if the number of maladjusted children he has to deal with is excessive — a situation not unknown in some of the large secondary schools in disadvantaged areas.

To help the teacher in his task of identifying a child at risk, some of the undermentioned signs and symptoms are worth bearing in mind.

1. Reluctance to attend school and/or to truant.
2. Preoccupation with problems located in the house, the neighbourhood, or even the school.
3. Passive or indifferent attitude towards studies, school affairs, and peers (few, if any friends).
4. Aggressiveness — sometimes with disastrous consequences. The aggressiveness may be inhibited and reveal itself in role-playing, drawings, and non-co-operation (bloody-mindedness).
5. Withdrawal or depression — this might be a passing phase due to temporary inability to cope with lessons or companions.
6. Inconsistent behaviour — great care must be exercised here to avoid confusing such behaviour with that which is characteristic of normal adolescent development. It might well be a symptom of drug abuse!
7. The child at risk is inevitably insecure and seeks attention in many ways — exaggerated behaviour, *petit mal*, lying (when not necessary i.e. trying to avoid, or to get out of, trouble) being noisy, disruptive. The first reaction towards a divergent pupil is to be critical, but make sure that the divergence is not due to circumstances which are threatening the child before taking action. Compassion and understanding are required for the pupil at risk.

APPENDIX TWO

Signs of Teachers at Risk

It is surprising that so many people, especially those in authority, do not appear to recognize the fact that a teacher may also be at risk. Perhaps the undermentioned circumstances, signs and symptoms might be noted.

1. Working in a school in a disadvantaged area (social, psychological, and educational problems are very acute in these areas).
2. Large classes
3. Classes with an undue percentage of disturbed pupils
4. Remoteness of head teacher
5. Not being included in consultations concerning the policy and organization of the school.
6. Poor internal communications
7. Unresolved intimate personal problems.
8. Unsuitable temperament
9. Personal health

Signs and Symptoms

1. Frequent short absences and/or late coming.
2. Starting a lesson late and finishing early.
3. Deterioration in general attitude to pupils and to school affairs.
4. Preoccupation; undue shouting; persistent or unjustified criticism; irritability; apathy, indigestion, migraine, and other physical disturbances.
5. Deterioration in class management and routine matters, e.g. preparing lessons, marking work etc.

REFERENCES

1. Department of Education and Science. (1972). *Health of the School Child.* Report of the Chief Medical Officer: 1969-70. London: HMSO.
2. Landon, J. (ed.) (1954). *The Epidemiology of Health.* Report by the Research Committee of the Kent Paediatric (now the Child Health) Society. Health Department, Bexley, Kent (now London Borough of Bexley): Kent Paediatric Society.
3. Holland, W. W. and Elliot, A. (1968). 'Cigarette Smoking, Respiratory Symptoms and Anti-Smoking Propaganda'. *Lancet.* 1:41-3.

FURTHER READING

Bowden, D. E. J., Davies, R. M., Holloway, P. J., Lemon, M. A. and Rugg-Gunn, A. J. (1973). 'A Treatment Survey of a Fifteen-year-old Population.' *Brit. Dental J.* 134: 375.

Department of Education and Science. (1966). *Health in Education.* Educational Pamphlet No. 49. London: HMSO.

Department of Education and Science. (1967). *Children and their Primary Schools* (Plowden Report). London: HMSO.

Department of Health and Social Security. (1973). *First Report by the Sub-committee on Nutritional Surveillance.* (Reports on Health and Social Subjects). (This Report contains appendices on the history of the arrangements for the provision of school meals, milk and welfare milk, and other data concerning growth studies and 'reasons against mounting a milk-feeding trial in children').

Leff, S. and Leff, V. (1959). *School Health Service.* London: H. K. Lewis.

James, F. E. (1970). *Educational Medicine.* London: Heinemann.

Rutter, M., Tizard, J. and Whitmore, K. (1970). *Education, Health and Behaviour* (Report of a survey in the Isle of Wight). London: Longmans.

CHAPTER 15

Matters of public concern

The five topics selected for discussion in this section represent matters of public concern at the present day. In defining what may be a matter of public concern, the following criteria are used.

1. The topic is discussed publicly in the press, on television and radio.
2. There is a consensus that the problem involves the whole community and, in some cases, the future of the community.
3. Public spokesmen, including those self-appointed, give continual advice on the solution of the problem but usually based upon one aspect.
4. The areas involved have been extensively researched.

The ages at which problems begin to be experienced vary. Many school-children begin to smoke at the age of eleven. Schofield's researches indicate that the age of inception of sexual activity is fifteen in the case of boys. The peak age at which unwanted pregnancies and sexually transmitted disease occur is between 18-24. Heavy drinking is now observed in teenagers who also experiment with certain drugs, but heroin addiction is hardly ever a school problem. The cancers, included here purely under the category of matters of public concern, are predominately a problem of middle adult life and the later years. The prevention of cancer however is already a matter of personal responsibility for young adults e.g. co-operation in cervical cytology screening programmes as well as preserving a high standard of personal hygiene in the sexual relationship, and — of course — refraining from smoking.

However, as we have already pointed out, school health education should not confine itself only to matters of the moment. There is a particularly vulnerable period of life after leaving school and before marrying (a step that involves necessary contact with the social services) which offers the social services an opportunity to give further guidance and counselling. This vulnerability increases greatly between seventeen and twenty-four, for example, in the case of sexually transmitted infections, the peak age of incidence, judged by attendance at clinics, is between eighteen and twenty-four.

The five topics under discussion are a preoccupation of health education at the present day which is sometimes unfortunate in that unnecessary emphasis is given to problems to the detriment of fundamental health education which, if carried out thoroughly, should tend to reduce the incidence of problems. It is generally agreed however that at the secondary level of education all these five topics should be included in a general programme. Some of them are highly emotive, for example, the subjects of birth control and drug-taking, and this makes it all the more important that they should not be given undue emphasis and treated in isolation. All the topics involve human behaviour and deliberate choice of action; four have legal sanctions attached to them, and all are the subject of governmental activity and interest in all countries.

Birth Control

This term is preferable to family planning, because the latter, by definition is concerned with the development of a family by spacing out births so that undue economic and social stress is not incurred. 'Birth control', on the other hand, not only affects all sexually active people, whether married or not, but allows us to include abortion under this heading. The methods of birth control range from abstinence from sexual intercourse, a factor which is seldom mentioned at the present day, control of sexual intercourse by withdrawal, or by choosing infertile periods during the menstrual cycle, the provision of mechanical barriers to prevent the sperm reaching the ovum, chemical attack on the sperm, the I.U.C.D. to prevent implantation of a fertilized ovum, and the most ingenious and scientific of all, the use of contraceptive pills. Further to this, there is sterilization both for males and females, and, as a last resort, abortion.

Some will doubt the wisdom of going into details of these methods with schoolchildren, lest it should encourage them to experiment with promiscuous sexual activity. There is no clear evidence of this, neither on the other hand is there any evidence that such education does make young people more cautious about their sexual relationships. Michael Schofield's study showed that the sexually active proportion of the sample were aware of contraceptive methods, but seldom used them, and the motives for not using them were entirely emotional, and, in the case of boys, were associated with the desire for toughness and the exhilaration of taking risks, although, in this case, they were taking risks with other people's lives.

AN INTELLECTUAL EXCERCISE
Nevertheless, most authorities accept that discussion about birth control should be included in a general programme of sex education which again should emphasize the importance of personal relationships. We have already mentioned how every child is exposed at the present day to information of all kinds through the mass media. They will have heard about birth control, they will have read about it, and they will have discussed it amongst themselves.

The subject can in fact become an intellectual exercise, and perhaps this is the first instance where a working knowledge of the menstrual cycle is of equal value to boys, as it is to girls. The idea that boys should be included in the instruction about menstruation was based on rather vague idealistic principals of equality between the sexes. It is clear, however, that boys, when confronted with problems of birth control, should understand the nature of the menstrual cycle and how fertility can be controlled by various methods. There is evidence too that young married couples are extremely ignorant about contraception, and are unable to make a choice of a method suitable to them without some guidance.

SOCIAL FUNCTIONS OF BIRTH CONTROL
The social functions of birth control can be summarized as, first, to limit population growth, secondly, to prevent illegitimacy and, third, to separate the function of sexual activity as part of a relationship and personal enjoyment from the function of pro-creation. Moral issues are obviously involved, and there is a by no means small, and vocal section of the community which objects to the widespread use of contraceptive methods by those other than married people, while the Roman Catholic Church disapproves of any method of contraception, save the restriction of intercourse to the infertile period.

Considerable alarm has been evinced all over the world about population growth. Attention has been drawn to the problem of providing sufficient food, shelter, transportation, and amenities to a population that could easily out-distance its economic resources. For once, Malthus is not discredited, despite ideological gestures, for Malthus seems to offend particularly Marxist views. This concern with population growth has led to views expressed by many public spokesmen that married couples should be rationed as to the number of children they should have. Some have even suggested penalizing them by reducing or removing child allowances, and forecasted that in the future married couples would require a licence to produce children. Such views are repugnant to many people and a counter-view has been put forward that excessive population growth is concerned only with unwanted pregnancies, occurring both outside and inside marriage. [1] Hence the slogan that every child should be a 'wanted child', which is being used at the present time in health education for birth control.

There is also an inevitable association between high population density and a low standard of living. It has been pointed out however that the Netherlands is very highly populated, but also enjoys a high standard of living, although it is true that in undeveloped countries an improvement in the standard of living is usually followed by a fall in birth-rate. Another problem in the undeveloped and developing countries is that water supplies cannot keep pace with the growth in population; there is widespread malnutrition, and also illiteracy. It is difficult enough to practice health education amongst literate populations, but the problem in the case of illiteracy is formidable.

A POPULATION POLICY

Figures have been calculated for an optimum birth-rate to ensure replacement of the population without an undue preponderance of old people and, at the same time, to provide a safeguard against overpopulation. For this country a figure of 13.5 per thousand has been calculated as the optimum birth-rate, and in 1971, the birth rate was 16.2 [2]

The population panel set up by the government in the United Kingdom to advise on population policy has produced a four-point plan which includes the development of comprehensive family planning services as part of the National Health Service; the appointment of a Minister of Population; a rejection of the idea that changing tax allowances or social benefits should be employed as a population policy; and a proposal that there should be no element of compulsion in any measures undertaken. Nevertheless, for the first time, it is suggested that Britain should have a governmental policy regarding population. The panel's observations on the birth-rate in Britain since 1965 when the birth-rate began to fall imply that the population might rise from about fifty-four million at the present day, to about sixty-four millions in forty years time. Nevertheless the panel believes that this country could accommodate any likely increase during the next forty years and that the present situation does not require dramatic action.

CHOICE OF METHOD

When we turn to the second and third possible aims of birth control, they are involved with the individual and with considerations of emotions and mental health. One might ask why there are so many different methods of birth control, and why one only is not applied, and most people would suggest that the contraceptive pill was the ideal method. It is interesting to find, however, that according to the Birth Control Campaign for Britain's report, [3] the numbers of married couples choosing the pill which has been available on medical prescription for many years is almost the same as those who prefer a male method, the use of the sheath.

Substantial proportions of the population using contraceptives choose some of the other methods, and this is an area of personal health in which choice has to be made according to circumstances, emotional attitudes, aesthetic attitudes, and in many cases, medical considerations. [4] Four of the methods only are used without reference to medical advice. These are abstinence, withdrawal, the sheath, and chemical pessaries. With the exception of abstinence, all of them have a high failure rate, although the sheath when combined with a chemical pessary is, on the whole, satisfactory.

Other methods, insertion of a cap or diaphram over the cervix of the uterus, I.U.C.D., and the use of the contraceptive pill, all require medical advice and frequent supervision. It is often objected that the restriction of these methods to prescription by doctors constitutes an unnecessary formality and barrier, and that they should be freely available across the counter in shops. In the case of the cap and the I.U.C.D. the problem is one of the individual anatomy of the woman concerned, and the need for her instruction in the use of this device. In the case of the contraceptive pill, this makes a deliberate readjustment of the hormonal homeostasis which is the mechanism of regulating the development and production of fertile ova. There are also side-effects which, although they affect a small minority of women and have decreased since the introduction of more refined products and adjustment of the content of oestrogen and progesterone, still include a small but definable risk of thrombosis which is not shared by husbands or male consorts. This risk will be reduced by the use of the new 'pill' with a lower oestrogen content.

STERILIZATION

Sterilization, both of men and women, is now legal in this country. In the case of men, it can be carried out by a minor operation in which the tube that conveys the sperms from the testicle to the seminal fluid is divided and the ends tied off. As this is irreversible, the decision to have this operation is one that is not entered into lightly. In the case of women, the surgical intervention involves opening the abdomen and the operation traditionally has been carried out with the consent of the woman and her husband at the end of some other abdominal operation undertaken for gynaecological conditions. A new surgical approach via the vagina can now be used in appropriate cases. Sterilization for married women has usually been carried out on grounds of the threat to health as the result of further child-bearing and after a woman has had several children. Vasectomy, the operation for male sterilization, is now available on the National Health Service.

ABORTION

Abortion was legalized in the United Kingdom by the Abortion Act of 1967 which came into operation in 1968. This Act does not operate in Northern Ireland. Abortion is not 'on demand', but can be obtained legally after certification by two doctors that one or more of four grounds for abortion have been shown to be present. These are: that to allow the pregnancy to continue would be a threat to the woman's life, or that it would cause injury to her physical or mental health. The third ground for abortion is that the continuation of the pregnancy would cause injuries to the physical or mental health of any existing children in the family, and the fourth ground is that there is a substantial risk that if a child was born, it would be defective.

The figures for legal abortions in England and Wales in 1971 show that of 126,774 abortions, 97,114 were performed solely on the ground of the risk to the woman's health. It must be remembered that this includes a risk to mental health, and that the interpretation of this risk is a matter for the medical practitioners

Table 16. Abortions performed in England & Wales in 1971 under the provisions of the Abortion Act, 1967

Total legal abortions performed in 1971	126,777
In NHS hospitals	54,000
On women resident in England and Wales	95,000
Residents from other regions	2,000
European or other foreign residents, total	30,000
French residents	12,000
German residents	13,000
Single women resident in England and Wales	53,000
Single women with no live children born (mean age 24 or less)	43,000
Married women	42,000
Married women with no live children born	7,000
Sterilization carried out	14,000
(includes 343 single women)	
Method of abortion	
Dilatation and curettage (i.e. surgical per vaginam)	58,000
Vacuum extraction (pregnancies of thirteen weeks or less)	53,000
Abdominal hysterotomy (i.e. surgical by opening abdomen)	11,000
Hysterectomy also performed	1,000
Total deaths, all methods	11

Source: Registrar-General's *Statistical Review of England and Wales.* (1973). Supplement on Abortion. London: HMSO. (Adapted from the *Brit. Med. J.*'s leading article, 26 May 1973).

Note: A scrutiny of these figures will show how decisions on abortion, including the choice of method, call for expert judgment and also counselling of the patients.

granting the certificate. The numbers of abortions performed on married and single women were about equal, 55,520 in the case of married women, and 60,926 in the case of single women.

PERSONAL AND ENVIRONMENTAL FACTORS

The figures published by the British Pregnancy Advisory Service referring to cases handled by that agency provide a breakdown of age-groups involved, as well as indicating whether the women concerned were sexual novices, or had had sexual experience. [5] Of the total of 16,244 cases, 10% were under the age of 16 and were sexual novices. The total number of sexual novices in this series was only 647, compared with 15,572 who had had sexual experience. The highest rate for abortion of girls under the age of twenty occurred in the age group 16-17 in the case of sexual novices where 32% of the abortions were in this category with 10% occurring amongst those who had had sexual experience. It is also interesting to find that amongst sexual novices 79% lived at home, 19% away from home and 1% were 'don't knows'.

There is scope for discussion and interpretation of these figures. Suffice it to say that our contention that the age-risk rises after leaving school is supported by the fact that the highest proportion of abortions as carried out on girls aged 16-17 as regards sexual novices. The peak age-incidence of those with sexual experience on the other hand was over twenty-five. It is also significant that living with parents does not seem to have had any effect on sexual behaviour and that sexual novices of all age-groups living away from home seem less vulnerable to this hazard than others.

A beneficial effect of the Abortion Act has been the reduction of illegal abortions performed often by unskilled operators under unhygienic conditions. This has led to a reduction in the deaths due to abortions which occurred mainly due to scepsis. Abortion has always been a widespread practice in every society, and in the writer's experience, forty years ago the gynaecological departments of general hospitals regularly admitted women with the results of incomplete and unskilled abortions. No prosecution was ever suggested in such cases, and these women were treated as sick in the ordinary way.

NEED FOR COUNSELLING

Another beneficial effect of the Abortion Act is that the formalities required to obtain a certificate offer the opportunity of personal counselling. Abortion on demand sounds attractive to people with liberal views who are not personally involved. It is not unknown for girls to change their minds, or to be profoundly regretful and depressed when they have had an abortion. They certainly need psychological support after the operation, and this is a problem of particular significance in implementing a policy of 'day care' in which women are not kept in hospital after abortion.

Legal abortions are carried out in hospitals under the National Health Service or in private nursing homes which have been specially licensed under the Act. It is important that women who become aware that they are pregnant and who do not wish the pregnancy to continue should consult their doctors as early as possible. As pregnancy advances, it becomes more difficult to perform an abortion, and at some later point it might be completely impossible. In early pregnancy, the abortion can be performed simply by the technique of vacuum extraction in which the foetus is literally sucked out of the uterus. Later in pregnancy it may be necessary even to open the uterus by a surgical operation through the abdomen.

GOVERNMENTAL INTEREST

Although birth control might be considered to be an entirely private concern, it has always attracted the attention of governments which in turn reflect the public concern. In some countries, the importation of contraceptives is illegal. This is either on religious grounds or in the case of some developing countries, because it is felt that they need to increase the size of their population to maintain an economically viable unit. In the United Kingdom early pioneers in contraception were brought to court and imprisoned. Later on, Marie Stopes succeeded in her campaign to set up birth control clinics despite public opposition and hostility. The Family Planning Association pioneered the operation of clinics in which general medical and personal advice was given, as well as the prescription of contraceptive appliances. Governmental sanction of contraceptive methods has been extremely cautious and gradual. In the 1930s, local authorities were empowered to offer contraceptive advice to women whose health might be endangered by future pregnancies. Contraception was therefore not regarded as an amenity of positive health, but rather as a preventive against disease, or further deterioration of those already diseased.

The needs of the unmarried were recognized by Mrs. Helen Brook who set up the Brook Centres at which advice, not only on contraception, but general counselling on sexual matters and personal relationships, is offered to unmarried girls. This voluntary activity was a forerunner of final governmental action in the National Health Service Reorganization Act of 1973. This allows the prescription of contraceptives under the National Health Service, but imposes a prescription charge. Nevertheless, this represents considerable saving in personal expense in the case of contraceptives such as the pill. It can be interesting to observe the operation of this clause of the Act, as it will be an indication of attitudes and behaviour with regard to contraceptive practices. It will also determine whether expense was a deterrent, or whether there are still substantial numbers of people as at present, who prefer not to use contraceptives. This is not confined to those who object on religious grounds. Whereas the saving in expense will be considerable in the case of the contraceptive pill and the diaphram, it will probably not be a great saving in the case of the sheath, even if men do ask for the sheath to be prescribed under the National Health Service. The contraceptive pill and the diaphram are in continual use, the use of the sheath is more influenced by the frequency of intercourse and it is known that this varies considerably, showing the characteristic normal curve of frequency distribution through the sexually active population.

INCLUSION IN THE SCHOOL HEALTH EDUCATION PROGRAMME

There is ample literature available for studying the technical details of contraceptive practice. In the case of school health education, if pupils have a sound grasp of the biological principles of conception, it should not be difficult for them to work out for themselves the ways in which conception can be prevented. This heuristic method should in fact be preferred to that which merely gives a list of contraceptive appliances without reference to the personal problems involved, and to the decision-taking that individuals must accept if they are to achieve the maximum benefit from contraception.

The ethics of abortion can be discussed alongside the ethics of contraception as to which the community prefers. It should not be necessary to remind teachers that in their classes they will have children whose own opinions and those of their parents differ from the majority, and minority opinions must not be allowed to be rejected as unscientific or reactionary. The emotive character of this subject has led to excessive zeal by many pressure-groups and this should be countered by a cooler approach to those who are about to enter adult life.

QUESTIONS

1. What are the arguments in favour of birth control and how may the general public be best informed about these?

2. What are the advantages and disadvantages of a free contraceptive service?

3. Should the response of the public be unsatisfactory, do you think that some form of compulsory control on the birth-rate is likely? Give your reasons.

Smoking

Tobacco smoke contains not only nicotine, but also volatile and non-volatile substances present in the millions of droplets that constitute smoke and which condense as the smoke cools to form the tar which collects in the last third of a cigarette. The effects of nicotine on the nervous-system and on the circulation have already been described; briefly they are that of stimulation, the production of excess adrenalin, and the consequent rise in blood-pressure, increase in heartrate and fall in skin temperature due to the contraction of the peripheral blood vessels. There is also a rise in blood cholesterol. In the tobacco tar, about 1,000 identifiable substances are present, and then in addition, in the volatile part of the smoke, there is carbon monoxide which enters into combination with the haemoglobin in the red cells of the blood.

CHEMISTRY OF TOBACCO SMOKING

Of the thousand identifiable substances, a few stand out as having specifically harmful effects. Thus, there is benz pyrene which is a known carcinogenic agent, polonium which is radio-active, phenols, which are irritating to the lining of the bronchial tubes, and acrolein which is believed to be the substance that causes the paralysis of the cilia, lining the bronchial tubes. Therefore, apart from the effect of nicotine, the other harmful effects of tobacco smoke are due to direct irritation of the lining of the bronchial tubes, causing the out-pouring of an excess of mucus in response, and incidentally, lowering the resistance to infection, as well as the specific carcinogenic effects, although it is not certain that these lie only in benz-pyrene, but may be due to the exposure of the lung to a mass of hydrocarbons.

Tobaccos vary in the nicotine content, ranging from as low as one per cent to eight per cent in the dried leaf, and when made into cigarettes, range at about one to eight milligrammes of nicotine per cigarette which will be inhaled by a smoker during ordinary smoking. Inhalation of tobacco smoke increases the absorption of nicotine, as well as exposing the deeper parts of the lung to the irritating effects of tar.

The recognition in recent years that non-smokers can be harmed by exposure to cigarette smoke converts the whole problem into one affecting the community. Whereas it has been said — and some will say with justification that once smokers have been warned of the dangers they run then it is up to them to take the advice, it is now a matter of public conscience not to expose non-smokers to hazards. Children living in smoking households tend to suffer a significantly greater degree of respiratory illness causing absence from school. There are irritating effects on nose, throat and eyes, and people with allergies have their complaints aggravated by exposure to cigarette smoke. Carbon monoxide is absorbed into the blood from other people's smoke and children who are exposed to a heavy concentration of cigarette smoke in an ill-ventilated room or car inhale as much carbon monoxide as if they themselves had smoked a whole cigarette. This was the basis of a 'shock' poster issued by the Health Education Council in 1973. It has also been shown that adults have a materially increased chance of lung disease if they are exposed to cigarette smoke by smokers. The practical policy that should emerge is the restriction of smoking to areas which can be avoided by those who do not wish to run this risk. The Victorian practice of confining smoking to a special room and even the wearing of special clothing (the 'smoking jacket' and 'smoking cap') now seems to have been sound.

MORTALITY ASSOCIATED WITH CIGARETTES
The most publicized effect of smoking cigarettes is lung cancer, of which 98% of cases occur directly in association with cigarette smoking. In terms of mortality, this disease accounts for nearly 30,000 deaths a year in England and Wales, but the division between men and women is unequal; the bulk of the cases occurring in men, that is about 24,000, and those occurring in women, about 5,500. Two-fifths of all cancer deaths in men are due to lung cancer, and one tenth of all cancer deaths in women. The occurrence of lung cancer in women is a comparatively recent event and reflects the fact that women are now catching up with men as regards the amount smoked. In 1971 for the first time since lung cancer has been prominent in national mortality statistics, there is a slight decrease in mortality in men under the age of sixty. Cases occur in men as young as thirty. This is a picture which is found in all countries in the world, although there are variations which maybe due to differences in smoking behaviour, or possibly due to differences in the tobacco and the products of its combustion.

SMOKING AND PREGNANCY
In addition to lung cancer, cigarette smoking is also responsible for the aggravation of bronchitis, ischaemic heart disease, including coronary thrombosis, and cancer of the bladder. It aggravates conditions such as gastric ulcer, presumably because nicotine has a stimulating effect upon the smooth muscle of the stomach and intestines. Smoking in pregnancy is now known to be harmful to the developing foetus, and in cases where women smoke heavily during pregnancy, there is a tendency to a lower birth-weight and to a higher rate of perinatal mortality. Further than this, there is evidence to show that there is retardation of reading age, observed as late as the age of seven in the case of children whose mothers smoked during pregnancy.

PIPES AND CIGARS
So far, reference has been to cigarette smoking only. Smoking of pipe tobacco carries a hazard of lung cancer, although slightly lower than that of smoking cigarettes, while the smoking of cigars does

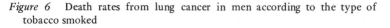

Figure 6 Death rates from lung cancer in men according to the type of tobacco smoked

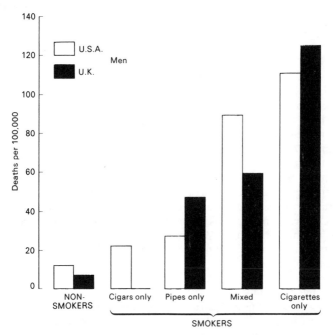

Source: Royal College of Physicians of London. (1971). *Smoking and Health Now: Report.* London: Pitman Medical Books.

Note: These figures are taken from the prospective study of British doctors aged 35 and over by Doll and Hill and the American study of men aged 40–79 by Hammond. Only in the American study were there enough men who smoked only cigars to estimate their death rate, which was only twice that of non-smokers. Pipe smokers had two or three times the risk of non-smokers. Smokers of cigarettes together with pipe and cigar smokers (who smoke relatively few cigarettes) had six to eight times the risk, and smokers of cigarettes only between eleven times (USA) and twenty times (UK) the risk of non-smokers.

not at present appear to carry any hazard of lung cancer at all. However, the inhalation of nicotine and of other substances contained in tobacco tar still occurs, and one could not say that smoking pipes and cigars is exactly healthy, although it is less hazardous than the smoking of cigarettes.

IMMEDIATE EFFECTS OF SMOKING
The hazards so far mentioned apply to the adult section of society, and therefore have no appeal at all to children and adolescents. However, there are immediate effects of smoking cigarettes both on

the heart and circulation and on the lungs, causing a diminution of airway and an effect on general physical well-being and performance. Recent studies of smoking behaviour which reveal that schoolchildren may start smoking as early as the age of eleven suggest that concentration should be upon the immediate effects, as these are more meaningful.

MEDICAL ATTITUDE TO SMOKING

Smoking has never had the whole-hearted approval of the medical profession and in Victorian times the majority of doctors appeared to advise against it. The earliest published statement of this kind was in *The Lancet* in 1857 when the writer of a leading article exhorted the 'young of this country' to give up the habit. It was in fact the immediate effects which were observed by physicians as causing ill health, which were the main concern, and lung cancer did not make its appearance in epidemic form until the twentieth century and then mainly after the Second World War, reflecting the great increase in the smoking of cigarettes, which built up from the time of the First World War and represented a change in smoking habits from those of the nineteenth century when cigars and pipes were mainly used.

SMOKING HABITS

Studies of smoking habits carried out during the last twenty years reveal various behavioural concepts, such as the desire to appear grown-up by adolescents, the desire to appear tough and rebellious in the case of young boys, rejection of adult standards and institutions, as a group phenomenon necessary in order to maintain personal prestige and to be accepted by a group, and so on. Strangely, none of them appear to have recognized the fact that smoking gives pleasure. Although no responsible person could do less than condemn the habit, it would be unreasonable to deny the fact that it has a strong pleasure element, quite apart from the effect of nicotine which produces an habituation, although not a true addiction in the ordinary sense. The aroma of burning tobacco is agreeable, the fashionable equipment that is used, that is lighters, cigarette cases, and the whole social background of smoking is undeniably attractive.

This fact was mentioned by McKennel and Thomas in their study of adult and adolescent smoking behaviour published in 1964. These authors urged against the policy of propaganda against smoking which concentrated on the unaesthetic aspects, i.e. stained fingers, the accumulation of cigarette ends, the smell of stale smoke on the clothes etc., and suggested that all health education efforts should take into account the acknowledged fact that many people derive ordinary pleasure from smoking, quite apart from other motives.

ECONOMICS OF SMOKING

The economics of smoking pose a considerable problem in the face of the need on health grounds to cut down the amount smoked and hope that smoking will eventually be phased out altogether. Figures produced by Peston at the second World Conference on Smoking and Health in London in 1971 showed that in 1970 consumers in the United Kingdom had spent £172 million on cigarettes and tobacco. 87% of this was on cigarettes and it represents an increase in expenditure in ten years of nearly £60,000,000 which in 1960 represented 88% of expenditure on cigarettes. At the same time the price of cigarettes and tobacco over the same period has risen by about 54%. Tax on tobacco realized £1,150 million in 1970 compared with £818 million in 1960, an increase of 41%. The Family Expenditure Survey in 1969 showed that people in the lower income-groups tended to spend relatively more on tobacco. Expenditure was shown to fall off fairly quickly above a level of £40 per week of general income. The Tobacco Research Council showed that, in 1969, 61% of men in unskilled occupations smoked, compared with 43% in the professions. In the case of women, the corresponding figures were 46% and 37%.

In every country of the world, tobacco is an important source of revenue for governments and therefore contributes to the general well-being of the community, and in some countries it is a part of the economy. In some cases, for example, tobacco is the principal crop that is farmed. Having contributed to the well-being of the community economically, tobacco then contributes to ill health and early mortality in its effects on those who smoke it. It is a paradoxical situation which makes it very difficult for governments to resolve.

INTERNATIONAL CONCERN

However the problem of smoking and its consequences to health exercises the mind of all governments, including the supra-national body, the World Health Organization. The World Health Assembly has passed resolutions on this matter, urging all member governments to take steps to reduce the amount of smoking by every possible means, including health education. The subject has also been considered of sufficient importance to merit conferences at world level. The first World Conference on Smoking and Health was held in New York in 1967, the second in London in 1971, while the third is planned for 1975. In the case of the United Kingdom the Government has financed campaigns for health education since 1957, the year in which the findings of the Medical Research Council, reviewing the literature showing the association between smoking cigarettes and lung cancer, was published. Since that time, efforts have been stepped up and increasing sums of money made available, although the amount of money available for publicity on this subject cannot be any more than a fraction of that used by cigarette advertisers.

ADVERTISING
The advertising of cigarettes on television was banned in 1965, and in 1971 manufacturers of cigarettes were obliged to include on the packet a government warning that smoking may harm health. In the same year, the first television advertising drawing attention to the dangers to health of smoking cigarettes was launched by the Health Education Council which produced a short television filler showing on the one hand the economic effects of smoking and the poor return one got, usually lung cancer for a fairly high expenditure, and on the other hand an appeal to the social and aesthetic sensibilities of people who might object to others smelling of stale tobacco smoke.

The Health Education Council also published several advertisements between 1970 and 1973 which appeared in mass circulation daily newspapers, as well as Sunday newspapers, drawing attention to the hazards of cigarette smoking, and in 1973, when the Government decided to publish comparative figures for tar and nicotine content of the various brands of cigarettes available, this subject also was covered.

TAR AND NICOTINE LEVELS
The decision to publish tar and nicotine values reflects the acceptance by official opinion that there are a large number of people who cannot give up smoking, but who could receive some benefit at least from relatively safer smoking. This includes the choice of cigarettes of a low tar and nicotine content, the taking of fewer puffs of a cigarette, smoking it more slowly, throwing away the last third of the cigarette (this is the fraction which contains the highest concentration of tar as the cigarette smoke has condensed on being exposed to room temperature), and the avoidance of inhalation. Although this is recommended as 'safer' smoking, the warning is also given that no cigarette can be regarded as safe.

SMOKING AMONGST SCHOOLCHILDREN
Since 1957 there has been a concentration on anti-smoking education amongst schoolchildren. The revelation that boys often smoke as early as the age of eleven shows that this is a topic suitable for the junior school, as well as for the secondary school. The World Health Organization stated that the prevention of the taking up of cigarette smoking among children is of great importance. They separated the factors that led to smoking from those that led to its continuation.

The evidence so far accumulated suggests that cigarette smoking should not be considered in isolation. This is an observation that applies to all specific health hazards that tend to attract public attention as being of general concern. It is also important to stress the immediate health hazards, for example, the cough, respiratory illnesses, impairment of physical performance, as well as the long-term health effects which will accrue eventually if children become habituated to smoking. This subject has been tackled in a variety of ways, and in the chapter on evaluation we have referred to the work of Watson who examined the relative effectiveness of five different methods of approach.

METHODS OF EDUCATION
In addition to classroom teaching, there are possibilities of the use of exhibition material and film while some kind of corporate activity, such as the formation of an anti-smoking league, an organization which started first in the Kingsdale School in Camberwell, has much to commend it. In a school in South Wales co-operation between the head teacher and the medical officer of health resulted in the members of the anti-smoking league making their own film (*'The Black Sheep'* see film list) which was then circulated to other schools in the country.

A SMOKING COMMUNITY
It has always been recognized that it is idle to make an approach to schoolchildren while ignoring the examples of smoking behaviour in the general community. Whereas we can have little influence generally in the adult world surrounding the child, apart from the use of mass media, the teachers and other members of the school staff have a direct obligation to support children in their determination not to take up smoking. It has already been pointed out that hospitals should be non-smoking communities showing an example to the remainder of the community, and certainly this should be true of schools.

In the case of doctors, only about 22% to 25% of practising doctors are smokers, and this is often cited as a possible example to their patients and to others which may have had an effect on the reduction of the total number of smokers in the community. Teachers also have to consider their personal position in this respect. The comments of the working group dealing with the control of smoking amongst children at the second World Conference on Smoking and Health are pertinent. This group suggested that teachers and educational administrators should be encouraged not to smoke cigarettes in front of children, and that smokers should be helped in their efforts to give up this habit. They also comment that a stressful school situation might adversely influence smoking behaviour, and in this respect it is necessary to dispel the myth that children preparing for examinations will be helped by smoking cigarettes.

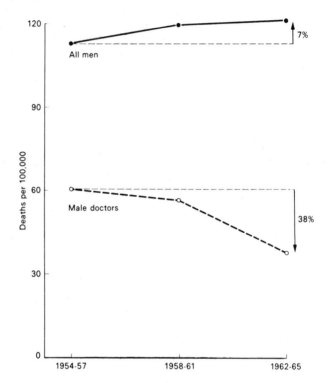

Figure 7   Death rates from lung cancer in male doctors and in all men in England and Wales

Source: Royal College of Physicians of London. (1971). *Smoking and Health Now: Report*. London: Pitman Medical Books.
Note: These figures are derived from the Registrar General's Mortality returns and from Doll and Hill's study of British doctors. The rates for the two groups of men have been standardised for age. During the last twenty years many doctors have stopped smoking and their death rate from lung cancer has declined by 38 per cent while in all men in England and Wales who have not changed their cigarette consumption the rate has increased by 7 per cent. This experiment which doctors have carried out on themselves is strong evidence of the benefits that would result if there was widespread discontinuance of smoking.

The law relating to tobacco and children is clear cut. Under the provisions of the Children and Young Persons Act, it is illegal to serve tobacco products to persons under the age of sixteen. There is a continual and widespread breach of this law which is well known and no doubt in many cases small shopkeepers are under undue pressure which causes them to break the law, sometimes even to the extent of selling single cigarettes. Enforcement of this law obviously depends upon the partnership between the shopkeepers, children, parents, and teachers.

RESTRAINTS ON SMOKING
By-laws allow public authorities to restrict smoking in public places, including railway-carriages and buses. It is interesting to observe that the popularity of non-smoking compartments in suburban commuter trains has increased enormously during the last fifteen years. Many large department stores forbid smoking by customers, and this can be justified also on the grounds of safety, but generally wherever the opportunities for smoking in public can be cut down, this will have a beneficial effect in that it will reduce the total dose taken in by individuals. There is also the question of when it is appropriate to smoke. People do not smoke in church, but neither do they usually smoke while dancing, or engaged in playing games. Nevertheless, people do smoke while driving motor vehicles, while performing manual tasks, whether these are part of their occupation or hobbies.

GIVING UP SMOKING
One of the results of publicizing the results of smoking has been that large numbers of people have asked for help in giving up the habit. There is no drug available that can guarantee that people will give up the habit of smoking, and in general this seems to be a psychological procedure undertaken either individually after counselling, or as a member of a group. Anti-smoking clinics have been set up, and these have relied upon group unity during the course of a series of consecutive sessions at which information has been given in the form of talks, films have been shown, and group discussion has been conducted on motives for smoking and attitudes to the habit. Unfortunately, the results of such clinics are equivocal, as are the results of other methods of helping people to give up smoking. About one third give up initially, one third make no change in their habits, and one third may even increase the amount of smoking. The difficulty that people encounter in attempting to give up smoking makes it all the more important that children and young people should not take up the habit. This should be stressed in information given to children pointing out that there will come a time when they wished they had never started, and that it will be extremely difficult for them to give up at that time.

THE EFFECTS OF ANTI-SMOKING EDUCATION
The amount of effort and the quantity of resources devoted to this aspect of public health during a period of nearly twenty years surely indicates that this is a matter of public concern. On the other hand, smoking continues, and although there has been a reduction

in the number of smokers during that time — it is estimated to be about one and a half million — we have yet to make a substantial impact. The reports of the Royal College of Physicians of London, the first published in 1962 and the second in 1971, had an immediate effect on smoking habits, which lasted for a matter of weeks. These reports summarized the evidence on the effect on health of smoking, and the public respect paid to the College and the considerable publicity which the press and mass media gave to these reports does seem to have had a temporary effect. Similarly, the report of the United States, Surgeon-General, which appeared between the publication of the two reports of the Royal College of Physicians was given publicity in the United Kingdom and, similarly, a temporary drop in the sales of cigarettes followed.

Surveys of public opinion and level of knowledge conducted as early as 1954 showed that as regards the penetration of the public mind by the message this had been successful. That is, 98% of people interrogated said that they had heard of the association between cigarette smoking and lung cancer. The majority of people also agreed that smoking was harmful, but few had given it up, although many mentioned friends and acquaintances who had done so.

Smoking differs from other health problems in that it is a deeply entrenched habit in all countries, it has had no moral sanctions against it with the exception of the small minority of those who object on religious grounds, and the arguments against smoking on grounds of health are based upon statistical evidence which as we have already noted has little impact on a public which has not been trained to think statistically. It is evident that it is extremely hard for the regular heavy smoker to give up the habit. Thus the compromise arrived at in 1973 when it was decided to use a new message — that of (relatively) safer smoker. The television fillers produced by the Health Education Council urged confirmed smokers to throw away one third of the cigarette, and not to inhale. At the same time, the publication of the tar and nicotine figures offered smokers the opportunity of choosing brands which were less likely to be toxic.

Nicotine is a drug and when smoking is used to overcome feelings of fatigue or frustration, or to ease tension, then smoking is on the same plane as other drugs which are similarly abused. For the smoker who relies upon tobacco as a crutch, some form of psychotherapy, which can even be self-administered, is probably the most effective way to help him to cut down smoking and eventually to abandon the habit. For example, it is recommended that smokers write down in a notebook all the occasions on which they take a cigarette, and then analyse them. The main hope for the future, however, will be for smoking to become unfashionable, as it once became unfashionable during the eighteenth century. The trend-setters in society are therefore the most important target.

QUESTIONS

1. Do you think that tobacco companies should be encouraged to produce a 'safe' cigarette? If they succeeded do you think that the lack of the element of danger would make smoking less attractive.

2. It is said that the tax revenue from tobacco is so great that if smoking ceased there would be a substantial rise in the rate of income tax? Is this true in the long run?

3. Is it a matter of trespassing on the private lives of people when anti-smoking pressures are forced upon them? If it is how do you propose to protect non-smokers from the inconveniences they suffer from others smoking?

4. What are your opinions on the decisions of some headmasters to allow senior pupils to smoke in the junior common rooms?

Drugs and Alcohol

At all times and in all parts of the world, man has always used certain chemical substances which cause an alteration of mood, the relief of pain or anxiety, to postpone fatigue, to promote social adequacy and performance, and to contrive illusory experiences outside reality. The type of chemical substance used has always varied according to the regions of the world. Such practices have impressed travellers who have then tended to bring the substance back into their own societies and to establish its use there. In some cases, the use of a substance by one society is the norm for that particular society, but when introduced into another society it becomes a social deviance. In some cases the chemicals used are also used in medical practice, but in other cases they have no medical use. In some cases too, the use of the substance has produced dependence, both psychological and physical, called loosely 'addiction,' a term which is still widely used, but which is discouraged by the World Health Organization which prefers the term 'dependence.' In other cases, the substance has a short-term effect and it does not produce dependence, although it may in time with continual use produce permanent psychological change in behaviour.

GEOGRAPHICAL VARIATION IN THE USE OF DRUGS
Practical examples of the foregoing generalizations are as follows. Alcohol and tobacco, tea and coffee are widely used in Europe and on the American Continent, both North and South America. In Moslem countries where alcohol has always been forbidden, hashish has been socially acceptable as a stimulant. In the Carribean, cannabis has been widely used and it is claimed that it was West Indian immigrants who first introduced cannabis into the United Kingdom. In some regions of Latin America, the taking of cocaine,

usually derived from chewing the coca leaf, is a widespread practice. Opium and its modern derivative, heroin, was widely used in China and the Far East and the opium trade was deliberately fostered during the nineteenth century. There were no laws against its use in this country in the nineteenth century and De Quincey could publish his account of his own experiences with opium without penalty, and it is significant to realize that Sherlock Holmes's apparently mild eccentricity of injecting himself with cocaine was accepted as part of the normal image of a man of his standing.

MEDICAL INITIATION OF ADDICTION

The use of certain substances in medical practice has often been the cause of addiction. In the United States, for example, the use of morphine injected by a hypodermic syringe, an innovation at the time, was part of medical practice in the Armed Forces medical services during the Civil War. Thus, many soldiers became addicted to morphine and on demobilization, large numbers of army veterans migrated to California. Thus it seems highly plausible that California should become an important centre of the modern drug scene.

This story illustrates two important aspects. One is that patients under treatment may become addicted, and this of course is a hazard of which all physicians are aware, and secondly that availability is one of the causes of drug abuse. Thus, morphine dependency has not affected large areas of the United States which were not colonized by the veterans of the American Civil War. Similarly, in the United Kingdom, 82% of heroin addicts on the Register of the Home Office live in Greater London. The problem is miniscule in many provincial centres.

Developments in the pharmaceutical industry itself have increased availability. The invention of the hypodermic syringe made the introduction of drugs into the system possible by a direct route causing immediate effect. So attractive is the principle of injection that drugs that were formerly taken by mouth, such as the amphetamines, have in recent years been produced in an injectable form which has been preferred by those who take them unlawfully. Towards the end of the nineteenth century synthetic drugs began to be produced in large numbers. Heroin was isolated from opium and the barbiturates were introduced into medical practice for the treatment of anxiety and for insomnia. Thus, the majority of people who are dependent upon the barbiturates are middle-aged women, but they have not deliberately chosen to use this drug, they have consulted their doctors who have prescribed it for them in order to relieve their symptoms.

In the twentieth century, the discovery of tranquillizers or drugs which could relieve anxiety without making people sleepy has given psychiatry important therapeutic weapons to use when dealing with psychoneurosis. In 1973 there was a 67% increase in the production of pharmaceutical products of this kind over production in 1963. In one representative year, 42 million prescriptions for psychotropic drugs were dispensed at a cost to the National Health Service of 21.5 million pounds.

BASIC PHILOSOPHY OF THE DRUG SCENE

There is therefore a general drug scene in society at the present day based on the popular idea that medical science has an answer for every human difficulty. Referring back to the chapter on mental health, it will be seen that this idea is an illusion. Problems of personality and social conflict, guilt and anxiety, must be handled at source and not by the treatment of symptoms. The cause for the anxiety or conflict or guilt remains the same, and the patient is no better off, and in many cases worse off, if he or she becomes addicted to one of the tranquillizing drugs.

HEROIN

Attention was drawn to this problem as it affects young people in the 1960s by the revelation that the numbers of people under twenty known to the Home Office as being dependent upon heroin had increased alarmingly. Fortunately, in the United Kingdom the problem is nowhere near as great as that in the United States. Although the numbers of those dependent on heroin has increased by ten times since records were kept, the original figures are very low, in hundreds, and at the present day, the figure is about 3,000. Of those under twenty, there are 350, but it is reassuring to record that in 1968 there was double this number; it dropped by a half in 1971. Once again, seventeen appears to be the age of inception and the chances of any one teacher encountering a case of heroin dependence in his classroom are extremely low. In the United Kingdom, we have a problem more of multiple drug abuse, that is the use of amphetamines, barbiturates, and of cannabis.

Table 17. Numbers of opioid addicts 1961−71 coming to the notice of the Home Office.

	1961−66	*1967*	*1968*	*1969*	*1970*	*1971*
All addicts	470−1349	1729	2782	2881	2661	2769
Number taking heroin	132− 899	1299	2240	1417	914	959
Number taking methadone	59− 156	243	486	1687	1820	1927
Number aged under 20 yr	2− 329	395	764	637	405	338
Number aged 20−34 yr	94− 558	906	1530	1789	1813	2010
Number aged 34−49 yr	95− 162	142	146	174	158	156

Source: Boyd, P. (1972). 'Adolescents, drug abuse, and addiction'. *Brit. Med. J.* 4:540.

MOTIVATIONS FOR DRUG TAKING

The motives for the illicit taking of drugs can be divided first into experimentation and a desire to compensate for some inadequacy or frustration. It has been estimated that between 10% and 40% of schoolchildren over the age of fourteen take drugs for this purpose. The use of cannabis reflects a different motivation. Cannabis can be used as alcohol is used for stimulation and excitement and for the social occasion. It is part of a group activity, and it may be a necessary practice if a boy or girl is to be accepted by the group. It is also identified with two modern images, the pop music industry and the 'alternative society'. There are therefore cultural and ideological undertones which are disturbing to the older generation, but which must be understood if young people are to be helped to avoid the use of this particular drug. It is certainly a very effective way of expressing one's dislike for established society with its beer, whisky, and cigarettes as socially acceptable drugs, and preference for an alternative society in which cannabis is socially acceptable.

There are important differences of personality involved in motivation for the illicit taking of drugs. The experimenter will usually try amphetamines and may have as his motive a desire to stay awake and alert during long protracted social occasions, and in fact these drugs have been used openly in the past by motor-rally drivers. If alcohol is consumed at the same time, then the effect of these drugs is enhanced and the consequences to behaviour and to accident-proneness can be very severe. In addition, people who take amphetamines in order to stave off sleep are denying themselves the rest which is essential for restoration of normal energy and if the practice is continued for too long, the cumulative effects of lack of sleep will soon become apparent.

AMPHETAMINES – 'THE PEP PILLS'

Amphetamines were taken without medical reason as early as the 1930s and medical students experimented with them in order to improve their performance during examinations. Unfortunately, this did not usually have the desired effect and the unusual excitement and tension and loquacity produced by these drugs actually detracted from examination performance. They have been used medically in recent years in cases of depression, and also in cases of obesity because they depress appetite. Many doctors have voluntarily bound themselves to abstain from prescribing them because the source of these drugs was mainly the surplus caused by excessive prescribing and they were frequently taken from household medicine chests by young people whose mothers were receiving these drugs. The practice of hoarding old medicines carries this as well as many other dangers.

PERSONALITY DIFFICULTIES

In the case of experimenters who use amphetamines for this purpose there are unlikely to be any personality difficulties and no doubt the majority abandon the habit when they find that the experience is not very rewarding. Nevertheless, it is estimated that there are about 100,000 users of amphetamines in the community at the present day.

It is a boy or girl with a personality difficulty who is at hazard. [1] They may take amphetamines in order to improve their social performance, but they may also take sedative drugs in order to shield themselves from reality which is too harsh for them. In some cases this may be merely an exaggerated form of the normal adolescent conflict with society and with himself, but in other cases there may be a more deep-seated personality disorder. It has been shown for example that the use of heroin is dependent upon a particular personality type, rather than an age-group. The use of hallucinogens, like L.S.D., introduces yet another motive. In some intellectual circles, L.S.D. is used deliberately to produce fantastic experiences to heighten sensory perception, so that, for example, ordinary objects acquire a greater significance, and in the terms of this particular group, to 'expand the mind'. Cannabis also has a certain hallucinogenic property and distorts perception, although it does not appear to be used deliberately for this purpose.

PUBLIC AND PROFESSIONAL INTEREST

The abuse of drugs is one of those matters of public concern which has brought together a number of professional and intellectual disciplines. This itself constitutes a problem insofar as it is possible to approach this matter from a number of avenues. In the 1960s when there was wide-spread public alarm about this matter, there was the tendency to approach it from the clinical aspect. There was concentration upon the identification of drugs used illicitly and their clinical effects, both immediate and long-term. It is beyond question that this general information should be part of general knowledge which is most usefully imparted during the course of a balanced health education programme.

Wigfield has found for example that when fifth and sixth-formers learn about the nature of drugs at school, they are less likely to experiment with them. [2] On the other hand, concentration upon the dramatic effects of heroin addiction with its progressive deterioration, drop out from society and eventual early death, only draws attention to the obvious. It is far more important to understand what first started the young addict on this road and to realize that when he first accepted the offer of the use of heroin he had no intention of ending up in five years time as a derelict on the point of death. The tendency now to concentrate on the reasons for drug taking, rather than the drugs themselves, is more helpful.

therefore have the psychiatric approach in which motivation
behaviour are analysed and closely allied to this is the
sociological approach in which the social environment is examined,
often very critically with the intention of changing this where
possible. Finally, there is the legal approach, that of magistrates and
police officers, who perhaps have figured too largely in many
well-intentioned health education projects in this field.

NO SINGLE CAUSE

The World Health Organization's expert committee on youth and
drugs has concluded that no single cause for drug dependence has
yet been demonstrated. [3] They list three main hypotheses:

1. The problems of the drug taker.
2. Mental or physical disorders.
3. Sociocultural pressures or social ills.

They believe however that most experimental drug use begins
during the pre-adolescence and adolescent years. Curiosity and the
need for acceptance and the desire for pleasure are the main
motives, and these are all perfectly normal. It is therefore more
important that teachers and parents should be aware of the need for
the achievement of satisfactions in these areas, that they should
offer a wide choice of alternatives to drugs than that they should
learn by heart the various clinical signs whereby they can detect
whether their children are taking drugs.

The idea of inspecting children regularly for needle pricks in their
arms or analysis of urine is neither practicable nor desirable. From the
epidemiological evidence, needle pricks due to heroin taking will
never be seen in schools, whereas needle pricks due to the injection of
insulin in the occasional diabetic child may mislead. Once a boy or girl
has got to the stage of injecting themselves with heroin, the
deterioration in their life-style would be so obvious that this is
something which attracts attention.

MANAGEMENT OF DRUG PROBLEMS IN SCHOOL

A school medical officer, L. M. Watson has offered advice on the
management of drug abuse in schoolchildren and has pointed out
that regular drug-users as well as pupils in general are remarkably
well informed about the ill effects of drug taking, and that this
knowledge is not likely to convert those to whom life is 'a bore or
weary burden'. [4] She also points out that experimenters even have
their interest heightened in flirting with danger and death.
Knowledge alone does not necessarily cause drug taking, cure it, nor
prevent it, but true prevention calls for a different priority, that of
a comprehensive programme of physical and mental health and
social education to all pupils from entry into school until
school-leaving age. This programme should be designed to produce

respect for self and others, a positive motivation, and an incentive for personal effort and achievement, a sound set of values, and a mature personality that can tolerate frustration. This fits in entirely with the programme for mental health education referred to earlier.

A practical difficulty is that such a programme is essentially adult, and middle class, and appears to reject the idea of an alternative society. The World Health Organization Expert Committee points out that modern youth is not interested in preserving the *status quo*. On the other hand, the adult point of view must have a hearing. Responsible adults are concerned about the fate of our civilization and culture, and the apparent rejection by young people of what is regarded by adults as their responsibility as carriers of that culture. They may of course be reassured by the large numbers of young people participating and enjoying traditional cultural activities (like classical music) as well as religious functions (like those connected with the Oecumenical movement). Nevertheless, young people who resort to drugs represent a threat and in this, as in other conflicts regarding life-style, a dialogue between the generations is essential.

LEGAL SANCTIONS

All governments have attempted to control the misuse of drugs by legislation. The history of legislation in the United Kingdom has been described in detail by Bradshaw.[5] He traces the history of the control of drugs back to the Pharmacy Act of 1868 which required all opium and derivatives to be labelled as poisons and the subsequent legal control over the misuse of dangerous drugs up to the Misuse of Drugs Act of 1971. It should be considered most important that all pupils before leaving school should be aware of the requirements of this Act and how they can be enforced and what penalties will ensue if the law is broken. The Act sets out to limit the availability of drugs, for example, to regulate their prescribing and supply, and also to tackle the problems of possession and trafficking. Drugs and dependents are also categorized into three categories according to their degree of harmfulness.

THE CANNABIS PROBLEM

Both in the United States and in the United Kingdom, there is a considerable body of opinion which believes that the use of cannabis should be legalized. In the present state of medical knowledge about this drug, however, and the uncertainty of long-term effects it may produce, the majority of medical opinion is against this. Readers should study the Wootton report on cannabis which it must be emphasized did not suggest that this drug should be legalized but that the very severe penalties for its possession should be reduced.[6] Similarly, the 1971 Act grades penalties for misuse, according to the degree of harmfulness of the drug. It is significant that cannabis has been classed as a category A drug, which category includes morphine, heroin and L.S.D.

ALCOHOL – EFFECTS ON NERVOUS SYSTEM

The immediate effects of alcohol are shown by the nervous system. Although erroneously believed to be a stimulant, alcohol is actually a depressant and it acts first on the highest levels of the brain which then relax their control of the centres below them. Thus judgment is impaired, people may become more loquacious, thus falsely believing that they are stimulated and as alcoholic intoxication progresses, there is an effect on the motor area causing staggering gait and eventually unconsciousness. The victim is then in the same position as a patient who has been heavily anaesthetized although in the case of modern anaesthetics, there are no unpleasant after-effects as occur inevitably following heavy drinking.

In serious cases of intoxication, death can ensue either from failure of the respiratory centre, or more frequently, due to inhalation of vomit, or a fatal accident, such as falling down a flight of stairs. Intermediate behavioural disorders are probably dependent upon the basic personality, some people becoming aggressive and violent, others sentimental. The effect on sexual prowess has been summarized as increasing the desire, but depressing the performance. (The original observation was Shakespeare's in *Macbeth*: 'it both provokes and unprovokes. It provokes the desire but unprovokes the performance.') Drunken behaviour is extremely distressing to other people and is no more appreciated by those who are regular drinkers than those who are teetotallers. The consumption of alcohol is directly related to road accidents and since the introduction of the breathalyser which has had a healthy deterrent effect, there has been some reduction of accidents due to this cause.

Figure 8   Consumption of potable spirits. Millions of proof gallons

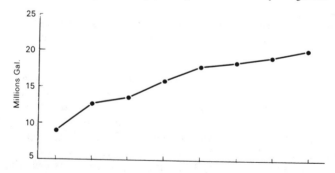

Comsumption of potable spirits. Millions of proof. gallons

Source: Dr H. D. Chalke, OBE.

Figure 9   Consumption of beer. Millions of bulk barrels

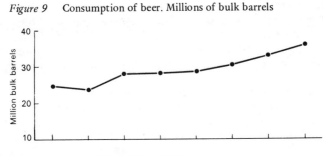

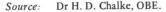
Consumption of beer. Millions of bulk barrels

Source: Dr H. D. Chalke, OBE.

Figure 10   Consumption of wine (imported and British)

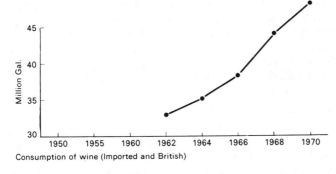

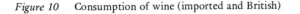
Consumption of wine (Imported and British)

Source: Dr H. D. Chalke, OBE.

ALCOHOLIC CONTENT OF DRINKS

Alcoholic drinks vary considerably in their alcohol content from beers up to spirits. The type of drink taken, the amount taken, and the size and weight of the person consuming the drink, are all factors which will affect the degree of intoxication. The taking of food before drinking or during drinking slows down the absorption rate and the most serious effects occur due to rapid absorption. Absorption starts even in the mouth and proceeds in the stomach but the majority of the alcohol, about 90%, is absorbed through the lining of the small intestines. The absorbed alcohol circulates in the blood and can be detected chemically, this being the basis of medico-legal tests, some is excreted in the urine where it can also be detected chemically, and a small proportion is contained in the expired air in the lungs. This is the basis for the breathalyser test. Alcohol absorbed into the body is de-toxicated by the liver.

EFFECTS OF PERSISTENT HEAVY DRINKING

After recovery from a bout of drunkenness, the body returns to normal, but with persistent heavy drinking, chronic effects begin to appear, some of which can still be reversed by abstention from drinking and medical treatment, but others which unfortunately are permanent.

Some of these chronic effects are indirect, for example, the alcoholic tends to neglect his normal diet because he obtains satisfying calorie intake from the alcohol. Calories obtained from alcohol however have no nutritive value in that they contain no amino acids or vitamins. This of course is referring to alcohol alone. Certain alcoholic drinks, such as beer, containing glucose, malt, and members of the vitamin B complex, and sweet wines which contain sugar provide energy-giving and protective foods, but obviously their contribution to a balanced diet must be minimal.

Instances have been described where because of dismay at the amount of drunkenness in African tribes, missionaries have made well-intended efforts to prevent brewing. This has resulted in vitamin B deficiency because the very poor and unbalanced diet consumed by the tribe did not supply these nutrients. This however is hardly a consideration in advanced industrialized societies. Heavy beer-drinking tends to produce obesity because of the excess of calories consumed over calories required, and in addition the heavy consumption of carbohydrates.

ALCOHOLISM

Alcoholism affects principally the middle-aged groups in society and mainly men. The effects of heavy drinking are shown in large-scale industrial absenteeism following weekends and public holidays, particularly New Year's Day. Drunkenness in public places is not so prevalent as it was at one time and is dealt with by the police and the Courts. Drunken driving leading to serious accidents has been reduced considerably by the threat of the breathalyser but the main concern is for the deterioration in social and work performance and in physical health caused by the disease of alcoholism itself.

The recognition of alcoholism as a disease has been a great step forward in combating this problem. A considerable amount of effort is now devoted towards the treatment and rehabilitation of the alcoholic, partly by voluntary organizations, such as Alcoholics Anonymous, and there are now regular medical conferences on national and international planes on this subject.

TEENAGE DRINKING

We have already mentioned that there is now concern about the increase of heavy drinking amongst teenagers. The legal age from which a person may be served liquor in a public place is eighteen. The recommendations of the Errol Committee [1] that the legal age should be lowered to seventeen has caused considerable criticism, but this recommendation should be looked at in the light of the findings of Davies and Stacey in Glasgow who pointed out that the main danger is clandestine drinking by people under the age of eighteen. [2] Once again we see the dangers of the generation gap and of the separation of the peer group from the reference group. In the case of boys the motivation for drinking is said to be the desire to appear tough and rebellious. However, if their early experiences of drinking were with responsible adults then their association of drinking with toughness might not arise.

AN ALTERNATIVE TO TEETOTALISM

Nineteenth century attempts to overcome alcoholism which was a very serious problem at that time were based on the teetotal principle. Teetotalism however has declined in popularity and is no longer identified even with nonconformist religious groups as used to be the case. There is a consensus that alcoholic drinks can be used sensibly by people of maturity and normal personality, and preferably in a social context. If young people are educated in the wise use of alcohol by their parents and other elders, there seems to be less chance that they may become heavy drinkers.

The difference between the use of alcohol and the use of cannabis is that alcoholic drinks have an attraction quite apart from any intoxication they may produce. Thus, the appearance, the flavour, and the sociability of alcoholic drinks belong to a life-style quite different from that of groups who share a reefer in secret gatherings.

ALCOHOL AND HEALTH EDUCATION

The relevance to health education in schools is that the subject of the use of alcohol should be presented in the context of a general health programme as we have reiterated several times in the case of other subjects, and that teachers should assume that the majority of their pupils will consume alcoholic drinks in their teens and throughout the rest of their lives. The dangers of excessive drinking however should be stressed, and this has been shown excellently in two films produced by the Medical Council on Alcoholism for use in schools.

Nowadays it is relatively easy to introduce this subject in a context that is meaningful and attractive to teenagers. For example, in the films referred to, the use of the breathalyser and urine test are demonstrated in the case of a boy who is arrested for drunken driving on a motorcycle and subsequently loses his motorcycle, his licence and, incidentally, his girfriend. Daphne Elliott (personal communication) has devised a method of demonstrating the breathalyser by an experiment in which pupils can inhale the fumes of methyl alcohol and then breathe into the apparatus.

QUESTIONS

1. Do you not think that the mass media, the press in particular, create unnecessary anxiety by exaggerating the reporting of cases? Give your concept of the current 'drug scene'.

2. Experimentation is a normal function in the process of growing up. How may this be interpreted in relation to (a) drugs as distinct from (b) alcohol (which is of course just another drug, but socially acceptable).

3. Why should the drinking of alcoholic beverages be of public concern?

4. From your personal experiences during your adolescent years, and afterwards, give a candid account of the drugs and alcohol 'scene' as you have seen it over the years.

5. Despite the publicity campaigns there has not been a decline in the consumption of alcohol — in fact drunkenness among young people is on the increase. How do you account for this?

6. It is alleged that a high proportion of accidents on the roads are associated with alcohol. What changes, if any, in the law relating to drinking and driving would you make?

7. Is the public really concerned?

The Sexually Transmitted Diseases

The ecology of man includes the ecology of animals and of micro-organisms with which he shares the world. Of the hundreds of thousands of species of micro-organisms, relatively few cause disease, and in each case, the disease is caused by their invasion of the body which is necessary in order for the species to continue its existence. The micro-organisms causing disease are bacteria, viruses, and protozoa, that is unicellular, animal-like, organisms. They are conveyed from the sick to the healthy by droplet infection from the nose and throat, contamination of food and water, by direct skin contact in an increasingly rare number of cases, by insect vectors as in the case of malaria, yellow fever, and sleeping sickness, by direct penetration of the skin, as in the case of hook worm, and through the mucous membranes of the genital tract.

Most of the major infections have now been controlled, and even virtually abolished by a combination of improved environmental hygiene, personal hygiene, and immunization where feasible. Infections of the genital tract however still remain resistant to these procedures, and they differ from the other infections in that they are contracted as a result of personal behaviour.

HISTORICAL INFLUENCES

Formerly known by the somewhat romantic and even sinister name of venereal diseases, a term which applied mainly to syphilis and gonorrhoea, it is now known that there is a wider range of infections of the genital tract, and the term 'sexually transmitted diseases' is becoming increasingly popular in medical circles. From the point of view of public relations and the encouragement of public discussion of these diseases, it is felt that the new term removes barriers to discussion and diminishes the unnecessarily sinister image which is of considerable antiquity.

No one can deny that the ravages of syphilis in Europe in the Middle Ages were terrible, being associated with diseases of the nervous system, including insanity and blindness due to infection of the optic nerve, as well as hideous deformities and the effects of congenital syphilis. It is hardly surprising that even today there is a carry-over of folk law about this group of infections.

Surveys of public opinion and attitudes taken in recent years indicate that 98% of the people interrogated in a quota sample in the age-groups eighteen to twenty-four are aware of the existence of sexually transmitted infections, but believe that they are in fact more frequent and prevalent than is actually the case. Information about symptoms, however, which could lead people to seeking diagnosis of treatment is vague, and only about 40% of samples interrogated have any idea of modern treatment.

BIOLOGY OF SEXUALLY TRANSMITTED DISEASES

The adaptation of the organisms responsible for these infections living only in the human genital tract is due to evolution. The organisms are extremely delicate, very difficult to cultivate outside the body, and do not survive unless offered the moisture, warmth, and nutrition provided by the body. In every community there is a so-called reservoir of infection, which means that there are numbers of individuals scattered at random throughout the community who are infected with these organisms and are therefore carriers. Sexual contact with one of these individuals will usually result in the infection being passed on to a new person. Thus the reservoir of infection will increase in size unless people newly infected recognize the symptoms and go at once to a special clinic for advice and treatment.

TYPES OF INFECTION

In the case of syphilis and gonorrhoea, the pool of infection is confined to people of promiscuous tendencies, that is those who have casual sexual relationships with more than one partner. It has now been recognized that the partner may include a person of the same sex. Promiscuous homosexuals are very liable to contract both syphilis and gonorrhoea. In the case of two people who have sexual relationships, but who have never had a partner beforehand and who are exclusive, no infection can occur. The ultimate prevention of syphilis and gonorrhoea therefore lies in the prevention of promiscuity which is itself a problem of mental health and personality.

In addition to the two infections mentioned, there is also a condition called non-specific urethritis. This is called 'non-specific' because up to the present it has not been possible to identify any one organism which is responsible for this infection, although there are now distinct clues. The symptoms appear predominantly in men, but bacteriological investigation of their women partners shows that similar organisms can be recovered from them. This condition, which has only been reported regularly since 1950 appears to be on the increase in the same way that gonorrhoea has increased. The diagnosis of non-specific urethritis is arrived at only after exhaustive bacteriological tests and physicians are at pains to exclude gonococcal infection. The problems of treatment are more complicated than in the case of gonorrhoea (*vide infra*). Authorities on this subject recommend the combined use of anti-biotics and sulphonamides and the treatment will involve both injections and the taking of tablets by mouth. As in the case of gonococcal infection patients should remain under observation for at least three months.

PROTOZOA, MOULDS, AND A VIRUS

There are two other infections of which the symptoms appear in women but where evidence can be obtained of their transmission to men. The first is *trichomonas vaginalis* which causes an irritating and sometimes offensive vaginal discharge in women and the presence of the organism can frequently be detected in the urethra of their male consorts. This is predominantly a sexually transmitted infection, but not necessarily a venereal one in the old sense, in that it can occur in married couples, and in a few cases it can appear to occur spontaneously quite apart from sexual intercourse. The trichomonas organism is a protozoal unicellular organism, but women are also subject to infection by a mould or yeast, *candida albicans*. This causes a troublesome discharge from the vagina and sometimes produces mild symptoms in male consorts. Treatment of both these conditions is specific and is undertaken after a diagnosis has been made by examining the discharge bacteriologically. Infection by candida albicans is treated by the use of pessaries containing an anti-biotic called 'nystatin'. Trichomonas infection is treated by another anti-biotic 'metronidazole' given orally. If possible, husbands or male consorts should also be examined and treatment offered if necessary. The discovery in the early 1970s that herpes virus can be transmitted sexually is important in that this infection causes damage to the covering of the cervix of the uterus and appears to be further confirmatory evidence of the way in which cancer of the cervix is related to long exposure to sexual intercourse, and to poor standards of personal hygiene.

Syphilis and gonorrhoea are matters of public concern, partly because they are indicators of sexual promiscuity, partly because of the carry-over of folk law regarding these diseases. Modern treatment using anti-biotics, coupled with careful surveillance of patients and follow up has resulted in a permanent cure, and prevention of transmission of disease to offspring. In the United Kingdom, the National Health Service maintains a chain of special clinics staffed by medical specialists in this group of diseases, supported by nurses, technicians, and social workers which provides free treatment without formality, and under conditions of strict confidentiality.

Fortunately, syphilis is not a large problem in the United Kingdom, although it is a very serious problem in the United States. There has been concern about the increase in the number of cases of gonorrhoea. In the middle 1950s the incidence of gonorrhoea in the United Kingdom sank to a very low level, and in fact there was some reason to believe that the disease was on its way out. There had been a high peak in its incidence during the war years which is consistent with our knowledge of the social causes of sexually transmitted infections. Where people are removed from their home environment and the social sanctions that go with it, when they are socially isolated, have time on their hands, or their inhibitions are released, these, coupled with fear of early death or of other misfortune, result in a tendency for sexually transmitted infections to increase. It is partly due to availability and partly to emotional conflicts precipitated by social pressures.

After the 1950s however, the incidence of gonorrhoea began to rise considerably.

SYMPTOMS OF INFECTION
The control of sexually transmitted diseases depends upon prompt treatment as soon as symptoms appear, and the follow up of contacts of the patient so that they too can be investigated and if necessary given treatment. In the case of the two major diseases, syphilis and gonorrhoea, the incubation periods and the symptoms are quite distinct. The incubation period of syphilis varies between ten days to ten weeks and the first symptom is the appearance of a sore, usually on the genital organs. If no treatment is given it is quite painless, it clears up in time, but the secondary stage makes its appearance later with fever, swollen glands and a skin rash. This stage is highly infectious and because there are syphilitic sores in the mouth and throat, this is one of the rare instances when syphilis can be transmitted by kissing. In the case of gonorrhoea, the incubation period is short — two to seven days, and in the male the symptoms are a thick discharge from the penis, accompanied by frequency and stinging or burning sensation on passing urine. These symptoms are usually so disturbing that it would be exceptional for anyone to ignore them.

IMPORTANCE OF CONTACT TRACING

Advertisements of special clinics where treatment can be obtained are posted in all public lavatories, and the institution of a telephone answering service, which also gives advice and addresses of various clinics, has made it certain that the majority of people who have contracted gonorrhoea obtain immediate treatment. The difficulty arises in the case of women in that, in 50% of cases, there is no vaginal discharge and no symptoms. Pain and frequency on passing urine may be ascribed to another cause. The follow up of the female contacts of patients with gonorrhoea therefore is most important and in this the responsibility is shared by the patient himself. Contact tracing is achieved either by the patient accepting a contact tracing slip with a clinic number on it and giving it to the girlfriend from whom he believes he contracted the infection and persuading her to attend the clinic, or by a welfare officer making a visit to the girlfriend or friends, and persuading them to come in for treatment.

EFFECTS OF SYPHILIS

From the point of view of the patient himself prompt treatment is essential in both syphilis and gonorrhoea. In the case of syphilis, the late results are very serious. Treponema pallidum, a motile corkscrew-like organism which causes the disease, multiplies rapidly in the primary sore, invades the bloodstream causing the secondary stage, and then enters many organs in the body causing permanent damage to the liver, heart, and nervous system We have now thirty years experience of treating primary syphilis by injections of penicillin as a result of which the late results of syphilis which colour the public's imagination with regard to this disease have virtually disappeared. It has been of great benefit also in the prevention of congenital syphilis in which the developing baby is infected by the mother. By the routine bloodtesting of all women in antenatal clinics the possibility of such infection being passed on has been eliminated. Penicillin can be given safely to women during pregnancy and this saves the baby.

EFFECTS OF GONORRHOEA

The organism causing gonorrhoea, the gonoccocus, behaves differently. It produces an acute inflamation at the site of entry causing the outpouring of pus following the destruction of cells lining the urethra. It too responds very well to penicillin although there are now drug-resistant strains appearing in all cities of the world and this may have come about through attempts at self-treatment, or through giving inadequate doses of penicillin, or where oral drugs have been used, through patients sharing these with their friends. Whatever the cause, penicillin resistance has to be accepted and the decision to use an alternative drug can only be taken by a physician specially experienced in this treatment.

If left untreated, gonorrhoea also can spread to other structures, causing local inflammation and abscesses in the structures related to the genital organs, however, the organism seldom invades the bloodstream. Inflammation of the testicle can produce sterility in the male and inflammation of the Fallopian tubes in the female causes sterility because the passage in the tube is obstructed and ova cannot be fertilized by the sperm. Chronic gonorrhoea causes a good deal of serious ill health, pain, and sickness in both sexes and in addition to the complications mentioned, arthritis also can occur.

From the point of view of individual well-being and for the well-being of the community, therefore, it is essential that all sexually active people who have casual relationships should be aware of the danger of infection and be able to recognize the symptoms, should go to the nearest special clinic if they suspect infection, should abstain from sexual intercourse until they have either been declared free from infection, or their course of treatment has been completed. They should co-operate with the welfare officers of the clinic in tracing contacts and should agree to remain under surveillance by the medical staff of the clinic until declared free from infection.

TREATMENT OF SYPHILIS AND GONORRHOEA

Syphilis is treated by a series of injections of penicillin over a few days, following confirmation of the diagnosis by examination of the primary sore, if present, supported by positive blood tests. When the treatment is completed, the patient should remain under surveillance for a period of two years during which time blood tests will be repeated and there will also be a test of the cerebro-spinal fluid in order to ensure that the nervous system has not been affected. The patient should not marry until pronounced free from infection, and in some countries indeed, the marriage licence is only granted on the production of a certificate declaring that a negative blood test has been obtained. This applies to all candidates for marriage, and in countries where syphilis occurs with considerable frequency, like the United States and in some European countries, this measure must have undoubtedly contributed to the decline in congenital syphilis. In the United Kingdom no such certificate is required, but it is a matter of personal responsibility for the individual concerned to put off marriage until free from infection.

Gonorrhoea is also treated by injections of penicillin, and in most cases a single injection is required only; the blood is tested to ensure that syphilitic infection has not occurred and the patient should be under surveillance at the clinic for a period of three months. Confirmation of freedom from infection can be obtained at the end of this period by bacteriological tests. In cases where the organism is resistant to penicillin, other anti-biotics may be necessary, or in some cases, very large doses of penicillin are used which, because of their bulk, are divided into two equal parts and injected separately.

Diagnosis of these infections is confirmed by isolation of the organism obtained by examination of material from the sore in the case of syphilis, and the discharge in the case of gonorrhoea, and subsequently cultured in the laboratory.

In the case of women, diagnosis may be difficult because the sore of syphilis may be hidden, and in the case of gonorrhoea, swabs must be taken repeatedly from the cervix of the uterus and the urethra, so that cultures can be isolated. Special clinics not only offer the technical skill for this kind of diagnosis, but their laboratory services also are specialized. It is significant that the figures published each year by the Department of Health and Social Security show that many patients attend the special clinics who are subsequently not found to be suffering from an infection. This is all to the good as it shows that an increasing number of people are aware of the risk of infection through casual contact and are prepared to accept the personal responsibility of obtaining medical advice. There is a tendency also for couples to attend together, and this does not mean married couples, and this reflects the greater frankness about these infections which has developed as a result of the softening up of public opinion by the continual stream of health education about these diseases through the mass media and the health education agencies.

RELEVANCE TO HEALTH EDUCATION IN SCHOOL

The relevance to health education in schools is that all school-leavers should be aware of the existence of the sexually transmitted diseases and of the symptoms that appear after infection. The subject can be approached from the general biological point of view during a consideration of the way in which bacteria and other micro-organisms cause disease. The teacher can then decide whether discussions on behaviour and morals can emerge after there is an understanding of the way in which the infections are contracted.

WHY THERE IS NO IMMUNIZATION AGAINST SEXUALLY TRANSMITTED INFECTIONS

Of the questions that are constantly asked, one concerns the effect on unborn children (which always excites the interest of girls) and the other is the question of immunization. Pupils will usually ask why there is no immunization against these grave infections when this is possible in the case of so many other diseases. Research has been in progress for many years towards the production of a vaccine that will protect people against syphilis. Progress is very slow, one difficulty being that the organism cannot be cultivated outside the body — an essential first step towards the production of an effective vaccine.

In the case of gonorrhoea, the nature of the organism appears so far to militate against a stable strain being available from which a vaccine could be made. No doubt these technical difficulties will eventually be overcome, but there then will remain the problem of how such a vaccine could be used. The present opinion amongst venereologists is that such vaccines, if effective, would best be used in the case of patients who are called 'repeaters', that is, those who are highly promiscuous and sexually active, and who come to the clinics repeatedly for treatment of further infection.

Care should be taken not to convey the idea that these diseases are very easily treated, as this may favour the development of the attitude that they are of little consequence as treatment is readily available. The World Health Organization reported in 1973 that there was an epidemic of gonorrhoea in Europe amongst young people. If the proportion of penicillin resistant strains increased, this could be a serious matter for the whole community and for the future. In some African countries, for example, as many as 30% of cases are resistant, and in some University populations in those countries as many as 60% and 70% of students are said to have gonorrhoea. If the control of gonorrhoea got out of hand, we might exhaust the range of other anti-biotics which could be used for treatment. There would therefore be a return to the days when chronic gonorrhoea and its attendant ill health and disability were common.

With regard to syphilis, it is fortunate that so far no penicillin resistant strains have appeared, but it would not be sensible for any community to rely entirely on the effectiveness of medical treatment. When we are dealing with ecology, we know that all organisms are remarkably adaptable in the race for survival of species. The history of myxomatosis in the rabbit population is an example. There is also the appearance of a strain of 'super lice'. There was also a race to eradicate malaria before mosquitoes became DDT-resistant. In other words, in the case of the sexually transmitted infections, the future health of the community lies in the hands of the sexually promiscuous section of the population. The tolerance of their sexual promiscuity by the community should be repaid by their own acceptance of their personal responsibility. At the same time, the whole community must accept the sexually transmitted infections as a community responsibility, particularly where consideration of personal welfare of young people in cities and social pressures are concerned.

QUESTIONS

1. 'Promiscuity is the major factor in the spread of sexually transmitted diseases yet the public appears to accept such practices — at least there is no real public outcry'. Comment on this statement.

2. Should more money be allocated to rearch on producing an immunization agent or on a more intensified campaign against promiscuity?

3. At what age would you, as a member of the public, suggest that education in personal relationships and personal responsibility should start and where?

4. There is widespread knowledge about sexually transmitted diseases and their spread — still the increase in some has been dramatic. How do you account for this

The Cancers — Specific Public Attitudes

Cancer is a matter of public concern for reasons quite unrelated to those we have discussed in respect of birth control, smoking, drugs, and sexually transmitted diseases. Malignant new growths have always been an object of particular fear, and public opinion has adopted a completely different attitude to diseases caused by such growths from that shown towards grave killing diseases, like for example, coronary thrombosis. It has been said that whereas coronary thrombosis is accepted as a cause of death, cancer is regarded with particular dread. This is probably because so many people have had personal contact with relatives and friends in the last stages of advanced cancers. There has been little or no publicity regarding the numbers of people who are cured each year as a result of surgery or radiotherapy. To say for example that 30,000 people were cured of cancer of different sites in the body during one year in England and Wales and that they have survived for a period of five years following the cure produces a completely different picture from the recital of statistics of death from cancer.

APPROPRIATE FOR SCHOOLS?

With the exception of rare cancers of the connective tissues (the sarcomata) and leukaemia, children and young people do not suffer from cancer and it might be argued that this subject is not appropriate for health education in schools. Bearing in mind that it has already been accepted that health education in schools could have a carry-over value into adult life and should anticipate problems that can be handled more effectively later on, it seems rational that the process of new growth should be studied as part of the study of biology itself. It is because malignant disease has appeared to be such a mystery, so inexplicable and threatening, that people have had such unreasoning fears that when they have suspected that they have symptoms which might be cancer, they have put off obtaining medical advice.

As long ago as 1802, an Edinburgh medical society studied the possibility of what we now call cancer education. They even circulated questionnaires to medical colleagues in different parts of the country, but the techniques of documentation and communication of information were so undeveloped at that time that they obtained little success. They were concerned with the recognition of the malignant process and with its early treatment, but at that period before even the invention of anaesthetics, the discovery of the principles of aseptic surgery, blood transfusion, and radiotherapy, there was virtually nothing that could have been done even in the early stages of a cancer.

MODERN TREATMENT

At the present day, we have highly developed techniques in surgery and radiotherapy, as well as diagnostic techniques involving X-rays and biochemical investigations, and techniques for the observation of individual cells which may show early stages of cancer. The setting up in 1973 of 'oncological centres' by the Department of Health and Social Security has resulted in the concentration of professional skill and technical resources which can all be brought to bear on the problem of the treatment of early cancer. At the same time, epidemiological investigations are throwing more and more light on the causation of certain kinds of cancer, the most classical example obviously is cancer of the lung, which one may say is almost entirely preventable. Industrial cancers caused by chronic exposure to various chemical substances can also be prevented by a total enclosure of the process, or by the substitution of non-carcinogenic chemicals for those previously used. This has been done, for example, in the rubber industry where certain chemicals used in processing rubber (betanaphthylamine) used to give rise to cancer of the bladder, and these are no longer used.

THE CANCER PROCESS

The secret to the understanding of the way in which cancers arise is the study of the growth process in the cell. The cells of all living organisms possess this unique property of growth by cell division. Growth of structures and organs does not take place by enlargement of cells, but by the increase in the number of cells. This is common to every living organism and Julian Huxley's book on cancer should be studied as it shows that new growth occurs as an abnormality in every type of living organism. Fossilized remains even of extinct species show evidence of what we would now call malignancy. Plants too show evidence of disorganized new growths.

During the life-cycle of the human being, growth is at its maximum from the time of fertilization and embedding of the fertilized ovum in the uterus. The rate of growth then is phenomenal — one has only to think of the increase in size from something of microscopical dimensions to a seven or eight pound baby at the time of birth. Growth continues towards maturity after birth, but its rate slows progressively and growth also occurs at different rates in different organs and systems. Once physical maturity is reached, the growth of cells is then related only to their replacement. In the case of the red blood cell, for example, its life is only about six weeks and the bone marrow is continually active in producing new red cells (as well as the granulocyte type of white blood cell). In the case of other organs, as cells become worn out and are shed, they are replaced by simple cell division of the remaining cells which then fill up with efficiency. This is going on quietly all the time and does not attract attention.

There are cases, however, where cell replacement becomes disorganized, resulting in disorderly growth, with rapid cell division and the production of cells which resemble the parent cell but which could be described as 'caricatures'. Growth which is irregular tends to invade the healthy cells in the immediate area, and also to spread through the bloodstream and lymphatic systems, first to glands draining the area of the new growth and later to distant organs. This is true malignancy.

In addition the tumour produces local effects according to its site. In tubular organs such as the stomach and the bowels it produces obstruction, and because the surface of the tumour tends to break down, bleeding also occurs. Tumours may press on nerves causing paralysis and also causing pain by pressure on tissues around them. Tumours may be felt with the fingers as in the case of surface organs, like the breast; they may produce alterations in the functions of an organ, for example, the thyroid gland or the pancreas, and in the case of the nervous system they produce paralysis, distortions of sensation or other disorders of function, according to the site in which the tumour occurs.

NOT A SINGLE DISEASE

For some years now, it has been the practice to talk about the cancers, and not cancer. Cancer is not a single disease, and there are several known causes. Over forty years ago, substances known as carcinogens were isolated from coal tar, and since that time there has been a vast amount of chemical research which has thrown light on the nature of carcinogens and the way in which they work. It is believed that there are two kinds, 'initiating substances', which may operate perhaps at the beginning of life, but which need the further action of 'promoting substances' which then set off the malignant process. Some cancers depend for their growth upon hormones, in particular, cancers of the breast and cancers of the prostate gland in the male. Of external causes, not only chemical substances, but also radioactivity appears to act as a promoting substance. For example, leukaemia in children has been associated with the too frequent X-raying of their mothers during pregnancy. Early pioneers in radiology suffered extensively from skin cancers, and the victims of the Hiroshima atomic explosion have suffered extensively from malignant disease.

The curability of cancers depends upon the degree of malignancy and the accessibility of the sites in which they occur. There are many types of cancer however in which early treatment provides a good chance of survival after a period of five years. It is particularly true of cancers affecting the lips, mouth, the tongue and the skin.

CANCER EDUCATION

Public concern about these diseases has been turned into constructive channels by the setting up of a number of voluntary agencies to promote so called cancer education. Cancer education, by explaining the nature of cancer, will diminish unreasonable fears about these diseases, and at the same time, by giving information about early symptons coupled with the provision of early diagnostic services which are now developing, will ensure that patients enjoy the best chances of survival. Symptons which require medical attention in any case, but which may be the signs of early cancer are:—

A sore on the skin or lip, which shows no tendency to heal.

Bleeding from bowel or bladder, or in the case of women, bleeding in between menstrual periods or following the menopause.

A sudden alteration of function, for example, the sudden onset of indigestion or abdominal pains, alternatively diarrhoea or constipation.

Loss of weight.

Hoarseness or cough.

The presence of a lump that can be felt with the fingers.

The last named symptom is most important in the case of cancers of the breast and for over forty years in the United States and more recently in other countries, self-examination of the breast has been taught so that women can take the advantage of reporting to their doctors at once, should they discover a lump in the breast. More elaborate techniques of tumour detection in the early stages in the breast have also been developed, including a special type of X-ray, and also a method involving the electrical estimation of local skin temperature. This subject has received a good deal of attention in the women's columns of newspapers and in women's magazines where well-informed articles have been presented to readers for several years.

EXFOLIATIVE CYTOLOGY

The discovery many years ago that abormalities can be detected in cells before they become malignant led to the organization of screening tests for cancer under the general heading of 'cytology'. This depends upon the fact that the surface cells continually exfoliate and can be collected and examined under the microscope. In another field, quite apart from cancer detection, the examination of the lining cells of the mouth has been used to study chromosomes and particularly the presence of abnormal sex chromosomes, this being the basis of the sex identification tests used in international athletic contests.

When examined under the microscope, it is possible to detect changes in the nucleus which will precede a malignant growth. This is a stage of a non-invasive new growth and if the test is positive thus a section of the tissue involved can be removed by a minor operation and looked at in more detail under the microscope. This offers the possibility of surgical treatment of cancer at the pre-invasive stage.

CERVICAL CYTOLOGY

The best known application of this method is in the case of cancer of the cervix of the uterus. Under the National Health Service, women over the age of thirty-five and those under the age of thirty-five who have had three children can obtain this service from either their own doctors, or from a clinic. In many cases mobile units have been organized so that the service can be taken to the women, thus removing any barriers that may inhibit women from asking for this service.

The surface of the cervix of the uterus is gently scraped with a wooden spatula, this is a completely painless procedure, a smear is made on a glass slide, 'fixed' and sent through the post to a laboratory. Laboratories have been organized to give special attention to this service and technicians, particularly skilled and experienced in the detection of early abnormalities, supervised by pathologists, can process a large number of slides at a time. At present it is recommended that the ideal situation would be that all women over thirty-five should have this test repeated at three yearly intervals.

Cytological examinations of this kind can also be carried out on sputum to detect lung cancer at an early stage, and in regions of the intestine accessible to instrumental examinations. However, the use of X-ray techniques of diagnosis are more common in the case of tumours in these sites.

CANCER RESEARCH

Research into the causation of cancer and its more effective treatment forms an important branch of medical science, and many medical scientists have devoted the whole of their careers to one aspect of this subject. The work involves not only pathologists, but also biochemists, biologists, physicists, and mathematicians.

Malignant tumours produce biochemical changes and these can be the subject of a study on their own. Surgeons whose practice is mainly in the field of treating cancer, and radiologists who organize radiotherapy centres are important partners in the research programmes. At the present time, one important area of research is to discover whether there is any immunity to the cancerous process. The growth of a malignant tumour is the only example of the failure of normal cells to respond to a foreign body. A malignant tumour is of course not truly a foreign body as it has developed upon the host's own cell. The suggestion is that in the case of malignant growths, there is no 'feed back' from the malignant cells to the host's cells, which then are unaware, so to speak, of the existence of the tumour. Nevertheless, in a small number of cases, there is evidence of some kind of immune action and cases of spontaneous disappearances of a malignant tumour of low-grade malignancy are not unheard of.

There is also an attempt to find a chemical treatment for cancer in place of, or to supplement radiotherapy and surgery. Unfortunately many chemical agents which destroy malignant cells will also destroy normal cells and the use of such chemical agencies is confined to treatment of advanced cases not suitable for other methods of treatment. The use of hormones in treatment however is interesting, particularly as it opens up a possibility of a deeper understanding of the nature of certain kinds of cancer. Thus in cancer of the breast, injections of male hormone will cause regression of the tumour, and in cases of cancer of the prostate in men, injections of female hormone will produce the same effect. The fact that these tumours are apparently dependent upon sex hormonal balance gives some idea of their possible causation, particularly as both tumours affect active glandular structures which are intimately connected with the sex life of the individual.

CANCER PREVENTION
However successful treatment of established malignant growths may be, as in other branches of medicine, prevention remains the ultimate ideal. Ideas for prevention are already emerging from epidemiological studies, and we have referred earlier to Burkitt's (see page 30) suggestion that the absence of roughage in modern diets has contributed to stagnation of movements of the large bowel, and is in some way associated with a tendency for cancer to occur in this site.

Comparative studies of the prevalence of cancer of various sites in the body show that there is great variation from region to region. Cancer of the liver for example is more common in Africa than in Europe, but in Europe and in the USA cancer of the intestines is frequent. A world picture shows that cancer of the colon (large intestine) is commonest amongst the Chinese population of Hawaii and that its incidence is about twice that in the UK. The incidence is very low in Japan and amongst the Bantu population of South Africa. It has also been observed that the prevalence of cancer in particular sites in migrant populations approximates to the pattern prevalent in the country to which they migrate and not to the country of origin. This has been found in respect of the mortality from cancer of the stomach in the USA. The incidence of this type of cancer in Japan is high but it is lowest amongst Japanese who have lived longest in the USA. This is an example of one of nature's controlled experiments which points to the operation of environmental factors in the causation of cancer.

The subject of the cancers therefore offer intellectual stimulation and interest for senior pupils in schools, and can be related to biological, geographical, and environmental studies. An opportunity can also be taken to dispel the unnecessary mystery and fear about this particular disorder, so that when they enter adult life, boys and girls will be prepared to accept screening procedures where appropriate, to take avoiding and preventive action where they are able to do so — here we would once again mention the case of the association of carcinoma of the cervix with poor personal hygiene — and to take prompt action if they suffer from any one of the symptoms outlined above, which may or may not be an early sign of cancer.

THE EFFECT OF THE COMMUNITY'S INTEREST
The collective emotionalism of the community is shown in the frequent appeals that are made on behalf of cancer research and the care of terminal cancer sufferers. This emotionalism has been channelled into constructive effort insofar as a considerable amount of research and care facilities are supported by voluntary effort, but it is time that the community began to think in terms of the prevention of cancer, rather than a cure. It has been said that whenever the community begins to take a collective interest in a problem and to discuss it widely, then the problem then begins to diminish. There has recently been a change of official opinion in that, whereas twenty years ago the idea that the facilities for the treatment of cancer should be concentrated in special centres was rejected, the decision to set up the oncological centres in different regions of the United Kingdom seems to follow this general principle that when there is a community concentration on a problem then it begins to resolve. This has been seen in the case of infant mortality and also in the case of tuberculosis. The position regarding the prevention and the control of the cancers is therefore now much more hopeful than formerly.

QUESTIONS

1. Why, in your opinion, should there be public concern about cancer?

2. Do you think that the public are well enough informed about the tests for signs of cancer? Why are so many people reluctant to seek medical advice if they suspect they have cancer?

3. Why is cancer so feared by the average person?

REFERENCES

Birth Control

1. Hawthorne, G. (1973). *Population Policy — A Modern Delusion.* Fabian Tract No. 418. London: Fabian Society.
2. Parsons, J. (1973). 'Population and Health' in *Population Growth and Control,* a supplement to the *Health and Social Services Journal.*
3. Birth Control Campaign. (1972). *A Birth Control Campaign for Britain.* London.
4. Woolf, Myra. (1971). *Family Intentions.* Office of Population Censuses and Surveys Publication. London: HMSO.
5. British Pregnancy Advisory Service. (1971). *Client Statistics, 1971. With Commentary.* Birmingham.

Drugs

1. Hindmarsh, I. (1972). 'Drugs and their Abuse: Age-groups particularly at Risk'. *Brit. J. Addiction.* 67(4):313—15.
2. Wigfield, W. J. (1972). 'Survey of Young People's Attitudes to Drug Abuse'. *Community Medicine* 129:139—41.
3. World Health Organization. (1973). *Youth and Drugs.* Report of a WHO Study Group. London: HMSO.
4. Watson, L. M. (1972). 'The Management of Drug Abuse in School Children'. *Publ. Hlth.* 86:10—19.
5. Bradshaw, S. (1972). *Drug Misuse and the Law.* London: Macmillan.
6. Advisory Committee on Drug Dependence (Chairman: Baroness Wootton). (1968). *Cannabis Report.* London: HMSO.

Alcohol

1. *Report of Departmental Committee on Liquor Licensing.* (Erroll Report). (1972). London: HMSO.
2. Davies, J. and Stacey, B. (1972). *Teenagers and Alcohol: A Developmental Study in Glasgow.* London: HMSO.

FURTHER READING

Birth Control

Alleson, Anthony (ed.) (1970). *Population Control.* Harmondsworth: Penguin.

Boyd, R. H. (1952). *Controlled Parenthood.* London: Heinemann.

Bull, David, (ed.) (1971). *Family Poverty.* London: Duckworth.

Cartwright, A. (1970). *Parents and Family Planning Services.* London: Routledge and Kegan Paul.

Dalzell-Ward, A. J. (1973). 'The Role of Health Education' in *Population Growth and Control,* a supplement to the *Health and Social Services Journal.*

Draper, E. (1972). *Birth Control in the Modern World.* Harmondsworth: Penguin.

Ferris, Paul (1968). *The Nameless: Abortion in Britain Today.* Harmondsworth: Penguin.

Gardner, R. F. R. (1972). *Abortion: The Personal Dilemma.* (Examines religious and ethical issues). Exeter: Paternoster Press.

Green, Shirley, (1971). *Curious History of Contraception.* London: National Magazine Co.

Hay, D. (1972). *Human Population.* Harmondsworth: Penguin.

Laing, W. (1972). *Costs and Benefits of Family Planning.* London: PEP.

McDougal, R. (1973). 'The Politics of Control' in *Population Growth and Control.*

McQueen, I. A. G. (1973). 'The Local Authority' in *Population Growth and Control.*

Munday, D. (1973). 'Abortion and Population' in *Population Growth and Control.*

Other papers published in *Population Growth and Control.*

Prosser, H. (1973). 'Family Size and Children's Development' in *Population Growth and Control.*

Taylor, L. R. (ed.) (1970). *The Optimum Population for Britain.* London: Academic Press.

Williams, J. M. and Hindle, K. (1972). *Abortion and Contraception: A Study of Parents' Attitudes.* London: PEP.

Smoking

Department of Education and Science. (1972). *Smoking and Health in Schools.* London: HMSO. (This publication contains a useful bibliography on the subject of smoking.)

Fletcher, C. M. (1965). *Commonsense about Smoking.* Harmondsworth: Penguin.

McKennel, A. C. and Thomas, R. K. (1967). *Adults' and Adolescents' Smoking Habits and Attitudes.* London: HMSO.

Richardson, R. G. (ed.) (1972). *Report of the Proceedings of The Second World Conference on Smoking and Health.* London: Pitman Medical Books (published for the Health Education Council). (This Report contains sections on the economics of smoking and the problems of prevention of smoking in children.)

Royal College of Physicians of London. (1971). *Smoking and Health Now: Report.* London: Pitman Medical Books.

Salzer, K. (1959). *Thirteen Ways to Break the Smoking Habit.* London: Duckworth.

Schroder, M. (1964). *Better Smoking.* London: Allen and Unwin.

Drugs

Association for the Prevention of Addiction. Various publications.

Aumonye, A. and McClure, J. L. (1970). 'Adolescent Drug Abuse in a North London Suburb'. *Brit. J. Addiction.* 1:25—33.

Birdwood, G. (1969). *The Willing Victim: A Parents' Guide to Drug Abuse.* London: Secker and Warburg.

Bradshaw, D. (1968). *The Drugs You Take.* London: Pan Books.

Cassens, James. (1970). *Christian Encounters: Drugs and Drug Abuse.* St. Louis: Concordia.

Chapple, P. A. L. (1970). 'The Spread of Drug Addiction in the UK'. *Roy. Soc. Hlth. J.* **90**(4):196.

Dawtry, F. (1968). *Social Problems of Drug Abuse.* London: Butterworth.

Family Doctor Series. Various publications.

McAthlone, Beryl (ed.) (1970). *Where on Drugs: A Parents' Handbook.* Cambridge: Advisory Centre for Education.

Mitchell, A. R. K. (1973). *Drugs — The Parents' Dilemma.* London: Priory Press.

Ripley, G. D. (1972). 'Drug Abuse Prevention through Education at School'. *Brit. J. Addiction.* **67**(3): *313—15.*

Schofield, M. G. (1970). *The Strange Case of Pot.* Harmondsworth: Penguin.

Wiener, R. S. P. (1970). *Drugs and School Children.* London: Longmans.

Wood, A. J. (1968). *Drug Dependence.* Bristol: Bristol Health Department

Wright, J. D. (1968). *About Drugs.* Wolverhampton: Wolverhampton Health Department

Alcohol

Al-Anon Family Groups. (1972). *Dilemma of the Alcoholic Marriage.* Available from Al-Anon Family Groups, c/o St Giles Centre, Camberwell Church Street, SE5.

Hatton, A. (1973). *Alcohol: Perspectives in Alcoholism.* Available from the National Council of Alcoholism 45 Gt Peter St, London SW1 P3LT.

Home Office. (1973). *Offences of Drunkenness.* (Statistics of the number of offences of drunkenness proved in England and Wales for the year 1972 compared with the number of offences proved in previous years.) Cmnd. 5380. London: HMSO. (This Report records offences by young people of both sexes in the age range under 14, 14—18, and 18—21, analysed according to geographical regions.)

Jahoda, G. (1972). *Children and Alcohol: A Developmental Study in Glasgow.* London: HMSO.

Kessel, Neil and Walton, Henry. (1965). *Alcoholism* Harmondsworth: Penguin.

Merseyside Council on Alcoholism (1972). *The Illness of Alcohol.* Liverpool: Merseyside Council on Alcoholism

National Council on Alcoholism (with Christopher D. Smithers Foundation Inc., New York). (1973). *Arresting Alcoholism.* (Including a questionnaire for self-completion.)

Office of Health Economics. (1970). *Alcohol abuse.* London.

Searle-Jordan, V. T. (1970). *Social Drinking and You.* (Pamphlet with Foreword by Dr A. D. C. S. Cameron.) London: London Borough of Hammersmith Health Education Service.

Zacune, J. and Hensman, C. (1972). *Drugs, Alcohol and Tobacco in Britain.* London: Heinemann Medical Books.

Sexually transmitted diseases

Catterall, R. D. (1967). *Venereal Diseases.* London: Evans.

Dunlop, E. M. C. (1973). 'Some Moral Problems posed by Sexually Transmitted Diseases'. *Brit. J. Ven. Dis.* **49**(4):203—208.

Hollins, F. R. and Dicks, S. (1968). 'A Personal Relationship Project in Senior Schools'. *Med. Officer,* **120**(19):261–4.

Holmes, M., Nicol, C. S. and Stubbs, R. (1969). 'Sex Attitudes of Young People'. *Hlth. Educ. J.* **28**(1):13.

Nahmias, A. J. Dowdle, W. R., Nash, Z. M., Josey, W. E., McClone, D. and Dimoshek, G. (1969). 'Genital Infection with Type Two Herpes Virus Hominis'. *Brit. J. Ven. Dis.* **45**(4):294.

Wells, B. B. W. and Schofield, C. B. S. (Jan. 1970). 'Target Sites for Anti-VD Propaganda'. *Scottish Health Bulletin.* London: HMSO. (This article gives the results of a study showing that there are specified venues in a city where male patients meet contacts from whom they contract a sexually transmitted infection.)

The Cancers

Bennette, Graham (ed.) (1971). *Cancer Priorities.* London: British Cancer Council.

Burkitt, D. P. (1971). 'Cancer and the Way We Live'. Chapter in Graham Bennette (ed.) *Cancer Priorities.* London: British Cancer Council.

Doll, R. (1967). *Prevention of Cancer – Pointers for Prevention.* (The Rock Carling Fellowship, Nuffield Provincial Hospitals Trust.) London: Whitefriars Press.

Harris, R. J. C. (ed.) (1970). *What we know about Cancer.* London: Allen and Unwin.

Higginson, J. (1972). 'Geographical Pathology and the Potential Prevention of Cancer'. *Roy. Soc. Hlth. J.* **92**(6):291.

Huxley, J. (1958). *Biological Aspects of Cancer.* London: Allen and Unwin.

PERIODICALS

Drugs and Society. A monthly magazine published by Macmillan Journals Ltd.

Monitor. A Teachers' journal on social problems published by the Teachers' Advisory Council on Alcohol and Drug Education, 437 Royal Exchange, Manchester M2 7EP. (This organization supplies lecture services to schools, colleges and PTAs, and teaching-charts and literature for pupils on the subject of drugs.)

FILMS

Title	Colour B/W	Running time	Distributor	Date
BIRTH CONTROL				
Family Planning (USA) (cartoon)	Colour	10 mins.	Educational Foundation for Visual Aids or Concord Film Council	1968
Happy Family Planning (USA; cartoon)	Colour	10 mins.	Educational Foundation for Visual Aids or Concord Film Council	1970

F I L M S (*continued*)

Title	Colour B/W	Running time	Distributor	Date
To Plan Your Family (USA)	Colour	10 mins.	Educational Foundation for Visual Aids or Concord Film Council	1968
Unmarried Mothers		30 mins.	Concord Film Council	1968

TAPE RECORDINGS (CASSETTES)

Title	Colour B/W	Running time	Distributor	Date
Interviews, tape No. 1 (suitable for all groups. Interviews with two girls, separately, aged 15 and 16. Views are expressed on relationships with parents and pre-marital sexual relationships.)			Birmingham Brook Advisory Centre	
A Matter of Life (cassette) deals with contraception		25 mins.	Infotape Productions, 50 Frith Street, London W1	1972

SMOKING

Title	Colour B/W	Running time	Distributor	Date
Dying for a Smoke (British; for 12—15 year-olds)	Colour	10 mins.	Central Film Library	1967
The Smoking Machine (British; for 9—12 year-olds)	Colour	16 mins.	Central Film Library	1964
The Black Sheep (this film was made by pupils at a secondary school)	B/W	12 mins.	Cancer Information Centre, College Bldgs., University Place, Splott, Cardiff	
The Drag (cartoon about pressures to conform)	Colour	9 mins.	Concord Film Council	1967

LUNG CANCER

Title	Colour B/W	Running time	Distributor	Date
This is Your Lung	Colour	16 mins.	Tenovus Cancer Information Centre	1963
A Time for Decision (USA)	Colour	16 mins.	Concord Film Council	1966

DRUGS AND ALCOHOL

Title	Colour B/W	Running time	Distributor	Date
Drugs and the Nervous System (American)	Colour	18 mins.	Boulton Hawker Ltd., Hadleigh, Ipswich, Suffolk	1967
One Way Ticket (British)	Colour	23 mins.	South Staffordshire Medical Centre, New Cross Hospital, Wolverhampton WV10 0PQ	1971

F I L M S (*continued*)

Title	Colour B/W	Running time	Distributor	Date
Alcohol and the Human Body	B/W	15 mins.	Rank Film Library	
The Choice is Yours (for 13—14 year-olds)	Colour	15 mins.	Concord Film Council (made by the Medical Council on Alcholism)	1973
What's Yours? (longer version of above for 16—20 year-olds)	Colour	30 mins.	Concord Film Council (made by the Medical Council on Alcholism)	

SEXUALLY TRANSMITTED DISEASES

Half a Million Teenagers (American)	Colour	16 mins.	Boulton Hawker Ltd., Hadleigh, Ipswich, Suffolk/N.A.V.A.L.	1965
VD — Don't Take the Risk (2 reels)	B/W	20 mins.	Central Film Library (adapted from TV World in Action)	1964
Shadow of Ignorance (3 reels)	B/W	25 mins.	Central Film Library (adapted from TV)	1963

TAPE CASSETTE

The X Factor (emphasises importance of contact tracing, dramatized recording of an actual case of infection)		24 mins.	Infotape Productions, Frith Street, London W1	1971

CANCER

What is Cancer? (USA) (intended primarily for medical audiences but included in BISFA/BMA catalogue)	Colour	21 mins.	Cancer Information Centre, Cardiff	
Time and Two Women (USA; deals with the value of cervical cytology)	Colour	18 mins.	Cancer Information Centre, Cardiff	1956
Cell Division (film loop) (this is helpful to understand the fundamental principle of the way in which normal cells can become malignant)			Macmillan, Brunel Road, Basingstoke (ref. BC/029)	

FILMSTRIPS
(referring to all topics in this chapter)

Pity the children	Concord
Problem Families (two parts)	Camera Talks Ltd.
Family Planning	Camera Talks Ltd.
Genital Diseases	Camera Talks Ltd.
Problems of Alcoholism (seven parts)	Camera Talks Ltd.
Drugs in Our Society	Camera Talks Ltd.
The Drug Problem — Marijuana Colour	Concordia
and L.S.D.	
Drugs and School Children (three parts)	Camera Talks Ltd.
1. Is there a Problem?	
2. Experience	
3. Why Drugs?	
Problem of Lung Cancer	Camera Talks Ltd.
Cancer Education	Camera Talks Ltd.
Air Pollution	Camera Talks Ltd.
The Air You Breathe	Diana Wyllie
Clean Air (two parts)	Camera Talks Ltd.
Mountain Safety (two parts)	Camera Talks Ltd.

CHAPTER 16

The learning environment

Health education employs all the methods and techniques which are used in the general educational field. Because of its separate development, health education outside the school — for example, that practised in child welfare centres by health visitors, or with groups of parents — has tended to consider the methods it uses as specific. Although this claim could not be justified, there are however various considerations related to the nature of the subject and the need for influencing attitudes and behaviour as well as communicating information. When one surveys the rich variety of aids for communication offered by modern educational technologists, the problem is to select those that are applicable to the situation and to define the objectives of the educational exercise beforehand.

Problems of Selection

We have already defined the aims and objectives of health education from the strategic point of view. From the tactical point of view, they can be defined as: giving information; changing attitudes where necessary; resolving anxieties and conflicts; and bringing about an alteration in behavioural patterns. The skill of the teacher lies in selecting that battery of aids which can stimulate the appropriate learning mechanisms to bring about this kind of result.

A convenient classification would be as follows:-

(a) methods involving organization in the classroom, for example, group discussion, buzzgroups, or projects.
(b) methods involving the use of non-projected visual aids.
(c) methods involving the use of projected aids.
(d) methods involving the use of electronic aids.
(e) programmed learning.

Involvement of Colleagues

We have already referred to the fact that health education involves team teaching and that some members of the team from time to time may not be on the teaching staff. This raises the problem of how most effectively to use colleagues, such as school medical officers or other doctors, health education officers, school nurses, and public health inspectors. The conventional approach is to ask one of these experts to visit the school to give a talk; the only information usually given is the age-group involved and the subject matter. This has several disadvantages.

First the selection of a particular topic, and it is usually something like sex education, venereal diseases, or drugs, isolates the topic from the general syllabus of health education and may confer on it an unnecessary importance. Secondly, the expert concerned, although he or she may be an extremely fluent public speaker and capable lecturer, has not received training as a teacher, and has no method at command, other than the didactic talk. Third, it is not possible for the outside expert to make a diagnosis of the need of the class concerned, or of the level of knowledge they already possess, or the quality of attitudes. Certainly experts who are working in the public health service will have had in-service training and considerable practical experience of health education, and nowadays would much prefer to be invited to take part in a team teaching effort in which they contributed their own particular expertise.

A better approach would be to explain the scope of the regular health education programme, the need for a contribution by an outside expert, and then to invite the person concerned to visit the school and to discuss the methods to be used with the class teacher. In this way, the guest speaker becomes involved in the life of the school, even if only for a temporary period and can discuss the scope of the content of the session and make suggestions as to ways in which it can be communicated. Amongst other things to be discussed are the kind of visual aids that will be available, and the apparatus needed to use them.

Partnership between Teacher and Health Profession

In place of a formal didactic talk, a learning situation can be set up with such a partnership which can involve the pupils to the maximum extent, and this process can often be initiated by a dialogue between the class teacher and the guest speaker. For example, a session may be broken up into a short introductory talk by the school medical officer, followed by a five minute session in which the class divides into small groups of six each to discuss the kind of questions that they would like to ask the doctor. A short film might then be shown and the final session would consist of class teacher and doctor conducting the discussion jointly. The class teacher may put questions to the guest speaker. In this way the teaching potential of the outside expert can be fully exploited and much more value will be gained from the visit than if he was merely asked to give a formal talk.

In the various in-service training experiences that are available to the staff of public health departments, this kind of advice is given to them. They are urged not to accept invitations to give talks, but rather to establish rapport with the school and to discuss the ways in which they can contribute to a team teaching situation. This method is appreciated by those who are able and fluent speakers and it becomes a necessity for those who do not enjoy this natural endowment or who have not had the experience that develops it. It is a matter of common experience that a quite ineffective and boring speaker can liven up to make an effective contribution when questions are put to him It is therefore only just to the invited guest that an opportunity should be taken of allowing him to demonstrate his particular expertise to the full.

With the close partnership that should exist between teachers and the school health service, such a dialogue should present no difficulties, and it is also an advantage that teachers attend meetings which are attended also by members of the school health staff where topics of common interest are discussed. In some areas of the United Kingdom, there are child health societies whose membership is multidisciplinary so that teachers and doctors, school nurses, psychiatrists and pyschiatric social workers involved with school children can meet regularly in the professional setting to listen to papers and to discuss them and to hold discussions on their joint problems concerned with the welfare of the schoolchild and health education.

Non-projected Aids

Health education outside the school has concentrated on the development of visual aids which encourage group participation. They are aids for communication of ideas which may be abstract to the group, but also they allow for the exercise of deductive powers when the group is invited to participate. The appearance of the sophisticated electronic aids which are fashionable at the present day has in no way supplanted simple devices such as the flannel-graph, which, when used in its 'multiple choice' form, provides the optimum situation for group participation.

Details of the design and construction of flannel-graphs can be learned from various technical works, some of which are listed at the end of this section. It is most important that flannel-graphs should be as simple as possible. Some well-meaning people construct flannel-graphs of so many small individual pieces that they are unmanageable and the teachers' attention is taken up with sticking the pieces on to the backcloth. The flannel-graph lends itself to symbolic representation of objects or ideas. For example, the conventional use of red, orange, and green can be used to signify danger, caution, and safety, and this will be applicable, for example, in a flannel-graph that dealt with the dangers of bacteria and the ways in which people can either avoid them, or be protected by immunization.

MULTIPLE CHOICE
The multiple choice system is particularly valuable where subjects are being dealt with which might cause embarrassment or offence when a pupil's life-style is compared unfavourably with the life-style being urged by the teacher. A multiple choice flannel-graph uses three columns with three main headings: 'Necessary', 'Desirable' and 'Unnecessary', Symbols of objects, for example, toilet requisites, or food, are handed out to a group which is then invited to come in a body to the blackboard and to place the objects with which they have been issued in the appropriate column. If handled correctly, it is impossible for anyone to identify an individual choice, and this hides the embarrassment of some people who might be uncertain or who might be conscious of some defect in their personal hygiene, choice of diet, and so on.

When the whole group has made its collective choice, the teacher can then discuss the pattern that is shown, and can invite the group to suggest the movement of some objects from one column to another. The leaders should avoid forcing or causing an individual to reveal his identity.

The writer found this device very helpful when asked to conduct a session with the domestic staff of a hospital on the subject of personal hygiene. The group were aged between seventeen and fifty, were all women, and might easily have been offended if they had received a didactic talk on how to wash and keep themselves generally clean. To set up the multiple choice flannel-graph, the group were invited to imagine themselves faced with a problem of having to undertake a journey immediately without notice, but with a few minutes which would allow them to pack a bag. They were invited to classify the objects issued to them as necessary, helpful, or unnecessary. The objects were the usual toilet requisites, including toothpaste, soap, toilet paper, in case this article was not supplied, towels, combs, sanitary towels, nail brush, handkerchiefs, and a change of underclothing.

The subsequent discussion when the pattern had been worked out by the group enabled the basic principles of personal hygiene and the importance of this in the prevention of the spread of harmful bacteria to other people to be discussed without embarrassment.

The multiple choice flannel-graph can be set up in a variety of ways, for example, 'which game, what age?' where, instead of the three standard columns, a number of columns can have headings according to different age-groups. In parentcraft teaching, it can be used to discuss the question of which toy at what age, and there would seem to be an infinite variety of ways in which a teacher could use this particular visual aid.

OTHER MOBILE VISUAL AIDS
The magnetic blackboard is another device which can be used for group participation. The principles of its use as a teaching aid do not differ from those of the flannel-graph. It is only the medium that is different. It has a disadvantage in being heavier and in requiring the attachment of symbols to magnets so that the preparation of a lesson necessarily takes longer. It can be said however to provide considerable job satisfaction to the teacher as the *panache* with which the objects can be almost thrown at the board to stick in the right place provides an element of excitement both for the teacher and the pupils.

Another device which has been used extensively in health education is the 'magiboard' which is really simply a 'blackboard' made of *white* formica on which drawings and writing can be done with coloured felt-tipped pens; in using this device, the same principles are applied as are necessary in using a blackboard. These can be summarized as using handwriting, rather than printing, in dividing the board into various areas so that the final result at the end of a lesson is a balanced pattern of words, drawings, figures, and diagrams. These of course are the general principles involved in classroom teaching, and are in no way specific to health education.

The use of coloured plastic materials, which can stick on to a sheet of black or coloured plastic, has been introduced under the term plastigraph. This has its uses if an attractive chart is to be produced that can be used as a teaching aid. It is not so useful as the flannel-graph or magnetic blackboard because the symbols cannot be readily moved; they have to be applied with deliberation and are not so easily moved for replacement.

The attractiveness of the plastigraph lies in the type of material and the bright colour contrasts possible. It should be mentioned here that in all colour contrasts, general physiological principles should be observed. White on black, black on yellow or yellow on black provide the best colour contrasts available. As the colour contrasts between the symbols and the background begin to fade, the visual perception becomes more difficult. Another problem is the question of glare, and this means that when shiny surfaces such as the magiboard or the plastigraph are used, the board to which they are fixed has to be arranged so that light does not fall on it directly, otherwise the reflected glare will prevent the class from seeing the symbols.

PUPPETRY

Puppetry can be used in health education for younger children, and has been so used to great effect, although mainly outside the school. The late Dr. Hoey who was a medical officer of health in Monmouthshire was a pioneer in the use of puppetry in health education and was able to attract audiences of over a hundred to evening shows at which puppet plays dealing with dental health, food hygiene, and immunization were presented.

There is a danger that if a pioneer is particularly successful with a method, then that method becomes automatically associated with the subject. All teachers will be aware of the use of puppetry in education, as well as for entertainment; some will have a particular liking and aptitude for this work, and will also have the necessary skill in design in making their own puppets. When used in health education, puppets must be made for the occasion, as it is unlikely that those available commercially will fit in to the characters required, or can even be adapted. The success of the use of puppetry depends entirely on the capacity for imagery of the teacher concerned, so that a drama can be written and presented which conveys real meaning in terms of the subject, as well as being entertaining.

EXHIBITS

Exhibition techniques also have an important place. Museums are by no means out of date and modern museum practice makes them lively and meaningful in terms of real life, keeping pace with change and developing attractive methods of presentation. A museum can be said to embrace a range of situations from the great museums of capital cities down to a small exhibit in the corner of a classroom. The museum is a place for the display of objects which may range in size from a complete aircraft or a locomotive, down to a printed circuit of microscopical proportions. The effectiveness of presentation depends on lighting, colour, background, accessibility, movement, and sound where possible. The use of expanded polystyrene and Letraset has provided teachers and health educators with a useful medium for the construction of exhibits. This is also an area in which the pupils themselves can participate, and projects involving the design, construction, and presentation of exhibitions can form a useful part of the health education programme.

Allied to this is the use of actual objects as teaching aids. In the experimental project in the infant school already referred to, (see Page 143) Boustead used actual X-ray plates borrowed from a hospital as well as several other objects and models to arouse the interest of these very small children. Where an object is portable, is not offensive, and can be used safely by a group of children, there is no point in making a model of it or showing a drawing or photograph. In the field of dental health education for example, local authority dental services have made available complete surgery equipment which children are allowed to handle. Thus, children can examine each other's teeth with a mirror, although perhaps it would be unwise to allow them to use a probe or any other instrument; they can amuse themselves by winding the chair up and down and they can use dental drills on model teeth or animal teeth embedded in soap.

Another useful teaching aid in this group of non-projected aids is the chart. The chart must not be confused with the poster, as the latter's function is to arrest attention, to give brief information, and to inspire to further action. A chart is more elaborate, contains more detail and is intended to be lingered over, discussed, and explained. Again in the field of dental health education, very many charts have been produced by the General Dental Council and other agencies for use in schools. A variety of charts can be obtained from commercial sources and an increasing number of educational publishers also now publish charts to be used as teaching aids.

Projected Aids

The aids available under this heading consist of the cinema film in 16 millimetre, 8 millimetre or super 8, slides, film strips, and the overhead projector. Once again it must be emphasized that none of these can be considered to be an alternative to the others — they all form part of a battery of visual aids from which selection should be made according to the subject.

USE OF CINEMA
Such a judgment tends to be most faulty in the case of the use of cinema in health education. Cinema is the most expensive as well as the most sensitive of the media that can be used in teaching. It performs *some* functions of communication exclusively. In other cases it does as well as other media, and in yet other cases it may not be as good as other media. Because of its great expense and the natural reluctance of education authorities to scrap films so long as they are usable, it calls for the greatest exercise of discretion, skill, and responsibility in its use. At one time the cinema film carried its own authority, but with the advent of television this authority is no longer enjoyed as of right. There is still a tendency however to think vaguely in terms of 'film shows' for, just as outside lecturers are often invited to come in and give a talk, so health education departments of local authorities may be simply asked to make films available.

CINEMA AT ITS BEST

This practice should be resisted, as a film can only be a teaching aid and must be selected in relevance to the topic and the situation. Generally speaking, the cinema is at its best when it is portraying human emotion and human behaviour. The series of films on child development produced by the Film Board of Canada illustrate this very well. There is no other way in which the uninhibited movements and behaviour of children in groups could be observed, save by filming them and then by producing an edited film.

The film is also an exclusive medium for contriving an experience which would not be possible in any other way. For example, in the world of the microscope, time-lapse photography has enabled cell division to be demonstrated, and the growth of plants. By the use of cinema techniques and radiology the working of internal organs in the body can also be observed. If the subject involves a geographical location which is not accessible, for example, in descriptions of the work of the World Health Organization, then it has an exclusive function. The cinema also has an importance in influencing motivation and now that camera techniques and editing are so much more sophisticated than in the days of the conventional documentary, perhaps the cinema is going to play its supreme role in health education in the field of mental health and the sociological approach.

SKILL IN USING FILM

Experience shows that there is also a considerable lack of understanding and skill in the use of the film as a teaching aid. It is best, where possible, to employ a separate projectionist, leaving the teacher free for comment and to conduct discussion. Even so, it is important that all teachers should be able to lace up a projector and to be aware of the way in which a film can be projected without damage, how to rewind the film after use, and so on. It is important to have adequate projection facilities, including blackout, as it is irritating and boring to a class to see a film that is barely visible, or where the sound is distorted.

There are many documentary films in the field of health education where the whole film is not really necessary, and where, by suitable planning, sections of the film or films can be shown to illustrate a particular point. Where a school has lavish provisions for audio-visual aids, more than one projector can be used for this purpose, each projector having a film laced up to the point at which a particular fragment needs to be shown. For example, on a lesson in the dangers of smoking, a film fragment could be shown which contains an animation illustrating the way in which the cilia in the bronchi are paralysed by the nicotine in the smoke.

Animated cartoon films lend themselves very much to this kind of use, but in preparing the lesson the teacher must be familiar with the whole of the film and should identify that particular fragment which .will suit his purpose when words or discussion cannot be sufficiently explicit.

Whenever a film is used, it should be introduced with some brief description of its content and an indication of particular features which should be observed in order that a discussion can be conducted afterwards. Where there are any misleading or ambiguous sequences, this should be anticipated. This is often necessary in the case of films which come from other countries, particularly the United States where the systems of medical care and education are different from those in the U.K. After the showing of the film, it is then essential to conduct a discussion which should be initiated by preparing suitable leading questions arising from incidents or sequences in the film. Health education films are usually supplied with teaching notes which provide the teacher with the shooting script, the references to background material, and also suggestions for leading questions for initiating the discussion.

THEMATIC FILMS

Cinema techniques can be used in ways which are designed to produce group discussion, rather than purely to communicate information. The first of these is the so-called thematic film. This was introduced first by Professor Cohen-Séat of Paris who used short filmed dramatized incidents as a kind of thematic apperception test. These films are silent and in black and white so that they are very cheap to produce. They run for two to three minutes: sufficient time to present a fragment of human behaviour involving two or more people in which communication is entirely by mime, gesture, posture, and the general scene which is presented. This technique has been used for example to open discussion on the problem of petting, a subject which it would be very difficult to approach with a mixed group without some embarrassment. It can also be used to illustrate problems of relationships between older and younger generations and various behavioural problems.[1] The group is prepared by a short explanation of what the film is intended to do, a warning being given that no information is imparted at all. When the film has been seen, the group is asked four questions. Who are these people? What is their relationship? What do you think has happened? What do you think will happen in the future?

This technique can be used by amateur film groups with whom teachers can co-operate by providing scripts and assisting in the direction. Some of these films are now produced commercially and are available with teaching notes and suggestions for introducing and discussion. Cohen-Séat believes that this technique is one of diagnosis of attitude, personality, etc. and that we have yet to arrive at a film which can actually intervene to influence behaviour. The only kind of film in this area at present is that used in the so-called behavioural therapy which belongs to the field of psychiatry and not to health education.

The recent development of the thematic film is the so-called 'trigger film,' which is longer, about fifteen minutes, and has a sound track in addition. The principle, however, remains the same and teachers may decide to use one or the other, according to the situation.

CONCEPT FILMS

The introduction of concept films and super 8mm loops for use in back projectors provides an opportunity for an individual learning situation where schools are sufficiently well equipped to provide pupils with the apparatus and the accommodation for looking at these films themselves. The film loop is particularly valuable in demonstrating biological phenomena like cell division, fertilization, and growth. It has the advantage of repetition so that the viewer becomes familiar with the movements and events and translates these into ideas or concepts.

FILMSTRIPS

The filmstrip is used extensively in health education, and there must be literally thousands of filmstrips on every subject in the field of human biology, medicine, and public health. Ideally, a filmstrip should not contain more than about twentyfive frames, although many contain as much as up to fifty. A filmstrip is one of those aids that stimulates the teacher as much as the pupil, and if it contains too many frames, it becomes unmanageable in the context of a single lesson. Once again the teaching notes will be found useful when first handling the filmstrip, although of course they will be dispensed with as the teacher becomes more familiar with the subject. Teaching notes usually contain references to background material and further reading, and often questions that can be discussed by the pupils. It is a useful exercise for a class to make its own filmstrip, and this could be on a subject pertaining to health, such as immunization or environmental control.

TALKIE-STRIPS

The use of disc or tape recordings in association with filmstrips is now a well-established method. There are two kinds of sound film strip. The first is where the recorded commentary is intended to supplant the teacher, and this may have limited use in the school. The second is where the filmstrip is used like the thematic film, in fact it was the precursor of the thematic film. In this device, the filmstrip has very few frames — there may be as few as a dozen or fifteen. It provides a series of snapshots of a human situation where the poses which suggest the relationships and the incidents are supplemented by a recorded dialogue. A commentator introduces the theme and then when the incident has been presented suggests certain questions for discussion.

The general educational principle behind this is the stimulating of the capacity to argue from the particular to the general, i.e. 'induction'. These filmstrips are 'problem-centred', but the ideal way in which they are used is not to solve the problem, but to stimulate discussion of the general principles that apply to the problem. In this way the group is able to identify its own lives with the situation and to become aware of general principles that could be used should they be in the same situation Despite the advent of thematic films and the introduction of the more sociologically based behaviour film, the talkie-filmstrip still has a place for the promotion of a structured group discussion. Experience has shown, however, that it requires considerable skill in use and that many people have found it disappointing as they have not undertaken the necessary preparation to use them effectively.

SLIDES
'Two by two' slides are tending to supplant the filmstrip as a teaching aid. The advantage of slides is that the order of presentation can be varied according to the teacher's wishes and his assessment of the situation. The use of the modern 'carousel' projector with remote control makes it easy for a teacher to use this device without the need for an operator to assist him, and the modern slide which has great clarity and which is pleasing to the eye is attractive to a class and holds its attention.

Slide collections can be purchased from commercial distributors in the same way as filmstrips, but there is also great scope for the making of slide collections by teachers themselves or by groups of pupils under the guidance of the teacher. A 35 millimetre, precision camera of good quality is required, and a very high degree of skill in photography and in processing film is also necessary These resources can usually be found in most schools today.

Making Effective Slides
It is unfortunate that many lecturers to scientific societies employ slides which although purporting to be visual aids are virtually invisible. Mistakes made are: to crowd far too much material into a slide, some examples of which have been aptly described as resembling bus time-tables, and the failure to recognize that for the purposes of photography bold firm lines are needed. The best results are obtained when a coloured background is used, for

example, blue, red, orange, or pink. White lettering on dark blue, for example, is extremely effective, or black lettering on orange. Where tabulated material is used, it should be simplified and if possible presented graphically, for example, piecharts, or histograms, or graphs, are preferable to tables which require much more concentration than is possible during the course of the talk.

The making of effective slides requires studio facilities and the skills of a graphic artist. Illustrations can either be photographs of actual objects or scenes, or photographs of charts and symbols.

Slide collections should be planned on systematic themes as in the case of filmstrips. There should be a general whole-part balance preserved, so that the various aspects of the theme receive sufficient treatment, but not too much in relation to the other parts of the theme. It is necessary therefore to write a treatment script of the theme, followed by a shooting script, as in the case of film scripts or of the film.

OVERHEAD PROJECTOR

The overhead projector provides flexible facilities for illustrating talks and lectures. As in the case of all visual aids, it requires practice before the necessary skill can be attained. Transparencies can be purchased commercially and there are a number in the health education field, but this medium lends itself very well to the preparation of one's own transparencies, or simply doing freehand drawings, or writing spontaneously as one addresses the class. With practice, the overhead projector offers great opportunities for job satisfaction, and for a brilliant performance. One might ask what is the difference in function between the use of 'two by two' slides and the overhead projector? The main difference lies in the fact that whereas slides lend themselves to the systematic presentation of the theme, the overhead projector is a rather more personal teaching aid for the illustration of the teacher's remarks as he proceeds through the lesson. Whereas the slide collection or the filmstrip has perhaps done the preparation of the lesson for the teacher, in the use of the overhead projector, the teacher will have the impression that the visual aid is following him.

Overhead projectors are expensive as an item of capital investment, and some schools may not have this instrument at all. Where an adequate budget is provided, an overhead projector is an essential part of the equipment that forms the battery of audio-visual aids.

Electronic Aids

CLOSED-CIRCUIT TELEVISION

Closed-circuit television has been established in the education field for many years. Some large local education authorities, for example, ILEA and Glasgow, have established closed-circuit tele-vision centres under full-time directors and staff with a link-up to all the schools in the authority's area. Health education programmes have been prepared by co-operation with the health department staff, and these have been viewed in the classroom under the class teacher's direction.

In the case of the ILEA, programmes on drugs and smoking have been relayed to schools in this way. It is also possible to obtain far less ambitious installations and with the growing popularity of this medium the price of basic equipment has been substantially reduced. In addition to programmes relayed live from a central studio, video-tape recordings can also be used either relayed to schools, or distributed to schools for use on their own apparatus.

Closed-circuit television has a considerable value as a communica-tion medium, quite apart from its present novelty or its resem-blance to domestic television, which seems to be regarded as an indispensable amenity for living at the present day. It is therefore far more than a toy or a diversion, and it does call for a very high level of experience and skill in the planning and presentation of programmes. Many colleges of education now have closed-circuit television which is used for a variety of educational and entertain-ment purposes.

PREPARATION OF PROGRAMMES

According to the number of cameras available an infinite variety of small objects can be visualized, for example, scientific experiments, giving the viewer a visual experience that would not be possible in any other way. It is also possible to use all the visual aids normally used in the classroom, and in addition, some which are not available for classroom use. In some cases, objects or books of great value and rarity have been displayed before the cameras, and by switching from camera to camera a build up of sequences of visual experience can be employed as a learning experience.

The use of portable television cameras, recording interviews or experiences out-of-doors combining these with the use of video-tape recording, enables producers of programmes to build up a selection of visual experiences which, when pieced together, form a con-tinuous narrative.

TALK-BACK FACILITIES

The ideal situation is where there is a talk-back link up between the classroom and the studio, enabling a discussion to be carried on between the pupils who viewed the programme and the presenters in the central studio. This can be used with very large groups of children. For example, in London in 1962 a programme on the effect of smoking on health was relayed from a temporary studio in County Hall on the Southbank to a cinema in Regent Street that accommodated 1400 schoolchildren at one session. In the course of one day, nearly 3,000 children were able to see this programme and to take part in a discussion by using the talk-back to the studio. Included in this programme were some experiments such as that showing the effect of the smoking of a cigarette on the blood-vessels of the hand, causing a lowering of skin temperature. The equipment used in this demonstration was highly specialized, not readily available to schools, and required a team of specialists to set it up and to use it. It was possible therefore to provide this unique experience for a substantial part of the school population susceptible to the dangers of smoking, at a considerable saving of time and cost. In this case, the Eidophor system of colour television was used, and the system was loaned for this occasion, free of charge by CIBA, the Swiss pharmaceutical firm who were using it in connection with medical conferences.

A more modest piece of equipment which could be used in an individual school would call for two cameras, one portable camera, a video-tape recording set, and play-back apparatus, and two or more monitor screens. The servicing and use of such equipment calls for special technical expertise, and this can be obtained at short training courses. In the case of a large fixed installation, a full-time technician is essential.

The production and presentation of closed-circuit television programmes requires a team in which the roles of director, producer, script-writer, commentator or presenter, and technician, are all represented. Broadcast television is of an extremely high quality and the schoolchild will not be impressed by anything that is amateurish, has awkward pauses, or breaks of continuity or which has not been well rehearsed. The use of closed-circuit television therefore involves a considerable amount of hard work and preparation but many will consider this to be well worth while.

Electro-video recording apparatus is also being widely used, but one difficulty is that there are at present insufficient programmes as an input. The apparatus is on the market, however, and if programmes can be designed, libraries can be built up of health education material that could be circulated by local education authorities to the schools in their areas.

BROADCAST TELEVISION

Broadcast television also forms part of the learning environment and there is an increasing number of programmes on health matters, not only in schools' broadcasts, but also in programmes broadcast to the general viewing public. Advanced information can be obtained from the broadcasting authorities about these programmes, and teachers can arrange for them to be viewed by groups and for discussion and follow up to ensue. An interesting account of an experiment conducted on these lines is given by R. L. Brown who evaluated the impact of school television programmes on venereal diseases, broadcast to children in the fifteen- and sixteen-year-old age-group. [2]

EVALUATION OF TV PROGRAMMES

Three classes of fifteen-year-old pupils containing boys and girls of average to below average intelligence were selected to watch the series and then using questionnaires, information was collected on what the children thought about the programmes and what changes in knowledge and attitudes each programme produced. Six programmes altogether were involved, dealing successively with the topics of puberty, childbirth, unmarried mothers, venereal disease, the sexual behaviour of young people, and, finally, the family and marriage. One of the questions asked of the pupils was the rating they would give to the individual programmes, and it was interesting to find that they all placed the programme on venereal diseases first in terms of giving information and correcting wrong ideas.

When the sexes were compared, the programme on venereal disease was found to be more informative for boys, but, when correcting wrong ideas was concerned, the impact was the same for both sexes.

Three questions were put to the pupils on venereal disease in order to assess the recall of information:

(a) One of the symptoms of venereal disease called gonorrhoea is the frequent passing of water.

(b) The number of people with venereal disease is rising quite fast.

(c) The signs of the venereal disease called syphilis appear at least nine days after a person gets infected.

It was found that the programme had led to a larger proportion of both boys and girls giving the right answer after the programme than before. Amongst other observations, it was found that boys had a weight of worry and guilt lifted from them, and the author suggested that it was the definite information contained in the programme which achieved this.

An interesting use of broadcast television to assess parental attitudes to sex education is described by Gill, Reid, and Smith working in Aberdeen. [3] These authors conducted a survey of public opinion by scrutinising a file of press cuttings compiled by a professional agency for Grampian television. This was an assessment of the response to a television series 'Living and Growing'. It was possible to find answers to the questions whether sex education should be given, who was the appropriate agent, at what age should instruction begin and how broad should the content be.

It was found in general that there was a statistically significant tendency for mothers who had not seen these programmes to provide less support for a policy of sex education than those who had seen them. Similarly, those who had not seen the programmes felt that if sex education was to be given, it should be given at a later age than that specified by the mothers who had seen the programmes. The important result of this survey was the conclusion that subjects coming under the heading of sexual education — for example, morality, sex and religion, birth control and family planning — would have different connotations in the various sociocultural groups which make up our society

GROUP VIEWING

It is interesting to note that although the use of television for group viewing is a very limited activity in this country, it is for example employed by the Halifax Association of Parents for the purposes of parent education. In some of the developing countries group viewing is used extensively for health education. One example is Kenya where communal television viewing is practical in rural areas, and an opportunity is taken to broadcast regular programmes on health subjects.

The general programmes broadcast to the adult viewing public can often be adapted for educational purposes in the case of senior pupils. Social documentaries dealing with such matters as population and birth control, venereal disease, abortion and artificial insemination, are the work of highly specialized and skilled teams and it is up to schools to make as much use of them as possible. Certainly no teacher can afford to ignore the fact that television is an essential part of the general learning environment of every child in his class, and this applies even to the youngest children. It is impossible to be sure that a child has not seen a programme which may have conveyed highly sophisticated and sometimes frightening information.

When discussing television with parents, too much emphasis should not be placed on the negative aspects, and teachers should seize the opportunity to discover if they can what is the pattern of viewing amongst their pupils.

CONTEMPORARY VIEWS ON TELEVISION

The importance of television for family education has been recognized by the International Federation of Parent Education which organized an international conference in Hungary in 1971. Cassirer, Director, Division of the Mass Media in Out-of-School Education, UNESCO, said that the use of mass media to enhance parent education was one of the new avenues worth exploring to meet the vast educational needs of society.[4] He said also that Unesco was particularly interested because changes in the educational system, including lifelong education, were focused on the role, the awareness, and the responsible initiative of parents and their family.

A French journalist, Dubois-Dumée, has pointed out that every person in Europe will soon have access to a television set, and that homes will start to have a second or even a third set, and that we are still only at the beginning of the television age.[5] He compared the three centuries' history of the press, the eighty years' history of the cinema, and the mere twelve years' history of television since the time when it began to have real influence. With the introduction of relay satellites the entire globe of the earth will be encircled, and this and other technical developments, he says, will do away with the characteristic box television; the screen will expand to cover the walls which will then become screens, and the differences between television and cinema will disappear.

This technical revolution will quickly lead to changes in behaviour. Dubois-Dumée warns that it is important to know how to use television, and not for human beings to become its slave. He suggests that the best place for doing this is in school, and that 'tele clubs' can be set up in the same way as cinema clubs. Audio-visual concepts should be integrated into teaching as a new discipline, not as a way of teaching, but as a subject to teach. This is a challenge which the whole world of education will have to face, but health education in the meantime would seem to have a particular role to play.

TAPE RECORDERS
Aids to Role-Playing
Tape recorders can be used for recording discussion, for play-back, or as a special modification of psychodrama and role-playing which are mentioned below. They can also be used to record short programmes which have been scripted by groups of the pupils themselves. The use of a tape recorder requires careful organization and preparation. It is best to assign a small group to each project, and then to allocate roles, such as script-writing, dramatization, production, and recording. Good acoustic conditions are required, otherwise the results will be disappointing and pupils will either lose interest in the technique, or regard it merely as a diversion.

A tape recorded discussion can be used as a follow up to seeing a film, particularly when thematic films are used, or the talkie filmstrips described above. It is useful to stand back from a discussion and to examine it objectively in this way and pupils will be assisted to obtaining insights into their own motivation.

PROGRAMMED LEARNING
Programmed learning using either teaching machines, mechanical or electronic, or linear programmes based simply on scoring responses in a printed programme, are now used in health education. There

are a number of commercially produced programmes on the market, a selection of which is included at the end of this section. In addition, teachers who are interested in programmed learning, and who have access to teaching machines, can write their own programmes on health subjects. Programmed learning of course takes us into the field of individual learning, and it can be combined in the elaborate piece of equipment, known as a teaching carrel. This is a console equipped with back projection apparatus for 8 millimetre film and slides, tape recorder, and a teaching machine. On a more modest basis, pupils can be issued with printed programmes to work out in their own time. Before attempting this technique it is recommended that a pupil's motivation and reaction to such an exercise should be assessed, e.g. by a few trial runs.

Method relying upon Group Organization

GROUP DISCUSSION

Group discussion was discovered by health educators outside schools over twenty years ago. At that time, there was a danger of it being used in a doctrinaire fashion i.e. slavishly without regard to circumstances, as some people suggested that this method would supplant all didactic forms of learning, and even formalized knowledge itself. Many papers were published showing the results of experiments in which group discussion was compared with formal teaching, or the issue of literature on the effect of behaviour. As a rule, the experiment showed statistically significant differences between those who had taken part in group discussion, and those who had received formal instruction. This was very useful in such areas as infant-feeding and child care, or in some environmental situations, such as taking appropriate action in the household to prevent the spread of an infectious disease, like dysentery.

SELECTION OF METHOD

However, group discussion should be considered as only one of the methods available for health education, and most teachers will in any case have been acquainted with the method which is used in education generally. It is fortunate that two experts, Dr. J. H. Kahn, a psychiatrist, and Mrs. Sheila Thompson, a psychiatric social worker, published a book in 1970 which surveyed the whole field of group work and clarified its relationship to health education. [6,7] They pointed out that knowledge about group dynamics has been derived largely from the practice of group psychotherapy, and there is no doubt that many health educators have confused the psychotherapeutic role of groups with that of education.

The method is particularly applicable in health education where one is dealing with abstract concepts, such as those involved in human relations and mental health, or areas where personal responsibility are involved. It is therefore particularly applicable to the secondary stage of education when it can exploit the well known tendency for adolescents to argue and to discuss.

AIMS

The aims of group discussion include the promotion of changes in behaviour or attitudes in the individual members, but as Thompson and Kahn point out, the members of groups are not intended to be converted or indoctrinated, nor even should they be instructed. They identify the agent of change as participation in the group itself. They also point out that changes in behaviour do not come about merely by willing them. 'The ways in which we habitually react are not usually within our conscious control. If members of a group are going to be able to behave in a different way, then they must feel that they are in a different situation; if they are to modify the defences they use in order to feel secure, then alternative sources of security have to be provided.'

ROLE OF LEADER

The organization of group discussion requires one member to play the role of a leader. Teachers may either take the lead themselves, or delegate this to one of the pupils by remaining in the circle of the group as a resource person, that is, someone with expert knowledge who can be asked to provide factual information when the group is in difficulty. It is unfortunate that training in the leading of group discussion is very difficult to obtain, and the only way in which one can acquire any skill is to undertake this task as often as possible. The role of a leader of group discussion is extremely difficult to define, because according to the rules, he should not direct the discussion or structure it in any way, and to the observer from outside, he might appear to play no part at all. It is however his responsibility, here we quote again from Thompson and Kahn, to see that the aims of the group are observed: 'These aims set bounds and limits to the proceedings, and any self-exposure should not overstep the limits set by the group's particular aim. Each member has to relinquish some part of his normal controls, and in doing so, he vests these controls in the leader.'

STRUCTURED DISCUSSIONS

In the educational field, group discussion obviously has to modify its aims in order not to waste time and so miss the opportunity of a learning experience for which, after all, it is designed in this situation. There is something to be said for structuring a group discussion beforehand, and that is done by defining certain questions and terms of reference for the discussion and making sure that these questions are covered before the end of the session. It is also useful to have some summing up which will leave ideas in the minds of the members, and may be influential in influencing their behaviour. Factual information will be communicated during a group discussion, but the discussion goes beyond this area, and it is particularly useful in dealing with topics in which there is personal anxiety, or conflict. The important thing is for the teacher to decide whether group discussion is the appropriate technique for any particular situation, a reinforcement again of the principle that there must be an educational diagnosis before embarking on a project. The active role of the leader is to liberate the discussion from the repetition of book knowledge, or conventional opinions, and also to prevent any individual members from monopolizing the discussion. It is most important that members of a group have a clear idea about its purposes and processes. It is necessary also to caution people in the use of group discussion, less they stray into the area of psycho-therapy or counselling, or cause such a disturbance of group dynamics that insecurity is generated. Experience has shown that this is likely to happen at conferences attended by adult professionals, and that when susceptible individuals are deprived of the security of the group on the termination of the conference, they tend to break down. In many cases the 'breakdown' takes the form of being unable to make an impact on colleagues in the normal working situation. To the stress of deprivation of the security of the conference group is added the stress of trying to battle alone against resistance to change — or prejudice. This situation supports the major argument in favour of in-service training experiences shared with accustomed colleagues.

In the field of health education outside the school, group discussion has been found useful in the case of people who are suffering from a chronic disorder with which they must learn to live. They can obtain great benefit from finding out that other people have identical problems and can suggest ways of solving them. It can also be used for counselling groups of parents with handicapped children.

BUZZGROUPS

We have already referred to the limited use of group discussion method in order that a teacher may make a diagnosis of the level of attitude, interest, and knowledge about health topics. This is the so-called buzzgroup method, which in English literature describes the spontaneous organization of small groups of about six pupils who are then invited to spend five or ten minutes discussing a theme and formulating questions to put to the teacher. In American literature, the term buzzgroup has a completely different meaning.

It is useful to introduce the buzzgroup technique at the beginning of a session after a short introduction. The groups can either be left to discuss topics of their own choice with a view to formulating questions, or they can be given a specific question to answer. Sometimes such a question can be used to diagnose value-judgments and motivation. For example, the class could have the following question put to them 'If you were about to sit down to an attractively prepared meal, and you were very hungry what incident would cause you to leave the table, and to postpone your meal?'

This apparently frivolous question can produce the most profound discussion involving value-judgments. Eating is a fundamentally emotional process, so close to life itself and to sensual pleasures, and also considered to be so justified, that it is interesting to see the kinds of incidents that would persuade young people to put off a meal. Amongst adults, the reasons offered after buzzgroup discussions have varied from straightforward ones, such as the house catching fire, or hearing a cry for help from the street, to realizing that a particular piece of music was being broadcast on the radio in another room. One can also judge the degree of frankness and of personal insight in the kind of responses one would get to such a question.

The value of group discussion lies in the fact that the frivolous answer, or the answer designed to draw attention to personal qualities of integrity or the dishonest answer, are eliminated by other members of the group. It is therefore a particularly useful technique when conducting a session on subjects that are emotive, like sex or drugs. It is a great temptation encouraged by the present day degree of permissiveness for pupils to ask the kind of question that can cause the class to break down into ribaldry. In most buzzgroups, there will be a feeling of collective responsibility which will tend to avoid this situation.

An experienced teacher with a thorough knowledge of the subject can use this method in order to conduct a 'spontaneous lesson'. The most experienced, however, will be wise to warn the class that it may not be possible to provide answers to every question, but that the questions will be noted and answers will be supplied as soon as they can be checked. If there are not too many groups, say a limit of eight, it may be useful to take all the questions en bloc and to answer them and to comment further on them without further interruption. It usually occurs that some questions overlap, so that it is as well to require all groups to report back their questions verbatim, whereupon they can be written down, overlap can be taken into account, and the final talk will deal with some of the questions.

ROLE-PLAYING

Role-playing, sometimes called psychodrama, is another technique, which originated in the practice of psychiatry, but which has been adapted for health education. In support of our previous statement that Shakespeare packed the whole of his extensive psychological knowledge into one play, it will be remembered that psychodrama appears in Hamlet. It was used on that occasion to secure insight into guilt and responsibility. This is hardly the purpose in either psychotherapy or health education, but role-playing is useful in order that people can experience the feelings of those in different situations and also test out their capacity to meet a psychological or social challenge.

Setting up a Role-Playing Situation
Role-playing is a guide to decision-taking, and when discussing the results of the role-playing, the teacher will be able to explain the need to obtain information and to assess the validity of information on which to form a judgment. When there is sufficient time, pupils playing the roles can be changed and the rest of the class can be invited to comment as to whether they think the role-playing pupils are really being successful. Those who criticise can then be invited to do better. An interesting modification to role-playing is the use of the tape recorder, so that the performance can be discussed by the whole class at greater length, an opportunity being taken to go back to various phases of the role-playing for further examination. Role-playing can be used in parent education, and should be particularly valuable in helping pupils to come to terms with the generation gap. It should also encourage pupils to abandon meaningless clichés like 'treating people like human beings', 'talking to someone like a father', and so on.

DEBATES AND GROUP DIALECTICS
The method of debate can also be used, using a technique devised by Pauline Collyer, to which this writer has given the name 'group dialectics'.[8] The term, dialectic is used because this kind of debate depends upon a thesis and an antithesis, following which the resolution of the argument should arrive at the truth. The thesis is deliberately an *anti-health* thesis, for example, the proposition that smoking is not harmful, or that to preserve one's own natural teeth is not important, or any other anti-health proposition drawn from attitudes that are displayed by people when they show hostility to health education, which tends to interfere with their personal choice.

Discipline is required of the pupil who is asked to propose such an anti-health measure, since he will usually know that the proposition can easily be demolished by reference to facts. On the other hand, it sets up a situation in which the pupils who answer the proposition with a counter-argument have got to marshal the facts in an orderly fashion. No one should be allowed merely to demolish a proposition on emotional grounds, but should have good reasons to answer every one of the points put by the proposer. Five to ten minutes would be sufficient to allow for the proposition and the counter-proposition, leaving the rest of the time for pupils to join in the debate as they wish.

PROJECT METHODS
Health education lends itself very easily to the method of learning by enquiry. In many schools, successful projects have been carried out by groups of pupils on such matters as atmospheric pollution, water supplies, protection of food, and dental health. For this purpose, the learning environment extends outside the school and we would direct the reader's attention once more to the account of the Health Seminar at the comprehensive school in the Medway towns. Here the partnership of the school medical officer, nurse, and public health inspector will be particularly fruitful as it will be through these officials that introductions can be made to other officials who are in charge of the administration of the local health services. Public libraries will be helpful also in the conduct of projects and librarians will readily co-operate in obtaining books or journals that are not normally available, and by providing assistance to pupils in carrying out their researches.

An Introduction to Research Methods
This is a useful introduction to the technique of documentation in research, and apart from its value in learning by doing, it may be the beginning of a future career in the research field. Tasks can be assigned to individual members of groups according to their particular aptitude and skills. For example, those who are good at draughtsmanship can be assigned to the tasks of preparing charts and diagrams, others can prepare models, and those whose bent is literary expression can undertake the writing up of records and commentaries. These are matters of which every teacher is aware when using the project method generally, and it only suffices for us here to remind teachers that health education provides a fruitful field for enquiry of this kind.

Mass Communication

The learning environment is reinforced by the mass media of communication and a considerable amount of health knowledge is now conveyed in newspapers and magazines, particularly in women's magazines. Pupils can set up a press-cutting service of their own and can undertake the task of monitoring the daily press and the magazines they usually read, as well as news items or documentaries on television and sound radio. All children are exposed to the mass media — one cannot be isolated, even if that was desirable — and it does serve to stimulate interest and curiosity which must necessarily be satisfied at school. The complete confidence with which young couples will discuss with a television interviewer before an audience of literally millions, as to whether they use the sheath or withdrawal as a method of contraception, is indicative of the greater environment outside the school which the teacher must take into account in health education as in liberal studies.

Extracting the Best from Mass Media

The aims are to extract the best from the work of the mass media, and to borrow its authority in order to help schoolchildren gain further knowledge and to formulate attitudes. One has only to compare the situation just described with that of forty or fifty years ago, in which schoolchildren made the acquaintance of contraception through vague, disturbing, and ambiguous advertisements in public lavatories and the occasional discovery of the used condom while rambling in the country. At least the psychological trauma involved in these experiences of those who were children half a century ago could be avoided now and in the future.

The mass media are now extensively used in national health education campaigns. The Health Education Council has been responsible for poster and advertising campaigns on the subjects of smoking, and health, and birth control. Television 'spots' have also been produced on smoking both in 1971 and 1973, and in 1973 an experimental campaign on contraception was organized for Yorkshire Television in conjunction with the Family Planning Association.

Such campaigns are based on communications research. This involves the pre-testing of material with samples of the population representative of the audience at which the message is aimed. There is also a 'before and after' attitude and knowledge survey so that a follow up can assess how far the messages have been perceived and understood, and also whether they have resulted in action. Communications research is concerned with the choice of language and imagery, and the overcoming of barriers to understanding. All the material produced by the Health Education Council — whether it is a simple single sheet leaflet, or a letterpress poster up to a television film — is based on research.

Health education agencies in all countries use mass media but it is usually agreed that it is complementary to face-to-face methods. The indiscriminate distribution of literature is not considered to be sound practice. Literature is used as an ancillary technique and its proper use calls for skill and judgment.

APPENDIX

Catalogues of Audio-Visual Aids

The Health Education Council. *Selected Book and Audio-Visual Catalogue.*
This had been compiled for the use of teachers by the Education and Training
Division of the HEC. It contains selected lists of films for both secondary and
primary schools, models and charts, background reading for teachers, names
and addresses of suppliers including catalogues, film strips, 8mm film loops,
and tape recordings. There is also a list of current projects by the Schools
Council. All items are accompanied by a short appraisal including indication
for suitability for a particular age-group. Obtainable from the Education and
Training Division, The Health Education Council, 78 New Oxford St, London
W.1.
Medical Films available in Great Britain, compiled by British Industrial and
Scientific Film Association and published for the British Life Assurance Trust
and the British Medical Association. Obtainable from BISFA, 197 Regent St,
London W.1. price: 95p.

The Educational Foundation for Visual Aids. 33 Queen Anne St, London WIM
OAC.

Encyclopaedia Britannica Instruction Materials Division.

National Children's Bureau. *An Index of Documentary Films about Children.*
Obtainable from Adam House, 1 Fitzroy Square, London WIP 5AP.

The Health Education Council. *Exhibition Aids from Various Sources.*
Obtainable from the Communications Division, the Health Education Council.

The Health Visitors' Association. *Health Education Index.* Compiled and
published for the Association by Brian Edsall Ltd., 36 Eccleston Square
London SW1.

This is a comprehensive, classified list of all material-publications, films, film
strips, loops, slide collections, overhead projector transparencies, tape recordings and exhibition material. The most recent edition contained over 3,000
items. A coding system enables all materials on a given subject to be found.

REFERENCES

1. Porter, D. Lynton. (1969). 'Behaviour and its Analysis through Thematic
   Film'. *Proceedings of the Royal Society of Health Congress.* Eastbourne.
   Page 45.
2. Brown, R. L. (1967). 'Some Reactions to a Schools' Television Programme
   on Veneral Disease'. *Hlth. Educ. J.* 26:108—16.
3. Gill, D. G., Reid, G. D. B. and Smith D. M. (1971). 'Sex Education, Press
   and Parental Perception'. *Hlth. Educ. J.* 30(1):2—9.
4. Cassirer, H. R. (Aug. 1972 issue entitled 'Television Power'). 'Television and
   the Education of the Family'. *Int. Child Welf. Rev.* Aug. 1972 issue: 32.

5. Dubois-Dumée, J-P. (Aug. 1972 issue entitled 'Television Power'). 'Television of the Future'. *Int. Child Welf. Rev.* Aug. 1972 issue: 6.
6. Thompson, S. and Kahn, J. H. (1970). *The Group Process as a Helping Technique.* (Commonwealth and International Library, Social Work Division). Oxford: Pergamon Press.
7. Thompson, S. and Kahn, J. H. (1972). 'Group Work — A Search for First Principles'. *Hlth. Educ. J.* 31(1):108.
8. Collyer, P. (1965). Personal communication to the author.

FURTHER READING

Hollins, F. R. and Dicks, S. (1968). 'A Personal Relationship Project in Senior Schools'. *Med. Officer.* 120(19):261–4. (This is an example of team teaching by a doctor and a health visitor.)

Appendix

Health education

Guild of Health Education Officers.
7 Sandringham Road,
Bromley, Kent. BR1 5AR.

Health Education Council,
78 New Oxford Street,
London. WE1A 1AH
Official Publication: *The Health Education Journal*

Institute of Health Education,
35 Victoria Road,
Sheffield. S10 2DJ.
Official Publication: *Journal of the Institute of Health Education*

Scottish Health Education Unit and Scottish Council for Health Education,
Health Education Centre,
21 Lansdowne Crescent,
Edinburgh. EH12 5EH.

Health Education Groups are attached to the following bodies:

Association of Teachers in Colleges and Departments of Education,
3 Crawford Place,
London. W1H 2BN.

Royal College of Nursing,
Community Health Section,
Henrietta Place,
London. W1M 0AB.

Royal Society of Health
13 Grosvenor Place
London, SW1X 7EN.

EUROPE:

Institute for Preventive Health Care,
2 Gärtnergasse,
Vienna,
Austria.

Institute for Health Education,
54 Sokolska,
Prague 2,
Czechoslovakia.

Danish Committee for Health
Information,
Kristianiagade 12A,
2100 Copenhagen Ø,
Denmark.

Finnish Council for Health
Education,
Toolonkatu 15 E 94,
SF − 00100 Helsinki 10,
Finland.

French Committee for Health
Education,
General Secretariat:
20 rue Greuze, Paris 16e, France.

Centre for Health Education Studies
and Projects:
44 Chemin de Ronde, 78-Le Vesinet,
France.

National Council for Health
Education in the Democratic
Republic of Germany,
Scharnhorststrasse 37,
104 Berlin,
Democratic Republic of Germany.

Federal Centre for Health Education,
Ostmerheimer Strasse 200,
5 Cologne-Merheim,
Federal Republic of Germany.

Ministry of Social Services,
Division of Education, Public and
International Relations,
17 Aristotelous,
Athens, Greece.

Central Institute for Health
Education,
Ministry of Public Health,
Nepkostarsasag utja 82,
Budapest VI, Hungary.

Experimental Centre for Health
Education,
via XIV settembre 69,
Casella postale 226,
Perugia, Italy.

Netherlands Association for Health
Education,
Potgieterstraat 37,
Utrecht,
Holland.

Institute of Hygiene,
Health Education Department,
str. Dr. Leonte Nr. 1−3,
Bucharest, Romania.

Health Education Section (HVUD),
Bureau of Information,
National Board of Health and
Welfare,
105 30 Stockholm,
Sweden.

Department of Health Education and
Medical Statistics,
Ministry of Public Health,
Ankara, Turkey.

Central Institute for Scientific
Research in Health Education,
42 Kirova Street,
Moscow, USSR.

Institute of Health Education in the
Socialist Republic of Serbia,
24 Skerliceva Str.,
Belgrade, Yugoslavia.

U.S.A.

Society for Public Health Education,
655 Sutter Street,
San Francisco,
California 94102,
U.S.A.
Official Publication: *Health
Education Monographs*

INTERNATIONAL:

International Union for Health Education,
Headquarters: 20 rue Greuze, Paris 16e, France.

European Regional Office: Bachstrasse 3—5, 053 Bonn-Bad Godesberg, Federal Republic of Germany.
Official Publication: *International Journal of Health Education.*

World Health Organisation, Health Education Section: Avenue Appia, 1211 Geneva 27, Switzerland.

Regional Office for Europe: 8 Scherfigsvej, DK-2100 Copenhagen Ø, Denmark.

Official Publications: *World Health: Bulletin of The World Health Organisation and WHO Chronicle.*

Associated Subjects

UNITED KINGDOM

ABORTION:

Abortion Law Reform Association,
22 Brewhouse Hill,
Wheathampstead,
Herts.

British Pregnancy Advisory Services,
1st Floor,
Guildhall Buildings,
Navigation Street,
Birmingham B2 4BT.
and
40 Margaret Street,
London, W1.

ALCOHOL:

Alcoholics Anonymous,
11 Redcliffe Gardens,
London, S.W.10.

British Temperance Society,
Stanborough Park,
Watford,
Herts. WD2 6JP.

The Carter Foundation,
34 Seymour Street,
London, W.1.

Medical Council on Alcoholism,
8 Bourdon Street,
London, W1X 9HY.

National Council on Alcoholism,
Hope House,
45 Great Peter Street,
London, S.W.1.
(*Note:* Alcoholism Information Centres have been set up in a number of cities in England in association with the Council.)

Teachers' Advisory Council on Alcohol and Drug Education,
437 Royal Exchange,
Manchester M2 7EP.

AUDIO-VISUAL AIDS

The British Film Institute,
81 Dean Street,
London, W1V 6AA.

The British Industrial and Scientific Film Association,
193—7 Regent Street,
London, W.1.

The Central Film Library,
Government Building,
Bromyard Avenue,
London, W3 7JB.

Centre for Educational Development
Overseas (CEDO),
Tavistock House South,
Tavistock Square,
London, WC1H 9LL.

Department of Audio-Visual
Communication,
(British Medical Association and
British Life Assurance Trust for
Health Education),
BMA House,
Tavistock Square,
London, WC1H 9JP.

Educational Foundation for Visual
Aids,
33 Queen Anne Street,
London, W1M 0AL.

Medical Recording Service
Foundation,
Kitts Croft,
Writtle,
Chelmsford,
Essex, CM1 3EH.

National Audio-Visual Aids Centre,
254–6 Belsize Road,
London, N.W.6.

The National Audio-Visual Aids
Library,
Paxton Place,
Gipsy Road,
London, S.E.27.

National Committee for
Audio-Visual Aids in Education,
33 Queen Anne Street,
London, W1M 0AL.

CANCER:

British Cancer Council,
2 Harley Street,
London, W1N 1AA.

Cancer Education Voluntary Service,
1 Colworth Road,
Croydon, CRO 7AD.

Cancer Information Association,
337 Woodstock Road,
Oxford OX2 7NX.

Manchester Regional Committee of
Cancer,
Kinnaird Road,
Manchester M20 9QL.

Merseyside Cancer Education
Committee,
9 Produce Exchange Building,
8 Victoria Street,
Liverpool L2 6QG.

Tenovus Cancer Information Centre,
111 Cathedral Road,
Cardiff CF1 9PH.

Women's National Cancer Control
Campaign,
44 Russell Square,
London, WC1B 4JB.

CHILD WELFARE:

British Association for Early
Childhood Education,
89 Stamford Street,
London, SE1 9ND.

British Toy Council,
Regent House,
89 Kingsway,
London, W.C.2.

Council for Children's Welfare,
183 Finchley Road,
London, N.W.3.

Institute of Child Health (University
of London),
30 Guildford Street,
London, WC1N 1EH.

National Association for Maternal
and Child Welfare,
Tavistock House (North),
Tavistock Square,
London, WC1H 9JG.

National Association for the Welfare
of Children in Hospital,
Exton House,
Exton Street,
London, S.E.1.

National Children's Bureau,
1 Fitzroy Square,
London, W1P 5AH.

National Society for the Prevention
of Cruelty to Children,
1 Riding House Street,
London, W1P 8AA.

Pre-School Playgroups Association,
Alford House,
Aveline Street,
London, SE11 5DJ.

CHILDBIRTH AND MATERNAL WELFARE:

National Association for Maternal
and Child Welfare,
Tavistock House North,
Tavistock Square,
London, WC1H 9JG.

National Birthday Trust Fund,
57 Lower Belgrave Street,
London, SW1W 0LR.

National Childbirth Trust,
9 Queensborough Terrace,
London, W2 3TB.

National Council for One Parent
Families,
255 Kentish Town Road,
London, NW5 2LX.

CONTRACEPTION:

Birth Control Campaign,
223 Tottenham Court Road,
London, W1P 9AE.

Brook Advisory Centres,
233 Tottenham Court Road,
London, W1.

Catholic Marriage Advisory Council,
15 Lansdowne Road,
London, W11 3AJ.

Family Planning Association,
Margaret Pyke House,
27–35 Mortimer Street,
London, W1A 4QW.

Jewish Marriage Council,
529b Finchley Road,
London, NW3.

Marie Stopes Memorial Centre,
106 and 108 Whitfield Street,
London, W1P 6BE.

DENTAL HEALTH:

British Dental Association,
64 Wimpole Street,
London, W1M 8AL.

British Dental Health Foundation,
3 Harcourt House,
19a Cavendish Square,
London, W.1.

British Dental Hygienists'
Association,
Dental Department,
Eastman Dental Hospital,
Grays Inn Road,
London W.C.1.

General Dental Council,
Dental Health Education Section,
37 Wimpole Street,
London W1M 8DQ.

Fluoridation Society,
40–43 King Street,
London WC2E 8JH.

Oral Hygiene Service,
Hesketh House,
Portman Square,
London W1A 1DY.

DISEASES AND DISABILITIES:

Arthritis and Rheumatism Council,
Faraday House,
8–10 Charing Cross Road,
London, WC2H 0HN

Asthma Research Council,
28 Norfolk Place,
London, W.2.

Association for Spina Bifida and
Hydrocephalus,
112 City Road,
London E.C.1.

British Diabetic Association,
3–6 Alfred Place,
London WC1E 7EE.

British Epilepsy Association,
3–6 Alfred Place,
London WC1E 7EE.

British Heart Foundation,
57 Gloucester Place,
London W.1.

British Leprosy Relief Association,
50 Fitzroy Street,
London W.1.

British Migraine Association,
6 Bryanstone Road,
Bournemouth.

British Obesity Association,
34 Weymouth Street,
London W.1.

British Polio Fellowship,
Bell Close,
West End Road,
Ruislip,
Middlesex HA4 6LP.

British Rheumatism and Arthritis
Association,
1 Devonshire Place,
London W1N 2BD.

Chest and Heart Association,
Tavistock House (North),
Tavistock Square,
London WC1H 9JE.

Coeliac Society,
P.O. Box 181,
London NW2 2QY.

Colostomy Welfare Group,
38/9 Eccleston Square,
London S.W.1.

Cystic Fibrosis Research Trust,
5 Blyth Road,
Bromley,
Kent BR1 3RS.

Haemophilia Society,
P.O. Box 9,
16 Trinity Street,
London SE1 1DE.

Ileostomy Association,
149 Harley Street,
London S.W.1.

Leukaemia Research Fund,
61 Great Ormond Street,
London WC1N 3JJ.

Leukaemia Society,
22 Springfield Park,
Twyford,
Berkshire.

Migraine Trust,
23 Queen Square,
London W.C.1.

Multiple Sclerosis Society,
4 Tachbrook Street,
London S.W.1.

Muscular Dystrophy Group of Great Britain,
26 Borough High Street,
London S.E.1.

National Society for Autistic Children,
1a Golders Green Road,
London N.W.11.

Parkinson's Disease Society,
36 Queens Road,
London SW19 8LR.

Patients' Association,
335 Grays Inn Road,
London W.C.1.

Phobia Information Centre,
109 Sheen Court,
Richmond,
Surrey.

Psoriasis Association,
22 Billing Road,
Northampton NN1 5AT.

Schizophrenia Association of Great Britain,
Port Dinorwic,
Llanfair Hall, Caernarvon.

Society for the Aid of Thalidomide Children,
28 Fouracres Walk,
Hemel Hempstead,
Herts.

Spastics' Society,
12 Park Crescent,
London W1.

The U and I Club (Urinary Infection),
8 Hopping Lane,
London N.1.

DRUGS

The Association for the Prevention of Addiction,
33 Long Acre,
Covent Garden,
London WC2E 9LP.

Institute for the Study of Drug Dependence,
Kingsbury House,
3 Blackburn Road,
London NW6 1XA.

Society for the Study of Addiction,
Tooting Bec Hospital,
London S.W.17.

Teachers' Advisory Council on Alcohol and Drug Education,
437 Royal Exchange,
Manchester M2 7EP.

National Addiction and Research Institute (CURE),
533A Kings Road,
London S.W.10.

THE ELDERLY

Age Concern (National Old People's Welfare Council),
55 Gower Street,
London WC1E 6HJ.

National Corporation for the Care of Old People,
Nuffield Lodge,
Regent's Park,
London NW1 4RS.

Pre-Retirement Association,
194 Clapham Park Road,
London SW4 7DU.

ENVIRONMENT

Council for Environmental
Education,
School of Education,
University of Reading,
24 London Road,
Reading RG1 5AQ.

Keep Britain Tidy Group,
76, Strand,
London WC2R 0DE.

National Association for
Environmental Education,
Environmental Studies Office,
Offley Place,
Great Offley,
Nr. Hitchin,
Herts.

National Society for Clean Air,
134–137 North Street,
Brighton BN1 1 RG.

Noise Abatement Society,
6 Old Bond Street,
London W1.

Town and Country Planning
Association,
Environmental Education Unit,
17 Carlton House Terrace, London
SW1Y 5AS.

EUGENICS

Eugenics Society,
69 Eccleston Square,
London S.W.1.

EYES

Eye Care Information Bureau,
55 Park Lane,
London W.1.

FIRST AID

St. John Ambulance Association and
Brigade,
1 Grosvenor Crescent,
London SW1Y 7EF.

British Red Cross Society,
9 Grosvenor Crescent,
London SW1X 7EJ.

FOOT HEALTH

Children's Foot Health Register,
9 St. Thomas Street,
London SE1 9SA.

Institute of Chiropodists,
59 Gloucester Place,
London W1H 3PE.

Society of Chiropodists,
8 Wimpole Street,
London W1M 8BX.

Society of Shoe Fitters,
9 St. Thomas Street,
London SE1 9SA.

HANDICAPS

Association for all Speech Disabled
Children,
6 Desenfans Road,
Dulwich Village,
London SE2.

British Deaf and Dumb Association,
38 Victoria Place,
Carlisle CA1 1EX.

British Disabled Drivers' Association,
4 Laburnum Avenue,
Wickford,
Essex.

Central Council for the Disabled,
34 Eccleston Square,
London S.W.1.

Disabled Living Foundation,
346 Kensington High Street,
London W.14.

Invalid Children's Aid Association,
126 Buckingham Palace Road,
London S.W.1.

National Association for Deaf/Blind
and Rubella Children,
61 Senneleys Park Road,
Northfield,
Birmingham B31 1AE.

National Deaf Children's Society,
31 Gloucester Place,
London W1H 4EA.

Royal National Institute for the
Blind,
224—229 Great Portland Street,
London W1N 6AA.

Royal National Institute for the
Deaf,
105 Gower Street,
London WC1E 6AH.

HOMOSEXUALITY

The Albany Trust,
32 Shaftesbury Avenue,
London W1.

Campaign for Homosexual Equality,
22 Great Windmill Street,
London W1.

The Gay Liberation Front,
5 Caledonian Road,
London N1.

HOSPITALS

Hospital Centre, (King Edward's
Hospital Fund for London),
24 Nutford Place,
Edgware Road,
London W1H 6AN.

Nursing and Hospital Careers
Advisory Service,
121—123 Edgware Road,
London W2.

LOCAL GOVERNMENT

Local Government Information
Office,
36 Old Queen Street,
Westminster,
London S.W.1.

MARRIAGE GUIDANCE

Catholic Marriage Advisory Council,
15 Lansdowne Road,
Holland Park,
London W11 3AJ.

National Marriage Guidance Council,
Little Church Street,
Rugby,
Warwickshire.

MENTAL HEALTH

National Association for Mental
Health,
39 Queen Anne Street,
London W1M 0AJ.

National Society for Mentally
Handicapped Children,
86 Newman Street,
London W1P 4AR.

Tavistock Institute of Human
Relations,
Tavistock Centre,
Belsize Lane,
London NW3 5BA.

NUTRITION

British Dietetic Association,
251 Brompton Road,
London SW3 2ES.

British Nutrition Foundation,
Alembic House,
93 Albert Embankment,
London S.E.1.

Food Education Society,
160 Piccadilly,
London W1.

Food Information Centre,
12 Park Lane,
Croydon,
Surrey CR9 3NX.

Nutrition Society,
Chandos House,
2 Queen Anne Street,
London W1M 9LE.

PARENTS/TEACHERS

Advisory Centre for Education
(ACE),
32 Trumpington Street,
Cambridge.

National Federation of
Parent-Teacher Associations,
1 White Avenue,
Northfleet,
Gravesend,
Kent.

PHYSICAL EDUCATION & SPORT

The Duke of Edinburgh's Award,
2 Old Queen Street, London S.W.1.

Institute of Sports Medicine,
Ling House,
10 Nottingham Place,
London W1M 4AX.

Physical Education Association of
Great Britain and Northern Ireland,
Ling House,
10 Nottingham Place,
London W1M 4AX.

Sports Council of Great Britain,
26 Park Crescent,
London W1N 4AJ.

RESEARCH

Centre for Educational Development
Overseas (CEDO),
Tavistock House South,
Tavistock Square,
London WC1H 9LL.

Medical Research Council,
20 Park Crescent,
London W1N 4AL.

National Foundation for Educational
Research in England and Wales,
The Mere,
Upton Park,
Slough,
Bucks.

Office of Health Economics,
162 Regent Street,
London W1R 6DD.

Social Science Research Council,
State House,
High Holborn,
London WC1R 4TH.

Schools Council,
160 Great Portland Street,
London W1N 6LL.

SAFETY

British Safety Council,
National Safety Centre,
62—64 Chancellors Road,
Hammersmith,
London W6.

Electrical Association for Women,
25 Foubert's Place,
London W1V 2AL.

Fire Protection Association,
Aldermary House,
Queen Street,
London EC4N 1TJ.

Firework Makers' Guild,
Information Office,
16 Bolton Street,
London W1Y 8HX.

Medical Commission on Accident
Prevention,
50 Old Brompton Road,
London SW7 3EA.

Royal Society for the Prevention of
Accidents,
Royal Oak Centre,
Brighton Road,
Purley CR2 2UR.

SEXUALLY TRANSMITTED DISEASES

British Social Biology Council,
69 Eccleston Square,
London S.W.1.

SMOKING

ASH (Action on Smoking and Health
Ltd).
11 St. Andrew's Place,
Regent's Park,
London NW1 4LB.

British Anti-Smoking Education
Society,
and

National Society of Non-Smokers,
125 West Dumpton Lane,
Ramsgate,
Kent.

British Temperance Society,
Stanborough Park,
Watford,
Herts. WD2 6JP.

See also under Cancer

VASECTOMY AND STERILISATION

Crediton Project,
West Longsight,
Crediton,
Devon.

Family Planning Association,
27—35 Mortimer Street,
London W1A 4QW.

INTERNATIONAL ORGANISATIONS

British Council,
65 Davies Street,
London W1Y 2AA.

International Federation for Parent
Education,
4 rue Brunel,
75017 Paris,
 France.
(*NOTE:* This is also the headquarters
of L'Ecole des Parents, Paris).

International Planned Parenthood
Federation,
Central Office: 18—20 Lower Regent
Street, London SW1Y 4PW.
European Regional Office: 64 Sloane
Street, London SW1X 9SJ.

Oxfam,
274 Banbury Road,
Oxford.

Save the Children Fund,
29 Queen Anne's Gate,
London SW1H 9DA.

United Kingdom Committee for the
Freedom from Hunger Campaign,
17 Northumberland Avenue,
London W.C.2.

United Kingdom Committee for the
World Health Organisation,
c/o London School of Hygiene and
Tropical Medicine,
Keppel Street,
Gower Street,
London W.C.1.

United Nations Association,
93 Albert Embankment,
London SE1 7TX.

War on Want,
2b The Grove,
London W.5.

Professional Bodies

Association of Public Health
Inspectors,
19 Grosvenor Place,
London S.W.1.

Association for the Study of Medical
Education,
150b Perth Road,
Dundee DD1 4HN.

British Dental Association,
64 Wimpole Street,
London W1M 8AL.

British Dental Hygienists'
Association,
Dental Department,
Eastman Dental Hospital,
Grays Inn Road,
London W.C.1.

British Medical Association,
BMA House,
Tavistock Square,
London WC1H 9JP.

Central Council for Education and
Training in Social Work,
Clifton House,
Euston Road,
London N.W.1.

Chartered Society of Physiotherapy,
14 Bedford Row,
London WC1R 4ED.

Council for the Education and
Training of Health Visitors,
Clifton House,
Euston Road,
London NW1 2RS.

General Nursing Council for England
and Wales,
23 Portland Place,
London W1A 1BA.

Guild of Health Education Officers,
7 Sandringham Road,
Bromley,
Kent. BR1 5AR.

Health Visitors' Association,
36 Eccleston Square,
London SW1V 1PF.

Institute of Health Education,
35 Victoria Road,
Sheffield S10 2DJ.

Medical Officers of Schools
Association,
Hon. Sec. Surgeon Captain P. de B.
Turtle, VRD,
Haileybury College,
Hertford.

National and Local Government
Officers' Association,
Nalgo House,
8 Harewood Row,
London N.W.1.

National Council of Social Service,
26 Bedford Square,
London WC1B 3HU.

Nursing and Hospital Careers
Advisory Service,
121—123 Edgware Road,
London W2.

Pharmaceutical Society of Great
Britain,
17 Bloomsbury Square,
London WC1A 2NN.

Queen's Institute of District Nursing,
57 Lower Belgrave Street,
London SW1W 0LR.

Royal College of General
Practitioners,
14 Princess Gate,
Hyde Park,
London S.W.7.

Royal College of Midwives,
15 Mansfield Street,
London W1M 0BE.

Royal College of Nursing,
1a Henrietta Place,
Cavendish Square,
London W1M 0AB.

Royal College of Physicians,
11 St. Andrews Place,
London NW1 4LE.

Royal Institute of Public Health and
Hygiene,
28 Portland Place,
London W1N 4DE.

Royal Society of Health,
13 Grosvenor Place,
London SW1X 7EN.

Royal Society of Medicine,
1 Wimpole Street,
London W1M 8AE.

Social Work Advisory Council,
26 Bloomsbury Way,
London W.C.1.

Society of Chiropodists,
8 Wimpole Street,
London W1M 8BX.

Society of Community Medicine,
Tavistock House South,
Tavistock Square,
London WC1H 9LD.

Index